The
Aging
Brain

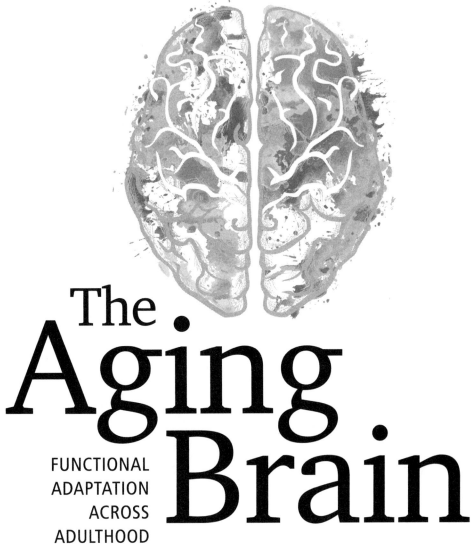

The
Aging
FUNCTIONAL
ADAPTATION
ACROSS
ADULTHOOD
Brain

Edited by
GREGORY R. SAMANEZ-LARKIN

AMERICAN PSYCHOLOGICAL ASSOCIATION
Washington, DC

Published by
American Psychological Association
750 First Street, NE
Washington, DC 20002
https://www.apa.org

Order Department
https://www.apa.org/pubs/books
order@apa.org

In the U.K., Europe, Africa, and the Middle East, copies may be ordered from Eurospan
https://www.eurospanbookstore.com/apa
info@eurospangroup.com

Typeset in Goudy by Circle Graphics, Inc., Reisterstown, MD

Printer: Sheridan Books, Chelsea, MI
Cover Designer: Naylor Design, Washington, DC

Library of Congress Cataloging-in-Publication Data

Names: Samanez-Larkin, Gregory R., editor. | American Psychological
    Association, issuing body.
Title: The aging brain : functional adaptation across adulthood / edited by
    Gregory R. Samanez-Larkin.
    Other titles: Aging brain (Samanez-Larkin)
Description: Washington, DC : American Psychological Association, [2019] |
    Includes bibliographical references and index.
Identifiers: LCCN 2018059461 (print) | LCCN 2019001920 (ebook) | ISBN
    9781433831157 (eBook) | ISBN 1433831155 (eBook) | ISBN 9781433830532
    (hardback) | ISBN 1433830531 (hardback)
Subjects: | MESH: Brain—physiology | Cognitive Aging | Cognition | Cognitive
    Dysfunction—prevention & control
Classification: LCC QP376 (ebook) | LCC QP376 (print) | NLM WL 300 | DDC
    612.8/2—dc23
LC record available at https://lccn.loc.gov/2018059461

http://dx.doi.org/10.1037/0000143-000

Printed in the United States of America

10 9 8 7 6 5 4 3 2 1

CONTENTS

CONTRIBUTORS

Alan D. Castel, PhD, Department of Psychology, University of California, Los Angeles

Lindsay B. Conner, MS, Department of Psychology, University of Central Florida, Orlando

Roger A. Dixon, PhD, Department of Psychology, University of Alberta, Edmonton, Canada

Audrey Duarte, PhD, School of Psychology, Georgia Institute of Technology, Atlanta

Kelly S. Giovanello, PhD, Department of Psychology and Neuroscience, Biomedical Research Imaging Center, The University of North Carolina at Chapel Hill

Angela Gutchess, PhD, Department of Psychology, Brandeis University, Waltham, MA

Mary B. Hargis, MA, Department of Psychology, University of California, Los Angeles

Briana L. Kennedy, PhD, Leonard Davis School of Gerontology, University of Southern California, Los Angeles

Elizabeth Kensinger, PhD, Department of Psychology, Boston College, Chestnut Hill, MA

Margie E. Lachman, PhD, Department of Psychology, Brandeis University, Waltham, MA

Nichole R. Lighthall, PhD, Department of Psychology, University of Central Florida, Orlando

Mara Mather, PhD, Leonard Davis School of Gerontology, University of Southern California, Los Angeles

Patricia A. Reuter-Lorenz, PhD, Department of Psychology, University of Michigan, Ann Arbor

Gregory R. Samanez-Larkin, PhD, Department of Psychology and Neuroscience, Duke University, Durham, NC

Alexander L. M. Siegel, MA, Department of Psychology, University of California, Los Angeles

R. Nathan Spreng, PhD, Montreal Neurological Institute, Department of Neurology and Neurosurgery, McGill University, Montreal, Canada

Gary R. Turner, PhD, Department of Psychology, York University, Toronto, Canada

Laura B. Zahodne, PhD, Department of Psychology, University of Michigan, Ann Arbor

PREFACE

GREGORY R. SAMANEZ-LARKIN

Many years ago as a first-year PhD student, I was sitting among about a dozen senior faculty members at the Stanford Center on Longevity, along with Jane Fonda. Ms. Fonda was at Stanford to talk to scientists doing aging research while working on an upcoming book. My advisor, Laura Carstensen, had invited me to the meeting to share my own emerging research on aging and decision making. In several studies, we had found a perhaps surprising lack of age differences in affective and motivational brain signals and decision-making behavior across adulthood. At one point in the discussion, Ms. Fonda turned to me and said, "What about you, young person, why are *you* interested in aging?"

Just a few years earlier, as a college student, I *hadn't* been interested in aging at all. When I first learned about the psychology and neuroscience of aging, it was fairly depressing. I learned about the steep and relatively linear declines in many aspects of memory and other fluid cognitive abilities. I learned about the similarly steep losses in gray matter and dopamine receptors in the brain. And I wondered how, with all of this consistently documented deterioration, does the aging brain function so well while making decisions?

Over the years, the view of brain aging as a period of deterioration and decline has been replaced with a more complex characterization of changes in brain structure and function. Not all cognitive processes decline with age; many remain stable, and some improve over adulthood. In my own area of research on decision making, this has been relatively well documented over the past several years. Younger and older adults often make similar decisions, but for different reasons or by using different strategies. As you will read throughout this volume, these sorts of findings are not limited to decision making. In nearly every chapter, there is discussion of how cognitive performance varies across different contexts, how different strategies are used at different ages, or how reorganization and plasticity of the brain supports behavioral function. Although there are undeniable losses in structure and function, the aging brain is more flexible and compensatory than research might have initially suggested.

A few years after the meeting with Jane Fonda, I was running a 92-year-old adult through a neuroimaging study and was shocked by the first whole-brain images we collected. I'd never seen so much atrophy in the striatum and sulci so expanded in the cortex. During the scan, I looked at the participant's neuropsychological test results, and they were normal. A few days later, I processed the neuroimaging data, and in that thin strip of caudate gray matter, there was fairly strong activation during our task. I was puzzled, and to some extent I still am. The aging brain continuously amazes me and is, in part, why I've dedicated my own career to studying adult development and aging. There are many unsolved mysteries of the aging brain, but as a field, we're making progress. You'll read about some of that progress throughout the chapters of this book.

The reason my interest in aging as a (formerly) young person was questioned so many years ago is likely because young people don't often learn about the complexities of aging. The hope is that this volume will provide a more comprehensive picture and, in doing so, inspire more emerging scientists to pursue aging research as well.

The
Aging
Brain

INTRODUCTION

GREGORY R. SAMANEZ-LARKIN

Historically, the scientific study of aging was focused heavily on deterioration and decline. Within psychology departments, for example, researchers studying aging were in clinical areas where their colleagues were focused on disease and disorder. Over the past 25 years, the historical view of brain aging as a decades-long period of deterioration and decline has been slowly replaced with a more complex characterization of changes—growth, decline, adaptation, selectivity, and reorganization—in brain structure and function across adulthood. This shifting view has been driven by research in both the behavioral and brain sciences. The research of psychologists and neuroscientists has revealed that not at all cognitive processes decline with age; some improve over adulthood, and often those that improve compensate for those that decline.

Being happy, healthy, and financially stable in old age depends on a wide range of psychological functions and behaviors across the life span. In response to recent demographic shifts (resulting from increased longevity

http://dx.doi.org/10.1037/0000143-001
The Aging Brain: Functional Adaptation Across Adulthood, G. R. Samanez-Larkin (Editor)

and low fertility rates), policymakers and private industry leaders across the globe are looking to psychologists and neuroscientists for advice on how best to promote and protect health and well-being in old age. Unfortunately, psychological research on aging is often too far removed from informing policy. A major reason for this is that aging research is not sufficiently integrative or translational, which significantly limits the potential for broader impact. The current within-area approach impedes cross-talk between disciplines and contributes to a fragmented understanding of aging. The recent rise in interdisciplinary research programs has potential for increasing translation of aging science for real-world impact. In the spirit of these recent developments in the field, this volume aims to combine multiple perspectives on aging from previously disconnected but complementary lines of research. Within most chapters of the volume, we invited contributors working in complementary areas but who had never worked together to coauthor a review of the literature. The hope was that this activity would not only provide a unique resource to the field in the near term but would also inspire new lines of interdisciplinary research that have greater potential for enhancing well-being in old age in the long term.

The primary goal of this volume is to present a more complete, nuanced, and modern view of brain aging by reviewing emerging behavioral and brain research from a broad range of areas across psychology and neuroscience. Although previous books have focused on what is known about cognitive losses with age, less attention has been paid to the broad range of psychological and neural functions (e.g., affective, socioemotional, motivational, cognitive, and decision-related processes) that decline, remain stable, or improve with age. The collection of chapters here aims to provide a more balanced perspective on our current understanding of normal human brain aging.

The book begins with a broad overview of regional and network-level brain structure and function (Chapter 1) to lay the foundation for the remaining chapters. A series of process-focused chapters follow (Chapters 2–6) that discuss attention, learning, memory, motivation, cognition in everyday life, and social function. The final two chapters (Chapters 7 and 8) are once again more general and deal with broader theoretical issues that are critical to our understanding of both the processes discussed in the focused chapters throughout the middle of the book and our understanding of the function of the aging brain overall. The majority of chapters begin by reviewing the brain functions being discussed, the brain structures involved, the current state of empirical research, and the topic's significance within the broader realm of brain-aging studies, then conclude by outlining future avenues of research.

Chapter 1 by Spreng and Turner provides a broad summary of age-related changes in the structure and function of the brain based mostly on evidence from in vivo human neuroimaging. Across studies, there is relatively consistent evidence that structurally, anterior cortical regions, including the prefrontal cortex, decline in early older adulthood, whereas posterior sensory–motor regions decline in later older adulthood. Functionally, older adults tend to display less network specialization, with greater recruitment of frontal and contralateral regions during cognitively demanding tasks. The chapter introduces a number of larger scale brain networks and individual brain regions that are discussed throughout the book.

Chapter 2 by Kennedy and Mather discusses emerging research on how attentional selectivity changes across adulthood and into older age. One of the most well-characterized cognitive deficits in older age is the difficulty in inhibiting attention to irrelevant information, even though there is relative preservation of other attentional processes. In this chapter, the authors detail how age-related changes in the frontoparietal network—slowing in alpha band activity, decreased GABAergic and dopaminergic densities, and impaired frontoparietal connectivity with noradrenergic release under arousal—play a critical role in age-related changes in attentional selectivity.

Chapter 3 by Lighthall, Conner, and Giovanello begins a series of three chapters that discuss elements of memory abilities. This chapter discusses how long-term nondeclarative (priming, classical conditioning, procedural, and reinforcement learning) systems and declarative (episodic and semantic memory) systems decline or may be partially preserved with age. The authors first introduce the distinct learning and memory systems for the acquisition, retention, and subsequent retrieval of information but go on to discuss evidence that these systems are highly interactive.

Chapter 4 by Duarte and Kensinger focuses specifically on episodic memory, the ability to encode and retrieve details that allow individual events to be distinguished from one another. They discuss both the neural declines that contribute to memory impairments as well as the relative preservation of older adults' emotional memories. They also highlight how memory can be preserved with age by staying mentally and physically active across adulthood.

Chapter 5 by Hargis, Siegel, and Castel is the third in the series related to learning and memory but focuses on the critical contributions of motivation and goals. Rather than focusing on findings from neuroimaging (of which there are currently few), the authors examine how younger and older adults selectively learn information, highlighting reward salience and the importance of attentional control during encoding. They also discuss how goals and extrinsic and intrinsic motivational factors may change decision-making and lead to preservation of function across adulthood. Overall, the chapter identifies many examples of how motivation can enhance learning and memory well into old age.

Chapter 6 by Gutchess and Samanez-Larkin examines the influence of aging on social processes, including thinking about the self and others, mentalizing and empathizing, and responding to stigmatized others. In addition to discussing the types of processes that are preserved or decline with age, they consider ways in which the impact of aging on socioemotional processes may differ from the ways in which aging impacts cognitive processes. They identify multiple interacting brain networks that have subcomponents that are preserved or decline with age that may account for these behavioral effects. Functional adaptation of these brain systems may account at least partially for some of the preservation of motivational and emotional function identified in Chapters 4 and 5.

Chapter 7 by Zahodne and Reuter-Lorenz introduces and discusses the concept of neural compensation in older age. They review emerging findings from the past couple of decades that identify alterations in neural function in response to age-related neural declines that preserve cognitive function. Many of the previous chapters identify aspects of preserved functional output from brain networks that show unquestionable losses with age. This chapter describes how these compensatory processes may work in both normal and pathological aging.

Chapter 8 by Dixon and Lachman discusses risk and protective factors and their independent and interactive effects on trajectories of cognitive change across adulthood. They discuss the contributions of both nonmodifiable factors such as genetics and modifiable factors such as lifestyle interventions that may contribute to preservation of function in both normal and pathological aging. On the basis of emerging research, the chapter identifies goals to potentially reduce or delay neurodegenerative cognitive declines and potentially prevent the onset of dementia.

This book is not intended to be comprehensive in its coverage of all areas of human cognitive function. There are important areas of research that are not covered. For example, although many chapters discuss issues of cognitive control, there is not a dedicated chapter on the topic. We also do not provide a comprehensive treatment of how the processes of normal aging and age-related diseases may diverge, although there is discussion of how compensatory function and modification of risk factors may slow or prevent the onset of serious cognitive decline in Chapters 7 and 8. This book is also quite focused on systems-level neural function as revealed by human brain imaging—mostly functional magnetic resonance imaging. A limitation is that there is little discussion of the specific lower level cellular and molecular changes across adulthood that influence function. Some discussion of declines and preservation in neuromodulatory (e.g., norepinephrine, dopamine) and neurotransmitter (e.g., GABA) function is provided in Chapters 2 and 6. This book would be an ideal companion to other books that provide broader coverage of cognitive change or lower level coverage of specific cellular and molecular mechanisms of brain aging.

The target readership for this book is primarily researchers working on the psychology and neuroscience of aging from graduate students and postdocs to faculty members. The collection of chapters could be used together in a graduate seminar on the psychology and neuroscience of aging. It also has the potential to be used in a focused, upper level, undergraduate seminar for students with a solid foundation in both psychology and human brain imaging. The individual chapters vary in their accessibility, so some of them may be used in more introductory courses at the undergraduate or graduate level. Individual chapters could also be used in a nonaging, topic-focused course that with the intent of exposing students to how these processes vary across adult development. For example, a course on attention might include Chapter 2, or a course on memory might include Chapters 3, 4, or 5.

In nearly every chapter, there is discussion of how cognitive performance varies across different contexts, how different strategies are used at different ages, or how reorganization and plasticity of the brain supports behavioral function. Although there are undeniable losses in structure and function, the aging brain is more flexible and compensatory than research might have initially suggested. The hope is that this book presents a more comprehensive picture of the functionally adaptive aging brain.

1

STRUCTURE AND FUNCTION OF THE AGING BRAIN

R. NATHAN SPRENG AND GARY R. TURNER

In this opening chapter of *The Aging Brain*, we set the stage for the contributions that follow by providing a broad overview of the latest advances in our understanding of how the brain changes, both structurally and functionally, across the adult lifespan. We leave domain-specific aspects of brain aging to the subsequent chapters, where contributors provide more targeted accounts of brain change germane to their particular focus on the aging brain. Here we review the extant, and rapidly expanding, literature to provide a brief overview and introduction to structural and functional change that occur with typical brain aging. We begin the chapter by looking back to review some of the early discoveries about how the brain changes across the adult lifespan. We close the chapter by looking forward, toward new discoveries that challenge our core assumptions about the inevitability or irreversibility of age-related brain changes. These sections serve as bookends for the core of the chapter where, we review the latest research advances that continue to uncover the mysteries of the aging brain.

http://dx.doi.org/10.1037/0000143-002
The Aging Brain: Functional Adaptation Across Adulthood, G. R. Samanez-Larkin (Editor)

INTRODUCTION: STUDYING THE AGING BRAIN

Whether in the lab or in the clinic, we now take for granted the ready access to measurement tools and the precision with which we are able to investigate lifespan changes in the structure and functioning of the human brain in vivo. However, the study of the aging brain is a relatively young endeavor. Early neuroscientific studies did not include, or perhaps even consider, systematic investigations of brain changes that may occur in later life. Indeed, a leading text on the history of neuroscience, *Origins of Neuroscience* (Finger, 1994), does not include a section on older adult brain development, and the term *aging* does not even appear in the subject index. Of course, this may be explained in part by the comparatively restricted range of the human lifespan before the turn of the 19th century. However, by the mid-20th century, researchers in the fields of medicine, neuroscience, and evolutionary biology began to recognize that the brain does not remain stable across the normal adult lifespan. Postmortem investigations began to report both gray and white matter volume loss as well as ventricular enlargement in older versus younger adults (for an early review, see Kemper, 1994). However, these early pathological and comparative neurological studies were plagued by small sample sizes and methodological constraints that affected measurement reliability (Good et al., 2001). By the latter decades of the 20th century, postmortem studies also began to identify broad topological patterns of age-related change in brain structure. Sensory cortices were seen be comparatively preserved, while more pronounced changes were evident in association cortices, including frontal and lateral parietal regions (Flood & Coleman, 1988). Following rapidly from these postmortem investigations, in vivo neuroimaging techniques, including computed tomography and two-dimensional magnetic resonance imaging (MRI), became more widely adopted. These methods were critical in advancing our understanding of the aging brain because they allowed the enterprise of brain research to essentially "scale-up," enabling the collection of brain volume measures from larger groups of participants that could then be more reliably compared across age cohorts. These imaging techniques, and in particular, the development of high-resolution, three-dimensional MRI neuroimaging methods in the late 1980s and early 1990s, as well as more sophisticated registration protocols necessary to spatially align individual brains to conduct group comparisons, opened the way for larger cohort and longitudinal studies that have become standard in the field today (Salat et al., 2004).

As with studies of structural brain aging, the earliest investigations of aging brain function in humans emerged in the middle decades of the 20th century. Indeed, as early as 1938, electroencephalogram (EEG) recordings were seen as offering "appreciable promise as a means to characterize significant deviations from the 'natural' aging found in Alzheimer and other dementias" (Berger, 1938, as reviewed by Rossini, Rossi, Babiloni, & Polich, 2007, p. 376). In the latter part of the century, increasingly sophisticated methods emerged to investigate age-related changes in brain function. These included single photon emission computed tomography, positron emission tomography (PET), functional MRI (fMRI), and magnetoencephalography (MEG) techniques. In the early decades of the 21st century additional techniques, including intracranial EEG or electrocorticography methods, have enhanced the spatial and temporal resolution of functional brain measurements. Transcranial magnetic stimulation (TMS) and transcranial direct current stimulation techniques now allow for the temporary modulation of brain activity, enabling researchers to more directly investigate how changes in brain function are associated with cognitive functioning in later life (e.g., Freitas, Farzan, & Pascual-Leone, 2013; Rossi et al., 2004). As we will see at the end of the chapter, these brain stimulation techniques are also offering considerable promise as interventions or treatments to potentially alter the course of cognitive aging (e.g., Zimerman et al., 2013).

In the following sections of the chapter, we survey findings drawn from each of these techniques to provide a comprehensive overview of the current state of research on structural and functional brain aging. As we have seen, the study of the aging brain remains in its infancy. Brain imaging, allowing us to measure and record from the brain in vivo, is barely half a century old. Yet despite this brief history, much is now known about the myriad ways in which our brains change as we move through adulthood and into older age—and of course much remains to be discovered.

STRUCTURAL BRAIN CHANGES IN OLDER ADULTHOOD

Age-related changes in the structure of the brain have been examined across multiple, interacting levels, from cells and synapses to regions or structures and, more recently, large-scale brain systems or networks. Although structural brain changes measured using in vivo techniques almost certainly reflect cellular changes including dendritic branching, synaptic density, and demyelination of local and long-range axonal fibers, here we focus our review on measures of parenchymal (gray and white matter) and cerebrospinal fluid (CSF) volumes, both globally and regionally, and how local changes converge at the level of whole-brain networks. Consistent with the vast majority of research literature in this field, we also limit our primary focus to changes primarily involving cortical structures. However, age-related changes to subcortical structures are of increasing interest in understanding age-related changes in cognitive and affective behaviors (e.g., Samanez-Larkin &

Knutson, 2015) or as early markers of atypical brain aging (e.g., Schmitz, Spreng, & Alzheimer's Disease Neuroimaging, 2016), and we highlight these where possible throughout our review. Whereas earlier studies measured structural change almost exclusively in terms of volumetrics, more recent work has emphasized other features, including topological variability, rates of change, and interindividual differences. In this section we provide an overview of the changing structure of the brain in older adulthood at each level of analysis and across these multiple features of brain aging. Although not the primary focus of the chapter, this evolving, multidimensional perspective on structural brain changes in older adulthood is gaining prominence in the search for sensitive neural biomarkers that signal transition from normal aging to brain disease, a topic we discuss briefly in the final section.

From Postmortem to In Vivo: Early Findings

Early in vivo neuroimaging studies of structural brain aging focused primarily on global changes in tissue compartments including gray and white matter and CSF volumes (for a review, see Raz, 1996). These studies confirmed postmortem investigations that had reported global volume loss and ventricular enlargement in older relative to younger adults (Kemper, 1994). In addition to confirming these ex vivo findings, early neuroimaging investigations provided the first indication of topological variability, with changes occurring at different rates for different brain regions and tissue types. This pattern has been described as a mix of declines and relative preservation (Raz, 2000), and suggested that not all brain regions demonstrate a similar extent or rate of decline across the lifespan. As we will see, more recent work suggests an even more complex picture of structural brain aging, with different regions demonstrating significantly different, and often nonlinear, trajectories of change (Fjell et al., 2014).

Investigations of structural brain aging using in vivo neuroimaging methods began to increase rapidly toward the end of the last century as MRI technology became more readily accessible and numerous groups began efforts to map the trajectory of age-related brain changes with increasing topological specificity. However, these efforts were not without controversy. Many of the earliest in vivo studies adopted a cross-sectional approach, comparing measures of brain structure between younger and older adults. However, cross-sectional designs have been criticized for providing purely chronologically based estimates of brain age. In other words, measurements at a single time point can only characterize brain structure at that time point. Single-point measures are unable to describe age-related changes in brain structure (Raz & Lindenberger, 2011). There are two primary criticisms of cross-sectional designs. First, they are contaminated by cohort effects, which confound group membership and age in difference calculations. Second, cross-sectional designs do not account for individual differences, which introduce significant variability in group-level estimates and likely deflate true estimates of structural brain change between age-groups. With the increasing accessibility of MR technology, research groups began to conduct longitudinal studies of age-related changes in brain structure. Although complex and costly, longitudinal studies hold the advantage of accounting for individual differences and controlling for cohort effects, providing what is arguably a truer estimation of age-related brain change. As a reflection of the differences in these two approaches, a recent study of age-related cortical thinning reported annualized rates of −0.30% using cross-sectional methods. This estimate stands in somewhat stark contrast to the estimated annualized rate of −0.59% using a longitudinal study method (Fjell et al., 2014). The difference represents a nearly twofold difference in annual change estimates. These results are consistent with an earlier study that used a combined cross-sectional and longitudinal design (Raz et al., 2005) and again reported deflated cross-sectional change estimates. Taken together, these studies urge caution in the interpretation of these estimated structural brain changes. Although cross-sectional studies of age-related brain change may be more feasible and cost-effective and may allow for larger study samples to be collected, these designs may nonetheless underestimate the magnitude of age-related brain changes.

Since the earliest in vivo investigations, the number of studies investigating structural brain changes associated with normal aging has increased exponentially. Taken together, the findings provide a complex picture, with often conflicting findings. In the following sections, we review the extant literature and distill the findings into the most commonly reported and replicated patterns of structural brain change in older adulthood. We begin by reviewing the most recent evidence for global changes in whole-brain and ventricular volumes and then summarize the current state of knowledge with respect to region-specific trajectories of change. The most common in vivo metrics for measuring changes in brain structure are volumetrics, cortical thinning, and surface area, and we limit our review almost exclusively to these measures. Because the health of cerebral white matter is assuming a place of increasing importance in the study of brain and cognitive aging, we review patterns of white matter change, including volumetrics, white matter integrity, and lesion burden in a separate section. Finally, we end this section of the chapter on structural brain aging with a brief review of structural brain networks. These covarying patterns of structural brain change appear to be potent predictors of the transition from normative to diseased aging and may in fact identify disease-specific structural network biomarkers.

Global and Regional Changes

Global Changes

Age-related changes in cerebral parenchyma and ventricular volumes have been reported from the earliest in vivo studies (reviewed in Raz, 1996). Interestingly, whereas gray matter, CSF and ventricular volume changes were consistently reported in these early studies, age-related changes in white matter volumes were generally not observed, although microstructural changes in white matter had been reported previously (Wahlund et al., 1990). Age-related changes in whole brain volumes were also reported in one of the first whole-brain, volume-based morphometry studies, with evidence that global gray matter volumes declined linearly and CSF volume increased linearly with age (Good et al., 2001). Again, consistent with earlier reports, no age changes were observed in global white matter volumes. In contrast, white matter volume changes were reported in an early longitudinal study from the Baltimore Longitudinal Study of Aging (Resnick, Pham, Kraut, Zonderman, & Davatzikos, 2003). Age-related declines on the order of 5.4, 2.4, and 3.1 cm^3 per year were reported for total brain, gray matter, and white matter volumes, respectively, whereas ventricular volume increased by 1.4 cm^3 per year. These findings were recently replicated in a larger sample from the same study cohort (Thambisetty et al., 2010).

Longitudinal investigations have characterized global (and regional) changes in brain structure in terms of annualized percent change estimates. Annualized percent change is a standardized metric for determining the rate and trajectory of age-related changes by calculating a per-year estimate of decline. Annualized percent change is typically calculated voxel-wise (volume-based morphometry) or vertex-wise (cortical thickness) for each participant across multiple time points, thus allowing for both global and regional estimates of change. Although different formulae for calculating annualized percent change have been reported, a typical approach involves calculating differences in volume (or thickness) between time points, which is then divided by the baseline volume (or thickness) estimate and the number of years between time points (e.g., M. E. Shaw, Sachdev, Anstey, & Cherbuin, 2016). Longitudinal studies of cortical thickness have reported annualized percent change ranging from −0.59 in a cohort with mean age of 75 (Fjell et al., 2014) to −0.35 for lifespan (Storsve et al., 2014) and young-old (60–66) samples (M. E. Shaw et al., 2016). In one of the few non-Western studies reported in the literature, annual change of −0.56% for total brain volumes were observed in the Singapore Longitudinal Aging Brain Study (Leong et al., 2017). These findings provide strong evidence that declines in parenchymal volume, and concomitant increases in CSF and ventricular volumes, are a hallmark of adult aging. Despite earlier cross-sectional reports, longitudinal studies demonstrate convincingly that both gray and white matter tissue compartments decline with age. Although estimates and measures vary widely across studies, there appears to be convergence around the extent of parenchymal change, with annual loss estimates ranging from −0.30% to −0.56% per annum. Further, this rate of global decline appears to accelerate in late life from young-old (60–66 years; M. E. Shaw et al., 2016) to middle-old (~75 years; Fjell et al., 2014) and old-old (+90 years; Yang et al., 2016). Finally, although a full review of sex differences in age-related brain change is beyond the scope of this review, it is important to note that the majority of published reports (whether cross-sectional or longitudinal) and across both global and regional measures, show a steeper and more rapid trajectory of decline for men than women (e.g., Driscoll et al., 2009; Good et al., 2001; Pfefferbaum et al., 2013; Raz et al., 1997; M. E. Shaw et al., 2016; Sullivan, Rosenbloom, Serventi, & Pfefferbaum, 2004; Thambisetty et al., 2010).

Regional Changes

The earliest in vivo imaging studies reported global, or nonspecific, brain changes in late life (Jernigan, Press, & Hesselink, 1990). However, evidence from animal and human postmortem studies (Flood & Coleman, 1988; Kemper, 1994) and later in vivo imaging studies (e.g., Pfefferbaum et al., 1994; Raz et al., 1997) observed regional variability in structural brain changes occurring in late life. Indeed, as noted earlier, the extent of regional variability was described in these early studies as a "patchwork" of age-related change across the cortical mantle (Raz et al., 1997). This distributed or "heterochronous" (Salat et al., 2004) nature of structural brain changes across the lifespan has been observed repeatedly in both cross-sectional studies (Dotson et al., 2016; Fjell et al., 2009; Fleischman et al., 2014; Salat et al., 2004; Walhovd et al., 2010; Yang et al., 2016; G. Ziegler et al., 2012) and longitudinal studies (Fjell et al., 2015; Pacheco, Goh, Kraut, Ferrucci, & Resnick, 2015; Resnick et al., 2003; Scahill et al., 2003; M. E. Shaw et al., 2016; Storsve et al., 2014; Sullivan et al., 2004; Thambisetty et al., 2010).

In a targeted investigation of regional differences in brain atrophy using region of interest methods, the most robust age changes were observed in prefrontal gray matter (Raz et al., 1997). The authors interpreted this finding in the context of earlier postmortem and in vivo imaging studies, suggesting that anterior brain regions, particularly prefrontal and temporal regions, may undergo accelerated changes with age (for a review of these early studies, see Raz, 1996). Subsequently, longitudinal studies appeared to confirm this finding of greater susceptibility of prefrontal and temporoparietal association cortices to age-related decline (Fjell et al., 2014, 2015; Pacheco et al., 2015;

Resnick et al., 2003; Salat et al., 2004; M. E. Shaw et al., 2016). We discuss network-level changes in more detail here, but several studies have specifically identified regions of the default network, a collection of functionally interconnected brain regions situated primarily along the brain's midline, as showing increased susceptibility to age-related changes (Fjell et al., 2015; Storsve et al., 2014). Explanations for these regional atrophy patterns include the "last-in, first-out" hypothesis (Raz, 2000), suggesting that brain regions such as the prefrontal cortex (PFC), which reach full maturation later in life, may be the most vulnerable to early decline in late adulthood. Similarly, the extended development–sensory hypothesis suggests that all heteromodal association cortices atrophy earlier, followed by declines in primary sensory-motor and paralimbic cortices in later older adulthood (McGinnis, Brickhouse, Pascual, & Dickerson, 2011).

On balance, existing research is consistent with these hypotheses, with frontal and heteromodal association areas most commonly identified as undergoing more rapid decline than sensorimotor regions (Pfefferbaum et al., 2013; Raz et al., 2005; L. M. Shaw et al., 2009; Storsve et al., 2014; Thambisetty et al., 2010). This leads directly to the conclusion that accelerated volume loss is not simply a global feature of structural brain aging. Support for this idea was recently provided in a large cross-sectional study, with a smaller longitudinal validation cohort (Fjell et al., 2015). Brain regions followed one of several trajectories with critical change periods, or inflection points, occurring in late adolescence or middle adulthood. Structures including the hippocampus, brain-stem regions, cerebellum, and cortical white matter, showed stability (or increases) in cortical thickness, followed by steep declines in later life. Structures including the amygdala, putamen, thalamus, nucleus accumbens, and cerebellar cortex showed a pattern of near linear decline across the lifespan. A third category, which included estimates of global parenchymal and cortical volumes, followed a quadratic function with accelerating decline in later life (Fjell et al., 2015). Regional variability in rates of brain atrophy was also reported in two recent studies of young-old (Shaw et al., 2016) and old-old (Yang et al., 2016). In young-old, greater annualized percent change was observed in heteromodal than in primary sensory motor cortices, with inferolateral temporal and inferior parietal cortices showing particularly pronounced changes. In contrast, for old-old adults, accelerated changes were observed in medial temporal and occipital cortices, particularly in the 10th and 11th decades of life (Yang et al., 2016). Structural declines have also been reported in primary sensory-motor and occipital brain regions in old-old adulthood (Salat et al., 2004; Storsve et al., 2014). Together these findings are consistent with the "retro-genesis" hypothesis (McGinnis et al., 2011), with prefrontal and heteromodal cortices developing later and declining earlier than primary sensorimotor regions.

White Matter Changes

A recent postmortem investigation of structural brain changes in older adulthood reported reduced cerebral white matter volume in both anterior and posterior brain regions while failing to find age-related changes in cerebral gray matter (Piguet et al., 2009). These results prompted the study authors to suggest that "healthy brain aging is a process affecting predominantly white, not gray, matter" (Piguet et al., 2009, p. 1294). These findings hint at the importance of considering white matter changes as a core feature of structural brain aging. Interestingly, changes in global white matter volume were not commonly reported in early cross-sectional studies, although subsequent well-powered cross-sectional and longitudinal studies did report reliable age-related declines in overall white matter volumes (Pfefferbaum et al., 2013; Raz et al., 2005; Resnick et al., 2003; Walhovd et al., 2011). Consistent with reports of regional specificity in cortical volume and thickness changes, white matter changes also appear to follow an anterior–posterior gradient with the most rapid atrophy occurring in frontal white matter (Raz, Ghisletta, Rodrigue, Kennedy, & Lindenberger, 2010; Raz et al., 2005; D. A. Ziegler et al., 2010). The vast majority of reports of white matter atrophy also describe a curvilinear pattern, with more rapid declines occurring in later older adulthood (Fjell et al., 2015; Maillard et al., 2009; Pfefferbaum et al., 2013; Walhovd et al., 2011; Yang et al., 2016).

Beyond volumetrics, white matter changes have also been characterized using diffusion imaging methods to assess the integrity of white matter fiber tracts in the brain. Several recent reports suggest that changes in white matter integrity may precede gray matter changes, thus providing a more sensitive marker of structural brain changes in normal aging (Arvanitakis et al., 2016; Hugenschmidt et al., 2008). Declines in white matter integrity have now been reported across numerous studies and again appear to follow an anterior to posterior gradient with the most rapid changes occurring in frontal white matter compartments (Bennett & Madden, 2014; Bennett, Madden, Vaidya, Howard, & Howard, 2010). A third metric for characterizing the health of cerebral white matter involves measuring the volume of white matter lesions. Lesions in the brain's white matter are thought to occur as a result of small cerebrovascular events, leading to alterations in axonal myelin and ultimately membrane permeability, resulting in axonal damage. White matter lesions are associated with cerebrovascular risk factors (Raz, Rodrigue, Kennedy, & Acker, 2007) and, given increasing rates of obesity and metabolic diseases in Western populations, likely represent one of the most rapidly growing forms of structural brain change in older adulthood. White matter lesion burden appears to rapidly increase in the oldest old with one recent report suggesting decelerating volume loss and accelerating lesion volumes in this cohort (Yang et al., 2016). Further, the presence of cerebral small vessel disease, including atherosclerosis, deep white matter lesions, or subcortical lacunar infarcts is strongly associated with Alzheimer's disease (Yarchoan et al., 2012) and a nearly two-fold increased risk of dementia onset (Snowdon, 1997).

Changes in Structural Brain Networks

Over the past decade research investigating structural brain change in older adulthood has expanded beyond global and regional changes to consider distributed patterns of structural decline. Structural covariance is observed as interindividual differences in regional brain structure covarying with other brain structures across the population (Alexander-Bloch, Giedd, & Bullmore, 2013; Evans, 2013; Mechelli, Friston, Frackowiak, & Price, 2005). Across individuals, intrinsically connected functional brain networks, such as the default network, can be topographically represented in the structural patterns of cortical gray matter. Patterns of covariance in brain structure were first identified in postmortem studies (Andrews, Halpern, & Purves, 1997), and changes in structural covariance networks with age have now been reported in whole-brain in vivo studies (Alexander et al., 2006; Brickman, Habeck, Zarahn, Flynn, & Stern, 2007; Chen, He, Rosa-Neto, Gong, & Evans, 2011; DuPre & Spreng, 2017; Meunier, Achard, Morcom, & Bullmore, 2009; Montembeault et al., 2012; Spreng & Turner, 2013; Zhao et al., 2015).

As with global and regional measures of structural brain changes, structural covariance changes with age are more prominent between frontal brain and posterior cortices, reflecting a loss of long-range covariance in favor of increased local processing (Montembeault et al., 2012; Wu et al., 2012; Zhao et al., 2015). Another prominent feature of network-level changes is declining structural covariance within the default network, a collection of functionally connected brain regions implicated in mnemonic and associative processing (Andrews-Hanna, Smallwood, & Spreng, 2014). In one report, structural covariance patterns were identified from seed regions showing maximal atrophy across various neurodegenerative diseases. Structural covariance with these seed regions in young adults reflected atrophy patterns in a disease specific manner (Seeley, Crawford, Zhou, Miller, & Greicius, 2009). As one example, structural covariance of the default network in young showed high spatial coherence with the pattern of neurodegeneration observed in Alzheimer's disease. We recently reported similar patterns of reduced structural covariance within the default network, with changes observable over as little as 2 years in a normal aging cohort. Further, we observed that changes in default network structural covariance reliably predicted the transition from mild cognitive impairment to Alzheimer's disease in a longitudinal sample (Spreng & Turner, 2013). Similar patterns of declining structural covariance have been reported in other large-scale distributed brain networks, including executive control networks, which have been implicated in those cognitive functions most affected by aging (Montembeault et al., 2012). Indeed, measures of structural covariance, when combined with estimates of cerebral blood flow, explained almost all age-related variance in cognitive performance in a recent report (Steffener, Brickman, Habeck, Salthouse, & Stern, 2013). This last observation speaks to the importance of measuring not simply independent trajectories of regional changes but covariance patterns describing how volume changes in distributed brain regions cohere across the across the lifespan.

Summary of Structural Brain Changes in Aging

With the advent of increasingly powerful in vivo neuroimaging techniques, the study of age-related structural brain changes represents a vast and expanding field. Given the scope of the review, we chose to focus on the broad trends that have been most reliably reported over the past 2 decades of structural neuroimaging research. Global changes in gray matter, white matter, and ventricular volumes are clearly a hallmark of normal brain aging. Heteromodal association cortices are more susceptible to late-life structural decline than primary-sensory motor regions, and rates of decline differ among cytoarchitectonic zones. Rapid declines occur in frontal and heteromodal association cortices in young-old, with comparatively shallow rates of decline observed in medial temporal lobe and primary sensorimotor regions. This is followed by more rapid changes in the medial temporal lobe and primary sensorimotor motor regions in old-old adulthood. White matter changes, whether measured as volume, integrity, or lesion burden, are also a prominent feature of brain aging and may in fact be a stronger predictor of cognitive decline and dementia than cortical changes. Finally, investigators are increasingly moving beyond region-specific metrics to identify whole brain patterns of structural brain change. Measures of structural covariance have proven to be powerful predictors of cognitive capacity in normal aging and as potent biomarkers of the transition from normal aging to neurodegenerative disease. Understanding these normative patterns of structural brain change is critical to expanding opportunities for detecting nonnormative brain aging using in vivo imaging methods. However, as we noted in our chapter introduction, age-related brain change is multidimensional, affecting both structure and function. In the next section, we turn our attention to changes in how the brain functions in older adulthood again considering how these are reflected globally, regionally, and at the level of interacting networks.

FUNCTIONAL BRAIN CHANGES IN OLDER ADULTHOOD

Functional neuroimaging methods have been used to study the aging brain for more than 3 decades. Much of the work over this period has used these methods to identify the neural correlates of cognitive functioning across myriad domains (e.g., sensory-motor, processing speed, memory, executive function). As with the research literature on structural brain changes, the findings characterizing functional changes in older adulthood are often varied and provide conflicting perspectives as to the nature and implications of observed differences in brain activation between age cohorts. In this section, we briefly review domain-specific brain changes, focusing on the findings of our recent meta-analytic reviews. We then review more domain-general patterns of functional brain changes in older adulthood and describe several of the leading theoretical perspectives in the field. As with our review of structural brain aging, we end this section by describing age-related functional brain changes at the level of large-scale, functionally connected brain networks. We have chosen to focus here on functional neuroimaging studies using MRI or PET measures of brain function. Although much research and numerous advances have been made using electrophysiological techniques, including EEG and MEG studies, we are unfortunately unable to cover these techniques within the scope of the review.

Domain-Specific Changes

The field of neurocognitive aging research has rapidly expanded over the past 2 decades. Although a comprehensive survey of the literature across this vast literature is beyond the scope of this chapter, we have published three meta-analytic reviews of studies investigating age-related functional brain changes. The first meta-analysis included 80 functional neuroimaging studies across four cognitive domains: perception, memory encoding, memory retrieval, and executive functioning (Spreng, Wojtowicz, & Grady, 2010). For perceptual tasks, older adults showed greater dorsolateral PFC as well as anterior insula and frontal opercular activation, whereas younger adults showed the predicted pattern of greater activity in sensory cortices, particularly occipital regions. For memory tasks, young adults showed greater right lateral PFC and medial temporal activity during encoding, whereas older adults preferentially engaged right PFC regions during memory retrieval. Age differences during executive control tasks were primarily observed in prefrontal brain regions. Specifically, older adults showed greater activation in more dorsal aspects of PFC bilaterally, whereas younger adults showed greater recruitment of right ventrolateral PFC regions. Across all domains, older adults engaged prefrontal regions to a greater extent than young adults.

In contrast, younger subjects, particularly those showing poorer task performance, engaged posterior sensory regions. Further, the enhanced pattern of PFC recruitment observed in the older adult cohorts was performance-dependent. Higher performing older adults showed greater left lateralized prefrontal engagement, while lower performing subjects engaged regions of right PFC.

In two follow-up meta-analyses, we examined age differences specifically in the domain of executive control processing. We examined patterns of age-related brain change associated with discrete executive control processes including working memory, inhibition, and task switching (Spreng, Shoemaker, & Turner, 2017; Turner & Spreng, 2012). Consistent with the findings of the earlier review, we observed a general pattern of increased functional brain activity for older versus younger adults. However, the specific nature of this enhanced functional recruitment was process specific. Task switching and working memory were associated with increased prefrontal recruitment bilaterally. In contrast, inhibition showed a "young-plus" pattern with age-related increases localized to regions typically implicated in young. Again, the most robust age difference observed across all three control processes was enhanced recruitment of prefrontal brain regions for older versus younger adults. This age-related difference in PFC activity was greater at higher levels of working memory demand, suggesting that increased recruitment of these regions may reflect greater reliance on, or strategic engagement of, working memory resources in older adulthood (Spreng et al., 2017).

Domain-General Changes: Neural Dedifferentiation

As reviewed in the preceding text, early functional neuroimaging studies of cognitive aging typically adopted a domain-specific approach, with investigators enumerating age-related changes in the neural implementation of specific cognitive task performance using cross-sectional study designs (for reviews, see C. L. Grady, 2008, 2012; Greenwood, 2007; Hedden & Gabrieli, 2004; Park & Reuter-Lorenz, 2009; P. A. Reuter-Lorenz & Lustig, 2005; P. A. Reuter-Lorenz & Park, 2014; Spreng et al., 2010; Turner & Spreng, 2012). Taken together, these studies also identified domain-general patterns of functional brain changes in aging, suggesting that all age-related cognitive changes may share, at least in part, a common neural substrate. Perhaps the most ubiquitous pattern observed across studies has been referred to as *neural dedifferentiation*, increased and more spatially distributed patterns of neural activity in older versus younger adults during cognitive task performance (Park, Polk, Mikels, Taylor, & Marshuetz, 2001). In one of the earliest functional neuroimaging investigations of cognitive aging, PET scanning methods were used to measure changes in metabolism across brain regions while younger and older participants performed visuoperceptual tasks. Older participants displayed greater functional activation during task performance than younger participants. Moreover, unlike the lateralized pattern of functional activity within the prefrontal cortex observed in the young, older participants demonstrated greater bilateral activation (C. L. Grady et al., 1994). Since this seminal work, this pattern of decreased lateralization in functional brain response in aging has been replicated in numerous reports using both PET and fMRI methods, spanning a range of cognitive domains including memory encoding and retrieval (Cabeza, 2002; Cabeza, Anderson, Locantore, & McIntosh, 2002; C. L. Grady, 1996; McIntosh, 1999; Velanova, Lustig, Jacoby, & Buckner, 2007), visual attention (Cabeza, 2002; Cabeza et al., 2002; C. L. Grady, 1996; Madden et al., 2007; McIntosh, 1999; Velanova et al., 2007); working memory (Cabeza, 2002; Cabeza et al., 2002; Cappell, Gmeindl, & Reuter-Lorenz, 2010; C. L. Grady, 1996; Mattay et al., 2006; McIntosh, 1999; Reuter-Lorenz et al., 2000; Rypma & D'Esposito, 2000; Velanova et al., 2007), and selective attention and inhibition (Colcombe, Kramer, Erickson, & Scalf, 2005).

The finding that cortical activation patterns become increasingly differentiated is now a leading account of functional brain changes in older adulthood and indeed of neurocognitive aging. Dedifferentiation has been operationalized in a number of ways. It has been described simply as nonidentical brain activity patterns between younger and elder populations (Zarahn, Rakitin, Abela, Flynn, & Stern, 2007) or as more diffuse and distributed cortical representations of cognitive activities (Craik & Bialystok, 2006). Other researchers suggest that it reflects a failure to engage specialized neural mechanisms during cognitive performance (Cabeza et al., 2002; Li, Lindenberger, & Sikström, 2001). Three forms of dedifferentiation have been described (Park et al., 2001). Contralateral recruitment refers to the age-related recruitment of brain regions homologous to those recruited in younger participants (e.g., C. L. Grady et al., 1994). Unique recruitment describes the engagement of additional (nonhomologous) brain regions (e.g., Davis, Dennis, Daselaar, Fleck, & Cabeza, 2008; Madden et al., 2007; McIntosh, 1999). Finally, substitution reflects activation of entirely novel neural networks in older relative to younger adults, perhaps signaling strategy differences or functional reorganization (e.g., Rieck, Rodrigue, Boylan, & Kennedy, 2017; Turner & Spreng, 2015).

Evidence for dedifferentiated neural response in older versus younger adults suggests that reduced neural specialization may provide a neural marker of age-related cognitive decline. However, as a theory of neurocognitive aging, it is ambivalent with respect to whether these brain changes are compensatory or deleterious. In other words, does dedifferentiated neural response reflect compensatory functional responses or inefficient processing in older adults? In general, decreased lateralization of functional brain activity (i.e., greater dedifferentiation) has been considered compensatory for cognitive performance in older adulthood. In an early report, older participants who performed better on a verbal memory task showed greater bilateral PFC activation than those who performed more poorly, suggesting that dedifferentiated neural activity was indeed a compensatory functional response to degraded neural circuitry in healthy aging (Cabeza et al., 2002). Dedifferentiation through substitution has also been positively associated with cognitive performance. During an incidental encoding task, older adults recruited medial temporal lobe regions less, and lateral PFC regions more, than their younger counterparts (Gutchess et al., 2005). Moreover, recruitment of lateral PFC and medial temporal lobe structures were inversely correlated in older but not younger participants. The investigators concluded that because the analysis was only conducted on "remembered" stimuli, dedifferentiation was compensatory for recognition performance in the older adults. Perhaps the most compelling evidence that dedifferentiation is compensatory was provided by the application of repetitive TMS (rTMS) to older and younger participants during an episodic memory task. Although memory retrieval was disrupted by rTMS to a right PFC region in younger participants, older participant performance was disrupted by rTMS applied to both right and left PFC, suggesting that greater bilateral recruitment (i.e., dedifferentiation) supported cognitive performance in these participants (Rossi et al., 2004).

In contrast to these compensatory accounts, several functional neuroimaging studies have reported that dedifferentiated neural response is associated with poorer, not improved, cognitive ability in older adults. In one of the few studies to directly contrast these competing behavioral accounts of neural dedifferentiation, functional compensation and neural inefficiency hypotheses were directly contrasted in a sample of healthy older and younger adults during performance of a delayed recognition task (Zarahn et al., 2007). The authors observed evidence of inefficient neural responding (i.e., greater activity for equivalent performance) in older relative to younger participants across a large area of cortex during encoding and maintenance epochs of the task. Moreover, the spatial patterns of response in younger participants were more similar to the pattern observed in higher performing than lower performing older adults, which is inconsistent with a compensatory account.

Dedifferentiation of neural response in older relative to younger adults has been one of the most ubiquitous findings in the neurocognitive aging literature. Moreover, this account of functional brain changes parallels a similar pattern of dedifferentiation in behavioral performance across cognitive domains in older adulthood (Baltes & Lindenberger, 1997). Although there is strong empirical evidence demonstrating dedifferentiation of functional brain response in older adulthood, the data remain equivocal as to whether these changes are compensatory or associated with cognitive decline in later life. In the next section, we briefly review several leading theories of age-related changes in brain function that attempt to reconcile the compensation versus decline debate, while also providing more specific accounts of the topology and cognitive implications of age-related functional brain changes.

Theories of Brain Function in Older Adulthood

As with studies investigating structural brain changes, accounts of functional change across the adult lifespan are highly variable and report somewhat conflicting findings with respect to the patterns of change and their implications for cognitive function in later life. However, areas of broad convergence have emerged, and these have been characterized by several leading theories of neurocognitive aging.

Consistent with the evidence for functional dedifferentiation reviewed earlier, a series of studies investigating brain changes during episodic, working memory, and visual attention tasks, older adults demonstrated a robust pattern of reduced asymmetry in the pattern of activation across cerebral hemispheres (Cabeza, 2002). This pattern of overlapping, or dedifferentiated, neural response across cognitive tasks was described as *hemispheric reduction asymmetry in older adults* (HAROLD). Older adults demonstrating the HAROLD pattern of functional brain changes showed better performance on an episodic memory task than those who showed a more "young-like" pattern of asymmetry in the recruitment of prefrontal brain regions during the task, suggestive of compensation. Further, this pattern was observed across multiple cognitive domains including episodic memory, working memory, and visual attention (Cabeza et al., 2004).

Age-related functional brain changes have also been observed in response to increasing levels of task challenge leading to the *compensation-related utilization of neural circuits hypothesis* (CRUNCH) of cognitive aging (P. A. Reuter-Lorenz & Cappell, 2008; P. A. Reuter-Lorenz & Lustig, 2005). This theory posits that inefficiencies in neural processing may cause older adults to overrecruit neural resources to achieve the same level of cognitive performance as younger adults. As with HAROLD, increased, or dedifferentiated, recruitment patterns were seen as evidence for compensatory activity, necessary to overcome degraded or noisy neural signaling associated with broader neuronal tuning curves (e.g., Li & Rieckmann, 2014) or degraded signaling pathways (e.g., Bennett & Madden, 2014). The CRUNCH hypothesis predicts two patterns of functional brain change that are commonly reported in older adulthood. At lower levels of task demand, increased recruitment is observed in the context of equivalent cognitive performance for older and younger adults. However, as task demands increase, older adults demonstrate lower levels of brain activity than younger individuals, and task performance declines. Thus, although considered a compensatory account, by incorporating levels of task demand, CRUNCH suggests that older adults show poorly modulated and inefficient neural recruitment patterns, with greater brain activity required per unit of cognitive output.

A third theory of neurocognitive aging integrates both structural and functional brain changes when considering the behavioral implications of dedifferentiated patterns of brain activity in older adulthood. The *scaffolding theory of aging cognition* (STAC) argues that changes in cortical volume, white matter integrity, and neurochemical signaling may be counteracted, at least in part, by the construction of neural "scaffolds" (Park & Reuter-Lorenz, 2009; P. A. Reuter-Lorenz & Park, 2014). Conceptually similar to the CRUNCH hypothesis, these scaffolds involve the functional recruitment of additional neural resources to offset these age-related structural brain changes. In this model, dedifferentiated patterns of brain response in older adulthood reflect a scaffolding process wherein additional neural resources are engaged to supplement task-specific recruitment patterns observed in younger adults (P. A. Reuter-Lorenz & Park, 2014). As reviewed in the earlier domain-specific section, these scaffolds, or patterns of enhanced recruitment, in older adults typically involve activation of anterior brain regions bilaterally, consistent with the *posterior to anterior shift in aging* (PASA) hypothesis (Davis et al., 2008) and the HAROLD models (Cabeza, 2002).

The final theory we review in this section on domain-general theories of functional brain aging is *neuromodulation*. This account of age-related functional brain changes argues that declines in the goal-directed modulation of neural activity is a central mechanism of neurocognitive aging (Gazzaley, Cooney, Rissman, & D'Esposito, 2005; Gazzaley & D'Esposito, 2007). Consistent with this idea, reduced selectivity in neural responses in category-selective regions of visual association cortex in older relative to younger participants have been reported during a working memory task (Payer et al., 2006). Critically, this reduced selectivity in neural responses (i.e., noisier processing) was accompanied by enhanced activity in the PFC, suggesting greater PFC activity was necessary for older adults to modulate visual association regions in response to degraded perceptual representations. A similar pattern of age-related deficits in the modulation of neural responses based on task goals has been reported during selective working memory (Gazzaley et al., 2005). During the task, age-related reductions in goal-directed suppression of activity in the visual association cortex resulted in poor filtering of goal-irrelevant stimuli, and, critically, these brain changes predicted subsequent impairments on a recognition memory paradigm.

Consistent with this idea, impaired modulatory capacity, as seen in older adulthood, has been shown to attenuate neural responsiveness to afferent signaling in posterior brain regions, producing poorly regulated and noisy information processing as evidenced both in computational modeling (Li & Rieckmann, 2014) and functional neuroimaging (Schmitz, Dixon, Anderson, & De Rosa, 2014) studies. Resultant reductions in signal-to-noise ratios degrade the integrity of mental representations, thus reducing the quality of information throughput to higher cognitive processes. According to the neuromodulation account, reduced modulatory capacity should preferentially impact those domains dependent on the highest levels of representational complexity, including episodic memory, selective attention, and working memory. These are indeed among the most vulnerable to age-related decline and show robust patterns of dedifferentiated brain response in prefrontal brain regions (cf. Spreng et al., 2010, 2017; Turner & Spreng, 2012).

Changes in Functional Brain Networks

With the advent of whole-brain, in vivo functional neuroimaging methods, and recent advances in computational resources and multivariate analytical methods, neurocognitive aging is increasingly studied through the lens of large-scale functional brain networks (Damoiseaux, 2017). Commonly reported patterns of age-related changes in neural networks, or functionally connected assemblies of spatially distributed brain regions, include changes occurring within specific brain networks, as well as alterations in the dynamic interactions among networks.

Investigations of network changes associated with normal aging have typically implicated the default network, a collection of functionally connected brain regions including the posterior cingulate cortex (PCC), medial PFC (MPFC), inferior parietal lobule, and the medial and lateral temporal lobes (Andrews-Hanna et al., 2007; Damoiseaux et al., 2008; C. L. Grady et al., 2010; Hafkemeijer, van der Grond, & Rombouts, 2012; Persson, Lustig, Nelson, & Reuter-Lorenz, 2007; Sambataro et al., 2010; Sheline & Raichle, 2013; Turner & Spreng, 2012). The default network is activated during social or internally directed cognitive processes, including access to stored knowledge representations and experiences (Andrews-Hanna et al., 2014) and is typically suppressed during performance of externally directed tasks (Buckner, Andrews-Hanna, & Schacter, 2008). Age-related changes include reduced suppression (Hansen et al., 2014; Lustig et al., 2003; Persson et al., 2007) and decreased within-network connectivity during both task (Geerligs, Maurits, Renken, & Lorist, 2014; C. L. Grady et al., 2010; Sambataro et al., 2010) and rest (Andrews-Hanna et al., 2007; Chan, Park, Savalia, Petersen, & Wig, 2014; Damoiseaux et al., 2008; Geerligs, Renken, Saliasi, Maurits, & Lorist, 2015). Recent evidence also suggests that the default network is more functionally connected to other brain networks in aging (Chan et al., 2014; Geerligs et al., 2015; Muller, Mérillat, & Jäncke, 2016; Sambataro et al., 2010; Sheline & Raichle, 2013; Spreng, Stevens, Viviano, & Schacter, 2016), and this connectivity is poorly modulated by task context (C. L. Grady, Sarraf, Saverino, & Campbell, 2016; Rieck et al., 2017; Spreng & Schacter, 2012; Spreng et al., 2016; Turner & Spreng, 2015).

Although changes involving the default network have been frequently reported, there is mounting evidence to suggest that the global network architecture of the brain is altered across the adult lifespan. This has been characterized as reduced network segregation and increased integration (Chan et al., 2014). As with patterns of brain activity (reviewed earlier), interactions among spatially distributed brain networks become increasingly dedifferentiated in older adulthood. In the context of functional brain networks, this means that with age, interactions between networks increase (i.e., they become less segregated or differentiated), while within-network connectivity declines. Measured across the whole brain, older adults display a less discrete network architecture both during cognitive task performance (Chan et al., 2014; Gallen, Turner, Adnan, & D'Esposito, 2016) as well as during rest, suggesting these functional network changes are also manifest within the intrinsic network architecture of the brain (e.g., Geerligs et al., 2015).

Similar patterns of network differentiation with age have been reported in a more circumscribed set of brain networks, including the default, dorsal attention, and frontal parietal control networks both during task and at rest (C. L. Grady et al., 2016; Spreng et al., 2016). Specific changes include reduced anticorrelations between dorsal attention and default networks and increased network interactions across all three networks, consistent with a network dedifferentiation account. We have also reported poor modulation of network interactions based on task goals. Older adults fail to decouple default and frontoparietal control networks in response to changing task context (Spreng & Schacter, 2012) and control demands (Turner & Spreng, 2015). These observations led us recently to propose the *default-executive coupling hypothesis of aging* (DECHA; Spreng & Turner, in press; Turner & Spreng, 2015; see Figure 1.1). This network neuroscience model of neurocognitive aging suggests that with age, older adults fail to flexibly decouple brain regions implicated in control processes from the default network, implicated in more associative cognitive processes. We have recently shown that increased coupling of these networks, as predicted by the DECHA,

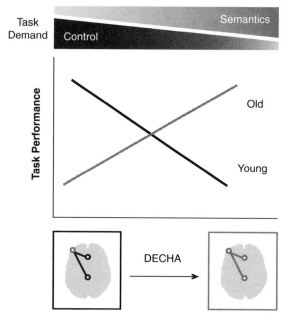

Figure 1.1. Default-executive coupling hypothesis of aging (DECHA): Integrated model of cognitive and brain aging. Behavior (top): Greater task demand for semantics impacts performance differently for younger and older adults. Brain (bottom): Default (midline circles) to executive (lateral circles) coupling increases from younger (black lines) to older age (lines). Data from Samanez-Larkin and Knutson (2015).

is associated with reduced fluid intelligence and increased reliance on semantic or crystalized knowledge in older adulthood (Spreng et al., 2018). Further, default coupling to the frontal–parietal control network defined more broadly, to include regions implicated in salience processing, may convey real-world benefits for older adults during tasks requiring access to prior knowledge such as creative problem solving (Adnan, Beaty, Silvia, Spreng, & Turner, 2019). Evidence both from cross-sectional (Rieck et al., 2017) and longitudinal (Ng, Lo, Lim, Chee, & Zhou, 2016) investigations provide support for this hypothesis and provide further evidence that these changes in network interactivity can predict individual differences in cognitive functioning. Taken together these network-based accounts of functional brain aging point to network neuroscience as an important new frontier in neurocognitive aging research.

Summary of Functional Brain Changes in Aging

In this section, we have reviewed the current state of knowledge with respect to changes in brain function that occur from younger to older adulthood. Domain-specific changes include greater recruitment of frontal brain regions during complex cognitive tasks, reduced hemispheric lateralization in anterior brain regions (e.g., Cabeza, 2002; C. L. Grady et al., 1994), and evidence for enhanced activation in regions typically engaged by young adults (Spreng et al., 2010, 2017; Turner & Spreng, 2012). Taken together, these domain-specific patterns of age-related brain changes reflect a global pattern of neural dedifferentiation, suggesting older adults have reduced capacity to recruit specialized neural circuits associated with discreet processing operations (Li et al., 2001). Leading theories of functional brain aging generally converge around the notion that these patterns of functional brain change are compensatory. Functional dedifferentiation reflects recruitment of additional neural resources, or scaffolds, to overcome the challenges posed by degraded neural signaling and communication associated with structural brain changes in later life. However, compensation comes at the cost of neural efficiency, with older adults expending greater neural resources per unit of cognitive output (cf. Zarahn et al., 2007). Finally, as with investigations of structural brain changes in older adulthood, researchers are increasingly studying age-related functional changes through the lens of distributed brain networks. Paralleling changes in regional activity, functional brain networks also appear to follow a dedifferentiation pattern in older adulthood, both with respect to the global network architecture of the brain and within more domain-specific cognitive networks. These network-level changes are marked by reduced within-network and increased between-network connections, as well as reduced modulation of network dynamics in response to changing task demands.

CONCLUSIONS AND NEW FRONTIERS

Summary of Structural and Functional Brain Changes

Over the past century we have learned much about the aging brain. With advances in in vivo imaging techniques, we now know that the cranial vault masks profound changes that occur in the structure of the brain across the adult lifespan. By some estimates, these changes may represent volume losses 0.3% per year through middle age, accelerating to almost 0.6% per year in older adulthood. We have also learned that these changes are not uniform across the cerebrum. The most profound and rapid losses occur in anterior and heteromodal association cortices, regions that are the last to reach maturation in early adulthood. Further, not all tissue compartments undergo similar rates of decline. Although earlier studies suggested that white matter was not affected in normal aging, more recent work demonstrates that changes in the volume, integrity, and overall health of the brain's white matter may be the most significant predictor of the transition from normal aging to neurodegenerative disease. Perhaps most surprising given the extent and pace of structural brain change, is the relative paucity of evidence linking these changes to cognitive abilities in later life. A central factor in this incongruity may be the role of altered brain function in mediating the impact of structural changes. Functional brain changes include both domain-specific and nonspecific alterations in neural activation patterns that together point to a generalized pattern of neural dedifferentiation. Theories of neurocognitive aging, although differing somewhat with respect to specific causes and consequences, coalesce around the idea that older adults recruit additional neural resources to sustain cognitive output at a level equivalent to young, but at the cost of neural efficiency. Finally, we observed a growing trend in the literature to consider brain aging not only in terms of local changes but as alterations in large-scale and spatially distributed brain networks. Network patterns appear to mirror local changes, with the greatest declines observed in nodal connections involving anterior and heteromodal association cortices as well as an age-related shift toward a more dedifferentiated functional network architecture.

Emerging Challenges and Opportunities

Despite significant advances in our understanding of the aging brain, many challenges remain. Foremost among these is characterizing the interdependencies between structural and functional brain changes across the lifespan, and how these interactions influence the trajectory of age-related cognitive decline. In our review, we addressed structure and function separately, mirroring the vast majority of the research literature in the field. However, mapping the interactions and contingencies between changes in brain structure and function across the lifespan is almost certainly a precondition for developing predictive biomarkers that can reliably differentiate healthy versus pathological brain aging (for a recent effort to develop an integrated computational model of senescence across the lifespan, see Naik, Banerjee, Bapi, Deco, & Roy, 2017). Advances in multivariate and machine learning analytical tools are now opening the door for the inclusion of an array of structural and functional brain metrics in a single analytical model to predict the trajectory of cognitive aging. These methods are allowing researchers to move beyond characterizing group differences to pursue the development of person-specific biomarkers of age-related cognitive change.

However, progress in this direction will require large-scale studies to develop normative data sets, a daunting challenge given that variability is increasingly seen as a hallmark of neurocognitive aging (Garrett et al., 2013).

The vast majority of research in the field still consists of cross-sectional, extreme group designs. As discussed earlier, this approach can mask individual differences, and tends to underestimate the extent of age-related change. Large-scale longitudinal studies, such as the Betula Project, the Baltimore Longitudinal Aging Study, or Singapore Longitudinal Aging Brain Study, are beginning to address this issue. Further, open data initiatives are allowing for the aggregation of brain data across studies and centers resulting in unprecedented sample sizes (e.g., Human Connectome, UK Biobank projects). Combined with exponential advances in computational resources, these efforts hold significant promise for overcoming challenges posed by heterogeneity to drive the development of person-specific biomarkers, mapping structural and functional brain changes to individual trajectories of cognitive aging.

Finally, while big data initiatives hold considerable promise for biomarker development, efforts to develop a more mechanistic understanding of structural and functional brain aging are also informing the design of targeted interventions to alter the course of cognitive aging. We have drawn on the neuromodulation theory of functional brain aging (D'Esposito & Chen, 2006; Gazzaley & D'Esposito, 2007) to develop a targeted behavioral intervention protocol to enhance goal-directed modulation of brain activity, and executive control capacity, in older adulthood (Adnan, Chen, Novakovic-Agopian, D'Esposito, & Turner, 2017). Researchers are also drawing from network neuroscience models of brain aging to guide neurostimulation interventions to alleviate symptoms of psychiatric and neurological diseases, including diseases of aging. In one recent report, brain network analyses were used to detect regions on the cortical surface that were functionally connected to subcortical brain structures typically targeted in deep brain stimulation treatments (Fox et al., 2014). These analyses open the possibility of stimulating surface nodes (e.g., using TMS) to activate or suppress subcortical nodes noninvasively to alleviate symptoms of neurological or psychiatric disorders. Although only two of many examples, these reports highlight the potential translational implications of our increasingly sophisticated understanding of the aging brain. As this review has clearly demonstrated, the first 100 years of research exploring the structural and functional brain changes that occur across the adult lifespan have proven remarkably fruitful, enhancing our knowledge of the aging brain and highlighting the limitations and pitfalls inherent to human brain mapping. Undoubtedly the next century will offer myriad advances—and surprises—as we continue the quest to map the topology and trajectory of brain aging and leverage these discoveries to sustain and enhance cognitive functioning in later life.

REFERENCES

Adnan, A., Beaty, R., Silvia, P., Spreng, R. N., & Turner, G. R. (2019). Creative aging: Functional brain networks associated with divergent thinking in older and younger adults. *Neurobiology of Aging, 75*, 150–158. http://dx.doi.org/10.1016/j.neurobiolaging.2018.11.004

Adnan, A., Chen, A. J. W., Novakovic-Agopian, T., D'Esposito, M., & Turner, G. R. (2017). Brain changes following executive control training in older adults. *Neurorehabilitation and Neural Repair, 31*, 910–922. http://dx.doi.org/10.1177/1545968317728580

Alexander, G. E., Chen, K., Merkley, T. L., Reiman, E. M., Caselli, R. J., Aschenbrenner, M., . . . Moeller, J. R. (2006). Regional network of magnetic resonance imaging gray matter volume in healthy aging. *NeuroReport, 17*, 951–956. http://dx.doi.org/10.1097/01.wnr.0000220135.16844.b6

Alexander-Bloch, A., Giedd, J. N., & Bullmore, E. (2013). Imaging structural co-variance between human brain regions. *Nature Reviews Neuroscience, 14*, 322–336. http://dx.doi.org/10.1038/nrn3465

Andrews, T. J., Halpern, S. D., & Purves, D. (1997). Correlated size variations in human visual cortex, lateral geniculate nucleus, and optic tract. *The Journal of Neuroscience, 17*, 2859–2868. http://dx.doi.org/10.1523/JNEUROSCI.17-08-02859.1997

Andrews-Hanna, J. R., Smallwood, J., & Spreng, R. N. (2014). The default network and self-generated thought: Component processes, dynamic control, and clinical relevance. *Annals of the New York Academy of Sciences, 1316*, 29–52. http://dx.doi.org/10.1111/nyas.12360

Andrews-Hanna, J. R., Snyder, A. Z., Vincent, J. L., Lustig, C., Head, D., Raichle, M. E., & Buckner, R. L. (2007). Disruption of large-scale brain systems in advanced aging. *Neuron, 56*, 924–935. http://dx.doi.org/10.1016/j.neuron.2007.10.038

Arvanitakis, Z., Fleischman, D. A., Arfanakis, K., Leurgans, S. E., Barnes, L. L., & Bennett, D. A. (2016). Association of white matter hyperintensities and gray matter volume with cognition in older individuals without cognitive impairment. *Brain Structure & Function, 221*, 2135–2146. http://dx.doi.org/10.1007/s00429-015-1034-7

Baltes, P. B., & Lindenberger, U. (1997). Emergence of a powerful connection between sensory and cognitive functions across the adult life span: A new window to the study of cognitive aging? *Psychology and Aging, 12*, 12–21. http://dx.doi.org/10.1037/0882-7974.12.1.12

Bennett, I. J., & Madden, D. J. (2014). Disconnected aging: Cerebral white matter integrity and age-related differences in cognition. *Neuroscience, 276*, 187–205. http://dx.doi.org/10.1016/j.neuroscience.2013.11.026

Bennett, I. J., Madden, D. J., Vaidya, C. J., Howard, D. V., & Howard, J. H., Jr. (2010). Age-related differences in multiple measures of white matter integrity:

A diffusion tensor imaging study of healthy aging. *Human Brain Mapping, 31,* 378–390.

Brickman, A. M., Habeck, C., Zarahn, E., Flynn, J., & Stern, Y. (2007). Structural MRI covariance patterns associated with normal aging and neuropsychological functioning. *Neurobiology of Aging, 28,* 284–295. http://dx.doi.org/10.1016/j.neurobiolaging.2005.12.016

Buckner, R. L., Andrews-Hanna, J. R., & Schacter, D. L. (2008). The brain's default network: Anatomy, function, and relevance to disease. *Annals of the New York Academy of Sciences, 1124,* 1–38. http://dx.doi.org/10.1196/annals.1440.011

Cabeza, R. (2002). Hemispheric asymmetry reduction in older adults: The HAROLD model. *Psychology and Aging, 17,* 85–100. http://dx.doi.org/10.1037/0882-7974.17.1.85

Cabeza, R., Anderson, N. D., Locantore, J. K., & McIntosh, A. R. (2002). Aging gracefully: Compensatory brain activity in high-performing older adults. *NeuroImage, 17,* 1394–1402. http://dx.doi.org/10.1006/nimg.2002.1280

Cabeza, R., Daselaar, S. M., Dolcos, F., Prince, S. E., Budde, M., & Nyberg, L. (2004). Task-independent and task-specific age effects on brain activity during working memory, visual attention and episodic retrieval. *Cerebral Cortex, 14,* 364–375. http://dx.doi.org/10.1093/cercor/bhg133

Cappell, K. A., Gmeindl, L., & Reuter-Lorenz, P. A. (2010). Age differences in prefrontal recruitment during verbal working memory maintenance depend on memory load. *Cortex, 46,* 462–473. http://dx.doi.org/10.1016/j.cortex.2009.11.009

Chan, M. Y., Park, D. C., Savalia, N. K., Petersen, S. E., & Wig, G. S. (2014). Decreased segregation of brain systems across the healthy adult life span. *Proceedings of the National Academy of Sciences of the United States of America, 111,* E4997–E5006. http://dx.doi.org/10.1073/pnas.1415122111

Chen, Z. J., He, Y., Rosa-Neto, P., Gong, G., & Evans, A. C. (2011). Age-related alterations in the modular organization of structural cortical network by using cortical thickness from MRI. *NeuroImage, 56,* 235–245. http://dx.doi.org/10.1016/j.neuroimage.2011.01.010

Colcombe, S. J., Kramer, A. F., Erickson, K. I., & Scalf, P. (2005). The implications of cortical recruitment and brain morphology for individual differences in inhibitory function in aging humans. *Psychology and Aging, 20,* 363–375. http://dx.doi.org/10.1037/0882-7974.20.3.363

Craik, F. I., & Bialystok, E. (2006). Cognition through the lifespan: Mechanisms of change. *Trends in Cognitive Sciences, 10,* 131–138. http://dx.doi.org/10.1016/j.tics.2006.01.007

D'Esposito, M., & Chen, A. J. (2006). Neural mechanisms of prefrontal cortical function: Implications for cognitive rehabilitation. *Progress in Brain Research, 157,* 123–139. http://dx.doi.org/10.1016/S0079-6123(06)57008-6

Damoiseaux, J. S. (2017). Effects of aging on functional and structural brain connectivity. *NeuroImage, 160,* 32–40. http://dx.doi.org/10.1016/j.neuroimage.2017.01.077

Damoiseaux, J. S., Beckmann, C. F., Arigita, E. J., Barkhof, F., Scheltens, P., Stam, C. J., . . . Rombouts, S. A. (2008). Reduced resting-state brain activity in the "default network" in normal aging. *Cerebral Cortex, 18*, 1856–1864. http://dx.doi.org/10.1093/cercor/bhm207

Davis, S. W., Dennis, N. A., Daselaar, S. M., Fleck, M. S., & Cabeza, R. (2008). Que PASA? The posterior–anterior shift in aging. *Cerebral Cortex, 18*, 1201–1209. http://dx.doi.org/10.1093/cercor/bhm155

Dotson, V. M., Szymkowicz, S. M., Sozda, C. N., Kirton, J. W., Green, M. L., O'Shea, A., . . . Woods, A. J. (2016). Age differences in prefrontal surface area and thickness in middle aged to older adults. *Frontiers in Aging Neuroscience, 7*, 250. http://dx.doi.org/10.3389/fnagi.2015.00250

Driscoll, I., Davatzikos, C., An, Y., Wu, X., Shen, D., Kraut, M., & Resnick, S. M. (2009). Longitudinal pattern of regional brain volume change differentiates normal aging from MCI. *Neurology, 72*, 1906–1913. http://dx.doi.org/10.1212/WNL.0b013e3181a82634

DuPre, E., & Spreng, R. N. (2017). Structural covariance networks across the life span, from 6 to 94 years of age. *Network Neuroscience, 1*, 302–323. http://dx.doi.org/10.1162/NETN_a_00016

Evans, A. C. (2013). Networks of anatomical covariance. *NeuroImage, 80*, 489–504. http://dx.doi.org/10.1016/j.neuroimage.2013.05.054

Finger, S. (1994). *Origins of neuroscience*. New York, NY: Oxford University Press.

Fjell, A. M., Westlye, L. T., Amlien, I., Espeseth, T., Reinvang, I., Raz, N., . . . Walhovd, K. B. (2009). High consistency of regional cortical thinning in aging across multiple samples. *Cerebral Cortex, 19*, 2001–2012. http://dx.doi.org/10.1093/cercor/bhn232

Fjell, A. M., Westlye, L. T., Amlien, I., Tamnes, C. K., Grydeland, H., Engvig, A., . . . Walhovd, K. B. (2015). High-expanding cortical regions in human development and evolution are related to higher intellectual abilities. *Cerebral Cortex, 25*, 26–34.

Fjell, A. M., Westlye, L. T., Grydeland, H., Amlien, I., Espeseth, T., Reinvang, I., . . . Alzheimer Disease Neuroimaging Initiative. (2014). Accelerating cortical thinning: Unique to dementia or universal in aging? *Cerebral Cortex, 24*, 919–934. http://dx.doi.org/10.1093/cercor/bhs379

Fleischman, D. A., Leurgans, S., Arfanakis, K., Arvanitakis, Z., Barnes, L. L., Boyle, P. A., . . . Bennett, D. A. (2014). Gray-matter macrostructure in cognitively healthy older persons: Associations with age and cognition. *Brain Structure & Function, 219*, 2029–2049. http://dx.doi.org/10.1007/s00429-013-0622-7

Flood, D. G., & Coleman, P. D. (1988). Neuron numbers and sizes in aging brain: Comparisons of human, monkey, and rodent data. *Neurobiology of Aging, 9*, 453–463. http://dx.doi.org/10.1016/S0197-4580(88)80098-8

Fox, M. D., Buckner, R. L., Liu, H., Chakravarty, M. M., Lozano, A. M., & Pascual-Leone, A. (2014). Resting-state networks link invasive and noninvasive brain stimulation across diverse psychiatric and neurological diseases. *Proceedings of the National Academy of Sciences of the United States of America, 111,* E4367–E4375. http://dx.doi.org/10.1073/pnas.1405003111

Freitas, C., Farzan, F., & Pascual-Leone, A. (2013). Assessing brain plasticity across the lifespan with transcranial magnetic stimulation: Why, how, and what is the ultimate goal? *Frontiers in Neuroscience, 7,* 42. http://dx.doi.org/10.3389/fnins.2013.00042

Gallen, C. L., Turner, G. R., Adnan, A., & D'Esposito, M. (2016). Reconfiguration of brain network architecture to support executive control in aging. *Neurobiology of Aging, 44,* 42–52. http://dx.doi.org/10.1016/j.neurobiolaging.2016.04.003

Garrett, D. D., Samanez-Larkin, G. R., MacDonald, S. W., Lindenberger, U., McIntosh, A. R., & Grady, C. L. (2013). Moment-to-moment brain signal variability: A next frontier in human brain mapping? *Neuroscience and Biobehavioral Reviews, 37,* 610–624. http://dx.doi.org/10.1016/j.neubiorev.2013.02.015

Gazzaley, A., Cooney, J. W., Rissman, J., & D'Esposito, M. (2005). Top-down suppression deficit underlies working memory impairment in normal aging [erratum at https://dx.doi.org/10.1038/nn1205-1791c]. *Nature Neuroscience, 8,* 1298–1300. http://dx.doi.org/10.1038/nn1543

Gazzaley, A., & D'Esposito, M. (2007). Top-down modulation and normal aging. *Annals of the New York Academy of Sciences, 1097,* 67–83. http://dx.doi.org/10.1196/annals.1379.010

Geerligs, L., Maurits, N. M., Renken, R. J., & Lorist, M. M. (2014). Reduced specificity of functional connectivity in the aging brain during task performance. *Human Brain Mapping, 35,* 319–330. http://dx.doi.org/10.1002/hbm.22175

Geerligs, L., Renken, R. J., Saliasi, E., Maurits, N. M., & Lorist, M. M. (2015). A brain-wide study of age-related changes in functional connectivity. *Cerebral Cortex, 25,* 1987–1999. http://dx.doi.org/10.1093/cercor/bhu012

Good, C. D., Johnsrude, I. S., Ashburner, J., Henson, R. N., Friston, K. J., & Frackowiak, R. S. (2001). A voxel-based morphometric study of ageing in 465 normal adult human brains. *NeuroImage, 14,* 21–36. http://dx.doi.org/10.1006/nimg.2001.0786

Grady, C. L. (1996). Age-related changes in cortical blood flow activation during perception and memory. *Annals of the New York Academy of Sciences, 777,* 14–21. http://dx.doi.org/10.1111/j.1749-6632.1996.tb34396.x

Grady, C. L. (2008). Cognitive neuroscience of aging. *Annals of the New York Academy of Sciences, 1124,* 127–144. http://dx.doi.org/10.1196/annals.1440.009

Grady, C. L. (2012). The cognitive neuroscience of ageing. *Nature Reviews Neuroscience, 13,* 491–505. http://dx.doi.org/10.1038/nrn3256

Grady, C. L., Maisog, J. M., Horwitz, B., Ungerleider, L. G., Mentis, M. J., Salerno, J. A., . . . Haxby, J. V. (1994). Age-related changes in cortical blood flow activation during visual processing of faces and location. *The Journal of Neuroscience, 14,* 1450–1462. http://dx.doi.org/10.1523/JNEUROSCI.14-03-01450.1994

Grady, C. L., Protzner, A. B., Kovacevic, N., Strother, S. C., Afshin-Pour, B., Wojtowicz, M., . . . McIntosh, A. R. (2010). A multivariate analysis of age-related differences in default mode and task-positive networks across multiple cognitive domains. *Cerebral Cortex, 20*, 1432–1447. http://dx.doi.org/10.1093/cercor/bhp207

Grady, C. L., Sarraf, S., Saverino, C., & Campbell, K. (2016). Age differences in the functional interactions among the default, frontoparietal control, and dorsal attention networks. *Neurobiology of Aging, 41*, 159–172. http://dx.doi.org/10.1016/j.neurobiolaging.2016.02.020

Greenwood, P. M. (2007). Functional plasticity in cognitive aging: Review and hypothesis. *Neuropsychology, 21*, 657–673. http://dx.doi.org/10.1037/0894-4105.21.6.657

Gutchess, A. H., Welsh, R. C., Hedden, T., Bangert, A., Minear, M., Liu, L. L., & Park, D. C. (2005). Aging and the neural correlates of successful picture encoding: Frontal activations compensate for decreased medial-temporal activity. *Journal of Cognitive Neuroscience, 17*, 84–96. http://dx.doi.org/10.1162/0898929052880048

Hafkemeijer, A., van der Grond, J., & Rombouts, S. A. (2012). Imaging the default mode network in aging and dementia. *Biochimica et Biophysica Acta, 1822*, 431–441.

Hansen, N. L., Lauritzen, M., Mortensen, E. L., Osler, M., Avlund, K., Fagerlund, B., & Rostrup, E. (2014). Subclinical cognitive decline in middle-age is associated with reduced task-induced deactivation of the brain's default mode network. *Human Brain Mapping, 35*, 4488–4498. http://dx.doi.org/10.1002/hbm.22489

Hedden, T., & Gabrieli, J. D. (2004). Insights into the ageing mind: A view from cognitive neuroscience. *Nature Reviews Neuroscience, 5*, 87–96. http://dx.doi.org/10.1038/nrn1323

Hugenschmidt, C. E., Peiffer, A. M., Kraft, R. A., Casanova, R., Deibler, A. R., Burdette, J. H., . . . Laurienti, P. J. (2008). Relating imaging indices of white matter integrity and volume in healthy older adults. *Cerebral Cortex, 18*, 433–442. http://dx.doi.org/10.1093/cercor/bhm080

Jernigan, T. L., Press, G. A., & Hesselink, J. R. (1990). Methods for measuring brain morphologic features on magnetic resonance images. Validation and normal aging. *Archives of Neurology, 47*, 27–32. http://dx.doi.org/10.1001/archneur.1990.00530010035015

Kemper, T. L. (1994). Neuroanatomical and neuropathological changes during aging and in dementia. In M. L. Albert & E. J. E. Knoepfel (Eds.), *Clinical neurology of aging* (2nd ed., pp. 3–67). New York, NY: Oxford University Press.

Leong, R. L. F., Lo, J. C., Sim, S. K. Y., Zheng, H., Tandi, J., Zhou, J., & Chee, M. W. L. (2017). Longitudinal brain structure and cognitive changes over 8 years in an East Asian cohort. *NeuroImage, 147*, 852–860. http://dx.doi.org/10.1016/j.neuroimage.2016.10.016

Li, S. C., Lindenberger, U., & Sikström, S. (2001). Aging cognition: From neuromodulation to representation. *Trends in Cognitive Sciences, 5,* 479–486. http://dx.doi.org/10.1016/S1364-6613(00)01769-1

Li, S. C., & Rieckmann, A. (2014). Neuromodulation and aging: Implications of aging neuronal gain control on cognition. *Current Opinion in Neurobiology, 29,* 148–158. http://dx.doi.org/10.1016/j.conb.2014.07.009

Lustig, C., Snyder, A. Z., Bhakta, M., O'Brien, K. C., McAvoy, M., Raichle, M. E., . . . Buckner, R. L. (2003). Functional deactivations: Change with age and dementia of the Alzheimer type. *Proceedings of the National Academy of Sciences of the United States of America, 100,* 14504–14509. http://dx.doi.org/10.1073/pnas.2235925100

Madden, D. J., Spaniol, J., Whiting, W. L., Bucur, B., Provenzale, J. M., Cabeza, R., . . . Huettel, S. A. (2007). Adult age differences in the functional neuroanatomy of visual attention: A combined fMRI and DTI study. *Neurobiology of Aging, 28,* 459–476. http://dx.doi.org/10.1016/j.neurobiolaging.2006.01.005

Maillard, P., Crivello, F., Dufouil, C., Tzourio-Mazoyer, N., Tzourio, C., & Mazoyer, B. (2009). Longitudinal follow-up of individual white matter hyperintensities in a large cohort of elderly. *Neuroradiology, 51,* 209–220. http://dx.doi.org/10.1007/s00234-008-0489-0

Mattay, V. S., Fera, F., Tessitore, A., Hariri, A. R., Berman, K. F., Das, S., . . . Weinberger, D. R. (2006). Neurophysiological correlates of age-related changes in working memory capacity. *Neuroscience Letters, 392,* 32–37. http://dx.doi.org/10.1016/j.neulet.2005.09.025

McGinnis, S. M., Brickhouse, M., Pascual, B., & Dickerson, B. C. (2011). Age-related changes in the thickness of cortical zones in humans. *Brain Topography, 24,* 279–291. http://dx.doi.org/10.1007/s10548-011-0198-6

McIntosh, A. R. (1999). Mapping cognition to the brain through neural interactions. *Memory, 7,* 523–548. http://dx.doi.org/10.1080/096582199387733

Mechelli, A., Friston, K. J., Frackowiak, R. S., & Price, C. J. (2005). Structural covariance in the human cortex. *The Journal of Neuroscience, 25,* 8303–8310. http://dx.doi.org/10.1523/JNEUROSCI.0357-05.2005

Meunier, D., Achard, S., Morcom, A., & Bullmore, E. (2009). Age-related changes in modular organization of human brain functional networks. *NeuroImage, 44,* 715–723. http://dx.doi.org/10.1016/j.neuroimage.2008.09.062

Montembeault, M., Joubert, S., Doyon, J., Carrier, J., Gagnon, J. F., Monchi, O., . . . Brambati, S. M. (2012). The impact of aging on gray matter structural covariance networks. *NeuroImage, 63,* 754–759. http://dx.doi.org/10.1016/j.neuroimage.2012.06.052

Muller, A. M., Mérillat, S., & Jäncke, L. (2016). Older but still fluent? Insights from the intrinsically active baseline configuration of the aging brain using a data driven graph-theoretical approach. *NeuroImage, 127,* 346–362. http://dx.doi.org/10.1016/j.neuroimage.2015.12.027

Naik, S., Banerjee, A., Bapi, R. S., Deco, G., & Roy, D. (2017). Metastability in senescence. *Trends in Cognitive Sciences, 21*, 509–521. http://dx.doi.org/10.1016/j.tics.2017.04.007

Ng, K. K., Lo, J. C., Lim, J. K. W., Chee, M. W. L., & Zhou, J. (2016). Reduced functional segregation between the default mode network and the executive control network in healthy older adults: A longitudinal study. *NeuroImage, 133,* 321–330. http://dx.doi.org/10.1016/j.neuroimage.2016.03.029

Pacheco, J., Goh, J. O., Kraut, M. A., Ferrucci, L., & Resnick, S. M. (2015). Greater cortical thinning in normal older adults predicts later cognitive impairment. *Neurobiology of Aging, 36,* 903–908. http://dx.doi.org/10.1016/j.neurobiolaging.2014.08.031

Park, D. C., Polk, T. A., Mikels, J. A., Taylor, S. F., & Marshuetz, C. (2001). Cerebral aging: Integration of brain and behavioral models of cognitive function. *Dialogues in Clinical Neuroscience, 3,* 151–165.

Park, D. C., & Reuter-Lorenz, P. (2009). The adaptive brain: Aging and neurocognitive scaffolding. *Annual Review of Psychology, 60,* 173–196. http://dx.doi.org/10.1146/annurev.psych.59.103006.093656

Payer, D., Marshuetz, C., Sutton, B., Hebrank, A., Welsh, R. C., & Park, D. C. (2006). Decreased neural specialization in old adults on a working memory task. *NeuroReport, 17,* 487–491. http://dx.doi.org/10.1097/01.wnr.0000209005.40481.31

Persson, J., Lustig, C., Nelson, J. K., & Reuter-Lorenz, P. A. (2007). Age differences in deactivation: A link to cognitive control? *Journal of Cognitive Neuroscience, 19,* 1021–1032. http://dx.doi.org/10.1162/jocn.2007.19.6.1021

Pfefferbaum, A., Mathalon, D. H., Sullivan, E. V., Rawles, J. M., Zipursky, R. B., & Lim, K. O. (1994). A quantitative magnetic resonance imaging study of changes in brain morphology from infancy to late adulthood. *Archives of Neurology, 51,* 874–887. http://dx.doi.org/10.1001/archneur.1994.00540210046012

Pfefferbaum, A., Rohlfing, T., Rosenbloom, M. J., Chu, W., Colrain, I. M., & Sullivan, E. V. (2013). Variation in longitudinal trajectories of regional brain volumes of healthy men and women (ages 10 to 85 years) measured with atlas-based parcellation of MRI. *NeuroImage, 65,* 176–193. http://dx.doi.org/10.1016/j.neuroimage.2012.10.008

Piguet, O., Double, K. L., Kril, J. J., Harasty, J., Macdonald, V., McRitchie, D. A., & Halliday, G. M. (2009). White matter loss in healthy ageing: A postmortem analysis. *Neurobiology of Aging, 30,* 1288–1295. http://dx.doi.org/10.1016/j.neurobiolaging.2007.10.015

Raz, N. (1996). Neuroanatomy of aging brain: Evidence from structural MRI. In E. D. Bigler (Ed.), *Neuroimaging II: Clinical applications* (pp. 17–55). New York, NY: Plenum Press.

Raz, N. (2000). Aging of the brain and its impact on cognitive performance: Integration of structural and functional findings. In F. I. Craik & T. A. Salthouse (Eds.), *Handbook of aging and cognition II* (pp. 1–90). Hillsdale, NJ: Erlbaum.

Raz, N., Ghisletta, P., Rodrigue, K. M., Kennedy, K. M., & Lindenberger, U. (2010). Trajectories of brain aging in middle-aged and older adults: Regional and individual differences. *NeuroImage, 51*, 501–511. http://dx.doi.org/10.1016/j.neuroimage.2010.03.020

Raz, N., Gunning, F. M., Head, D., Dupuis, J. H., McQuain, J., Briggs, S. D., . . . Acker, J. D. (1997). Selective aging of the human cerebral cortex observed in vivo: Differential vulnerability of the prefrontal gray matter. *Cerebral Cortex, 7*, 268–282. http://dx.doi.org/10.1093/cercor/7.3.268

Raz, N., & Lindenberger, U. (2011). Only time will tell: Cross-sectional studies offer no solution to the age–brain–cognition triangle: Comment on Salthouse (2011). *Psychological Bulletin, 137*, 790–795. http://dx.doi.org/10.1037/a0024503

Raz, N., Lindenberger, U., Rodrigue, K. M., Kennedy, K. M., Head, D., Williamson, A., . . . Acker, J. D. (2005). Regional brain changes in aging healthy adults: General trends, individual differences and modifiers. *Cerebral Cortex, 15*, 1676–1689. http://dx.doi.org/10.1093/cercor/bhi044

Raz, N., Rodrigue, K. M., Kennedy, K. M., & Acker, J. D. (2007). Vascular health and longitudinal changes in brain and cognition in middle-aged and older adults. *Neuropsychology, 21*, 149–157. http://dx.doi.org/10.1037/0894-4105.21.2.149

Resnick, S. M., Pham, D. L., Kraut, M. A., Zonderman, A. B., & Davatzikos, C. (2003). Longitudinal magnetic resonance imaging studies of older adults: A shrinking brain. *The Journal of Neuroscience, 23*, 3295–3301. http://dx.doi.org/10.1523/JNEUROSCI.23-08-03295.2003

Reuter-Lorenz, P. A., & Cappell, K. A. (2008). Neurocognitive aging and the compensation hypothesis. *Current Directions in Psychological Science, 17*, 177–182. http://dx.doi.org/10.1111/j.1467-8721.2008.00570.x

Reuter-Lorenz, P. A., Jonides, J., Smith, E. E., Hartley, A., Miller, A., Marshuetz, C., & Koeppe, R. A. (2000). Age differences in the frontal lateralization of verbal and spatial working memory revealed by PET. *Journal of Cognitive Neuroscience, 12*, 174–187. http://dx.doi.org/10.1162/089892900561814

Reuter-Lorenz, P. A., & Lustig, C. (2005). Brain aging: Reorganizing discoveries about the aging mind. *Current Opinion in Neurobiology, 15*, 245–251. http://dx.doi.org/10.1016/j.conb.2005.03.016

Reuter-Lorenz, P. A., & Park, D. C. (2014). How does it STAC up? Revisiting the scaffolding theory of aging and cognition. *Neuropsychology Review, 24*, 355–370. http://dx.doi.org/10.1007/s11065-014-9270-9

Rieck, J. R., Rodrigue, K. M., Boylan, M. A., & Kennedy, K. M. (2017). Age-related reduction of BOLD modulation to cognitive difficulty predicts poorer task accuracy and poorer fluid reasoning ability. *NeuroImage, 147*, 262–271. http://dx.doi.org/10.1016/j.neuroimage.2016.12.022

Rossi, S., Miniussi, C., Pasqualetti, P., Babiloni, C., Rossini, P. M., & Cappa, S. F. (2004). Age-related functional changes of prefrontal cortex in long-term memory: A repetitive transcranial magnetic stimulation study. *The Journal of Neuroscience, 24*, 7939–7944. http://dx.doi.org/10.1523/JNEUROSCI.0703-04.2004

Rossini, P. M., Rossi, S., Babiloni, C., & Polich, J. (2007). Clinical neurophysiology of aging brain: From normal aging to neurodegeneration. *Progress in Neurobiology, 83*, 375–400. http://dx.doi.org/10.1016/j.pneurobio.2007.07.010

Rypma, B., & D'Esposito, M. (2000). Isolating the neural mechanisms of age-related changes in human working memory. *Nature Neuroscience, 3*, 509–515. http://dx.doi.org/10.1038/74889

Salat, D. H., Buckner, R. L., Snyder, A. Z., Greve, D. N., Desikan, R. S., Busa, E., . . . Fischl, B. (2004). Thinning of the cerebral cortex in aging. *Cerebral Cortex, 14*, 721–730. http://dx.doi.org/10.1093/cercor/bhh032

Samanez-Larkin, G. R., & Knutson, B. (2015). Decision making in the ageing brain: Changes in affective and motivational circuits. *Nature Reviews Neuroscience, 16*, 278–289. http://dx.doi.org/10.1038/nrn3917

Sambataro, F., Murty, V. P., Callicott, J. H., Tan, H. Y., Das, S., Weinberger, D. R., & Mattay, V. S. (2010). Age-related alterations in default mode network: Impact on working memory performance. *Neurobiology of Aging, 31*, 839–852. http://dx.doi.org/10.1016/j.neurobiolaging.2008.05.022

Scahill, R. I., Frost, C., Jenkins, R., Whitwell, J. L., Rossor, M. N., & Fox, N. C. (2003). A longitudinal study of brain volume changes in normal aging using serial registered magnetic resonance imaging. *Archives of Neurology, 60*, 989–994. http://dx.doi.org/10.1001/archneur.60.7.989

Schmitz, T. W., Dixon, M. L., Anderson, A. K., & De Rosa, E. (2014). Distinguishing attentional gain and tuning in young and older adults. *Neurobiology of Aging, 35*, 2514–2525. http://dx.doi.org/10.1016/j.neurobiolaging.2014.04.028

Schmitz, T. W., Spreng, R. N., & the Alzheimer's Disease Neuroimaging Initiative. (2016). Basal forebrain degeneration precedes and predicts the cortical spread of Alzheimer's pathology. *Nature Communications, 7*, 13249. http://dx.doi.org/10.1038/ncomms13249

Seeley, W. W., Crawford, R. K., Zhou, J., Miller, B. L., & Greicius, M. D. (2009). Neurodegenerative diseases target large-scale human brain networks. *Neuron, 62*, 42–52. http://dx.doi.org/10.1016/j.neuron.2009.03.024

Shaw, L. M., Vanderstichele, H., Knapik-Czajka, M., Clark, C. M., Aisen, P. S., Petersen, R. C., . . . the Alzheimer's Disease Neuroimaging Initiative. (2009). Cerebrospinal fluid biomarker signature in Alzheimer's disease neuroimaging initiative subjects. *Annals of Neurology, 65*, 403–413. http://dx.doi.org/10.1002/ana.21610

Shaw, M. E., Sachdev, P. S., Anstey, K. J., & Cherbuin, N. (2016). Age-related cortical thinning in cognitively healthy individuals in their 60s: The PATH Through Life study. *Neurobiology of Aging, 39*, 202–209. http://dx.doi.org/10.1016/j.neurobiolaging.2015.12.009

Sheline, Y. I., & Raichle, M. E. (2013). Resting state functional connectivity in preclinical Alzheimer's disease. *Biological Psychiatry, 74*, 340–347. http://dx.doi.org/10.1016/j.biopsych.2012.11.028

Snowdon, D. A. (1997). Aging and Alzheimer's disease: Lessons from the Nun Study. *The Gerontologist, 37*, 150–156. http://dx.doi.org/10.1093/geront/37.2.150

Spreng, R. N., Lockrow, A. W., DuPre, E., Setton, R., Spreng, K. A. P., & Turner, G. R. (2018). Semanticized autobiographical memory and the default—executive coupling hypothesis of aging. *Neuropsychologia, 110*, 37–43. http://dx.doi.org/10.1016/j.neuropsychologia.2017.06.009

Spreng, R. N., & Schacter, D. L. (2012). Default network modulation and large-scale network interactivity in healthy young and old adults. *Cerebral Cortex, 22*, 2610–2621. http://dx.doi.org/10.1093/cercor/bhr339

Spreng, R. N., Shoemaker, L., & Turner, G. R. (2017). Executive functions and neurocognitive aging. In E. Goldberg (Ed.), *Executive functions in health and disease* (pp. 169–196). San Diego, CA: Elsevier. http://dx.doi.org/10.1016/B978-0-12-803676-1.00008-8

Spreng, R. N., Stevens, W. D., Viviano, J. D., & Schacter, D. L. (2016). Attenuated anticorrelation between the default and dorsal attention networks with aging: Evidence from task and rest. *Neurobiology of Aging, 45*, 149–160. http://dx.doi.org/10.1016/j.neurobiolaging.2016.05.020

Spreng, R. N., & Turner, G. R. (2013). Structural covariance of the default network in healthy and pathological aging. *The Journal of Neuroscience, 33*, 15226–15234. http://dx.doi.org/10.1523/JNEUROSCI.2261-13.2013

Spreng, R. N., & Turner, G. R. (in press). Shifting architectures of brain and cognition in older adulthood. *Perspectives on Psychological Sciences.*

Spreng, R. N., Wojtowicz, M., & Grady, C. L. (2010). Reliable differences in brain activity between young and old adults: A quantitative meta-analysis across multiple cognitive domains. *Neuroscience and Biobehavioral Reviews, 34*, 1178–1194. http://dx.doi.org/10.1016/j.neubiorev.2010.01.009

Steffener, J., Brickman, A. M., Habeck, C. G., Salthouse, T. A., & Stern, Y. (2013). Cerebral blood flow and gray matter volume covariance patterns of cognition in aging. *Human Brain Mapping, 34*, 3267–3279. http://dx.doi.org/10.1002/hbm.22142

Storsve, A. B., Fjell, A. M., Tamnes, C. K., Westlye, L. T., Overbye, K., Aasland, H. W., & Walhovd, K. B. (2014). Differential longitudinal changes in cortical thickness, surface area and volume across the adult life span: Regions of accelerating and decelerating change. *The Journal of Neuroscience, 34*, 8488–8498. http://dx.doi.org/10.1523/JNEUROSCI.0391-14.2014

Sullivan, E. V., Rosenbloom, M., Serventi, K. L., & Pfefferbaum, A. (2004). Effects of age and sex on volumes of the thalamus, pons, and cortex. *Neurobiology of Aging, 25*, 185–192. http://dx.doi.org/10.1016/S0197-4580(03)00044-7

Thambisetty, M., Wan, J., Carass, A., An, Y., Prince, J. L., & Resnick, S. M. (2010). Longitudinal changes in cortical thickness associated with normal aging. *NeuroImage, 52*, 1215–1223. http://dx.doi.org/10.1016/j.neuroimage.2010.04.258

Turner, G. R., & Spreng, R. N. (2012). Executive functions and neurocognitive aging: Dissociable patterns of brain activity. *Neurobiology of Aging, 33,* 826.e1–826.e13. http://dx.doi.org/10.1016/j.neurobiolaging.2011.06.005

Turner, G. R., & Spreng, R. N. (2015). Prefrontal engagement and reduced default network suppression co-occur and are dynamically coupled in older adults: The default-executive coupling hypothesis of aging. *Journal of Cognitive Neuroscience, 27,* 2462–2476. http://dx.doi.org/10.1162/jocn_a_00869

Velanova, K., Lustig, C., Jacoby, L. L., & Buckner, R. L. (2007). Evidence for frontally mediated controlled processing differences in older adults. *Cerebral Cortex, 17,* 1033–1046. http://dx.doi.org/10.1093/cercor/bhl013

Wahlund, L. O., Agartz, I., Almqvist, O., Basun, H., Forssell, L., Sääf, J., & Wetterberg, L. (1990). The brain in healthy aged individuals: MR imaging. *Radiology, 174,* 675–679. http://dx.doi.org/10.1148/radiology.174.3.2305048

Walhovd, K. B., Fjell, A. M., Brewer, J., McEvoy, L. K., Fennema-Notestine, C., Hagler, D. J., Jr., . . . the Alzheimer's Disease Neuroimaging Initiative. (2010). Combining MR imaging, positron-emission tomography, and CSF biomarkers in the diagnosis and prognosis of Alzheimer disease. *American Journal of Neuroradiology, 31,* 347–354. http://dx.doi.org/10.3174/ajnr.A1809

Walhovd, K. B., Westlye, L. T., Amlien, I., Espeseth, T., Reinvang, I., Raz, N., . . . Fjell, A. M. (2011). Consistent neuroanatomical age-related volume differences across multiple samples. *Neurobiology of Aging, 32,* 916–932. http://dx.doi.org/10.1016/j.neurobiolaging.2009.05.013

Wu, K., Taki, Y., Sato, K., Kinomura, S., Goto, R., Okada, K., . . . Fukuda, H. (2012). Age-related changes in topological organization of structural brain networks in healthy individuals. *Human Brain Mapping, 33,* 552–568. http://dx.doi.org/10.1002/hbm.21232

Yang, Z., Wen, W., Jiang, J., Crawford, J. D., Reppermund, S., Levitan, C., . . . Sachdev, P. S. (2016). Age-associated differences on structural brain MRI in nondemented individuals from 71 to 103 years. *Neurobiology of Aging, 40,* 86–97. http://dx.doi.org/10.1016/j.neurobiolaging.2016.01.006

Yarchoan, M., Xie, S. X., Kling, M. A., Toledo, J. B., Wolk, D. A., Lee, E. B., . . . Arnold, S. E. (2012). Cerebrovascular atherosclerosis correlates with Alzheimer pathology in neurodegenerative dementias. *Brain: A Journal of Neurology, 135,* 3749–3756. http://dx.doi.org/10.1093/brain/aws271

Zarahn, E., Rakitin, B., Abela, D., Flynn, J., & Stern, Y. (2007). Age-related changes in brain activation during a delayed item recognition task. *Neurobiology of Aging, 28,* 784–798. http://dx.doi.org/10.1016/j.neurobiolaging.2006.03.002

Zhao, T., Cao, M., Niu, H., Zuo, X. N., Evans, A., He, Y., . . . Shu, N. (2015). Age-related changes in the topological organization of the white matter structural connectome across the human lifespan. *Human Brain Mapping, 36,* 3777–3792. http://dx.doi.org/10.1002/hbm.22877

Ziegler, D. A., Piguet, O., Salat, D. H., Prince, K., Connally, E., & Corkin, S. (2010). Cognition in healthy aging is related to regional white matter integrity, but not cortical thickness. *Neurobiology of Aging, 31,* 1912–1926. http://dx.doi.org/10.1016/j.neurobiolaging.2008.10.015

Ziegler, G., Dahnke, R., Jäncke, L., Yotter, R. A., May, A., & Gaser, C. (2012). Brain structural trajectories over the adult lifespan. *Human Brain Mapping, 33,* 2377–2389. http://dx.doi.org/10.1002/hbm.21374

Zimerman, M., Nitsch, M., Giraux, P., Gerloff, C., Cohen, L. G., & Hummel, F. C. (2013). Neuroenhancement of the aging brain: Restoring skill acquisition in old subjects. *Annals of Neurology, 73,* 10–15. http://dx.doi.org/10.1002/ana.23761

2

NEURAL MECHANISMS UNDERLYING AGE-RELATED CHANGES IN ATTENTIONAL SELECTIVITY

BRIANA L. KENNEDY AND MARA MATHER

One of the hallmarks of cognitive aging is an increase in distraction from goal-irrelevant information (e.g., Hasher & Zacks, 1988; Lustig, Hasher, & Zacks, 2007). Hasher and Zacks's (1988) seminal chapter outlined age-related decreases in the ability to ignore irrelevant information—and to date, their chapter has been cited more than 3,500 times on Google Scholar. Age and inhibition has been one of the most prominent and explored research areas in cognition and aging in the past 30 years, and the deficit in ignoring irrelevant information in older adults compared with younger adults has now been demonstrated across many contexts and paradigms (see Weeks & Hasher, 2014).

However, despite this relatively intensive focus on age-related declines in this aspect of attention, it is not well understood which brain changes contribute most to these behavioral changes. In this chapter, we review evidence suggesting that age-related deficits in frontoparietal networks play a key role in older adults' impaired ability to ignore distracting information.

http://dx.doi.org/10.1037/0000143-003
The Aging Brain: Functional Adaptation Across Adulthood, G. R. Samanez-Larkin (Editor)

We discuss how these frontoparietal network impairments involve changes in alpha band activity, GABAergic processing, dopaminergic decreases, and changes in how noradrenergic release under arousal affects attention. In addition, we discuss alternative mechanisms of older adults' impaired attentional selectivity and directions for future research.

DISTRACTION, INHIBITION, AND AGING

The amount of information in our environment far exceeds what we can process and retain. We thus prioritize information that is most important to navigate our world (for a review, see Wolfe & Horowitz, 2017). For our attentional system, priority can be determined by several factors, including the bottom-up features of information in our environment (e.g., motion, contrast) or from top-down goals (e.g., items that share a feature being sought—such as blue items when searching for a friend known to be wearing blue). Top-down, goal-directed attention can be driven both by enhancing mental representations of stimuli that are more important and by inhibiting representations of stimuli that are less important.

Hasher and colleagues have proposed that older adults are less likely to actively inhibit representations and that this decrease in inhibition is responsible not only for the increase in distractibility among older adults but also for more general cognitive decline (Hasher, Stoltzfus, Zacks, & Rypma, 1991; Hasher & Zacks, 1988; Lustig et al., 2007; Weeks & Hasher, 2014). Across multiple tasks that require ignoring distracting stimuli (e.g., Stroop: West & Alain, 2000; Flanker: e.g., Zeef, Sonke, Kok, Buiten, & Kenemans, 1996; and Simon tasks: e.g., Kubo-Kawai & Kawai, 2010), older adults show slower reaction times and greater distraction by task-irrelevant features. Consistent with the hypothesis that inhibition of task-irrelevant information is the basis for these performance differences, older adults perform similarly to younger adults in many cognitive tasks when inhibition is not involved (Andrés, Parmentier, & Escera, 2006; Commodari & Guarnera, 2008; Madden, 2007).

Moreover, older adults spontaneously learn task-irrelevant information that younger adults usually inhibit (Healey, Campbell, & Hasher, 2008). For example, in an experiment in which participants were required to concentrate on a central task, younger adults failed to learn information about motion coherence that appeared in the background, whereas older adults performed well above chance in a later surprise test of the task-irrelevant information (Chang, Shibata, Andersen, Sasaki, & Watanabe, 2014). Similarly, when participants view common objects superimposed with task-irrelevant words, older adults are more likely than younger adults to demonstrate priming from the task-irrelevant words in a subsequent, surprise word completion task (Campbell, Grady, Ng, & Hasher, 2012; Rowe, Valderrama, Hasher, & Lenartowicz, 2006).

Functional magnetic resonance imaging (fMRI) data mirror behavioral findings. Gazzaley, Cooney, Rissman, and D'Esposito (2005) had participants view scene and face images and instructed them to do one of the following: (a) ignore scenes and remember faces, (b) remember scenes and ignore faces, or (c) passively view the images. Younger adults showed an increase in scene-selective activation (in the left parahippocampal/lingual gyrus) when remembering scenes and ignoring faces compared with passively viewing them and also showed a decrease in scene-selective activity when remembering faces and ignoring scenes. Although older adults also demonstrated an increase in scene-selective activity when remembering scenes and ignoring faces, they did not show any difference from passive viewing when they were remembering faces and ignoring scenes. The degree to which older adults demonstrated suppressed activation when ignoring scenes also correlated with their memory performance, suggesting that inhibition of irrelevant information helps determine what information is retained (see also Campbell et al., 2012; Lustig et al., 2007).

SELECTION PROBLEM OR SUPPRESSION PROBLEM?

To understand the underlying brain mechanisms involved in age-related attentional changes, it is helpful to identify the distinct cognitive processes involved. Could it be that older adults simply struggle to select and prioritize important information? Not all aspects of prioritization are impaired; activation of representations that are most important seems to remain intact. For example, older adults usually perform well in visual search tasks but struggle when the search requires a greater amount of effort because distractors need to be ignored in the search environment (e.g., Foster, Behrmann, & Stuss, 1995). More specifically, search performance is typically comparable between older and younger adults when they can use parallel search strategies—that is, when target items are distinctive from distractors due to a particular, single feature (Foster et al., 1995; Madden, 2007). However, when a visual search requires timely, serial search strategies (e.g., when task-relevant items are defined by a conjunction of features that make them similar to distractor items), older adults typically demonstrate greater impairments in search efficiency compared to young adults (Foster et al., 1995; Madden, 2007).

Because older adults can effectively search for single features but struggle when they have to actively disregard distractors to identify targets in a more complex serial search, the impairment in inhibition mechanisms in older adults could be due to their failure to use goal-directed attention and maintain an attentional set for the target over distractors (Hasher, Zacks, & May, 1999). Indeed, aging was associated with impaired inhibition when tasks required executive attentional control (i.e., Stroop, Stop Signal), as opposed to tasks that only required automatic attentional inhibition (i.e., Negative Priming; Andrés, Guerrini, Phillips, & Perfect, 2008). Consistent with this, older adults performed similarly to younger adults in search efficiency when a colored distractor or distractor with a surprise onset appeared in a search array (Colcombe et al., 2003; Kramer, Hahn, Irwin, & Theeuwes, 2000), but, unlike younger adults, older adults did not improve performance when specifically made aware of the distractors (Kramer et al., 2000). Thus, older adults seem less able to employ a goal-directed attentional set to ignore upcoming distractors compared with younger adults. However, this may be specific for harder tasks, as when identifying the target among distractors is easier (e.g., when knowing that a task-relevant target will likely be a color singleton), knowing about the target does improve older adults' performance (Whiting, Madden, Pierce, & Allen, 2005). In a similar vein, older adults show less object-specific activation in the lateral occipital cortex (LOC) when passively viewing objects imposed on scenes, but instructions to focus on objects enhance object-specific activation in the LOC in older adults (Chee et al., 2006). Taken together, these results suggest that (a) top-down control mechanisms may help overcome task-irrelevant distraction and (b) older adults do seem able to recruit some of these top-down control abilities, but that (c) older adults cannot override distraction with their goal-directed attention to the extent that younger adults can.

AGE-RELATED CHANGES IN THE FRONTOPARIETAL NETWORKS

The nature of these age-related deficits rules out any mechanisms that do not account for how selectivity can be coordinated across relatively distant brain regions. Thus, to understand these age differences, we need to focus on brain mechanisms that coordinate which stimuli representations are enhanced and which are suppressed—even when they are represented in different cortical regions, such as when someone is selectively attending to a scene and ignoring a face shown at the same time. Frontoparietal brain regions have been characterized as involved in a coordinated network that plays a key role in coordinating attentional selectivity (Hwang, Shine, & D'Esposito, 2018; Ptak, 2012; Scolari, Seidl-Rathkopf, & Kastner, 2015). These networked regions (see Figure 2.1) include areas in the posterior parietal cortex, the dorsolateral prefrontal cortex, and premotor cortex, including the anterior cingulate cortex, frontal eye field, and intraparietal sulcus

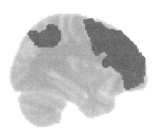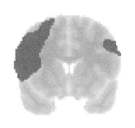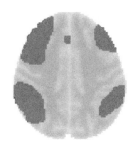

Figure 2.1. A mask of the right-lateralized frontoparietal network (FPN) based on data from Laird et al. (2011) overlaid on the Montreal Neurological Institute (MNI) template (Laird et al. ICA map 15; displayed at MNI coordinates x = 34, y = 14, z = 40).

(Ptak, 2012). Researchers posit that a frontoparietal network represents priority maps that identify and prioritize the spatial location of stimuli that are salient or important to the observer's top-down goals (Jerde, Merriam, Riggall, Hedges, & Curtis, 2012; Ptak, 2012; Treisman, 1998). Thus, a frontoparietal network plays a key role in distinguishing task-relevant targets from task-irrelevant distraction.

Researchers have posited that age-related decline in frontal regions can account for attentional inhibition changes in older adults (Allen, Bruss, Brown, & Damasio, 2005; Gazzaley & D'Esposito, 2007; Reuter-Lorenz & Cappell, 2008). There has been less focus on the potential role of frontoparietal networks in age-related decline in selective attention and inhibition. However, emerging research examining functional connectivity reveals age-related changes in frontoparietal networks (Campbell et al., 2012; Geerligs, Renken, Saliasi, Maurits, & Lorist, 2015; Goh, 2011; Madden, 2007; Sala-Llonch, Bartrés-Faz, & Junqué, 2015) that are associated with cognitive performance (Avelar-Pereira, Bäckman, Wåhlin, Nyberg, & Salami, 2017; DuPre & Spreng, 2017; C. L. Grady, Sarraf, Saverino, & Campbell, 2016; Mitchell, Ankudowich, Durbin, Greene, & Johnson, 2013; Nashiro, Sakaki, Braskie, & Mather, 2017; Siman-Tov et al., 2017; Zanto & Gazzaley, 2017). Of particular interest, older adults' reduced frontoparietal network activity was associated with poorer attentional selectivity in a study in which participants viewed task-irrelevant words during a picture 1-back task (Campbell et al., 2012). In this study, young adults showed greater brain activity in a frontoparietal network when they were trying to ignore distracting words. Older adults did not demonstrate such activation during the task and were worse at ignoring the words compared with young adults. Moreover, when participants were simply resting, parietal regions involved in ignoring stimuli correlated more strongly with regions of the rostral prefrontal cortex in young adults compared with older adults, suggesting that connectivity within the frontoparietal network is decreased in older adults (Campbell et al., 2012). Thus, both lowered brain activation and decreased network activity in frontoparietal regions suggest that impairments in cognitive control may stem from diminished integrity within a frontoparietal network involved in coordinating attention. Consistent with this, age-related decreases in brain volume in the frontoparietal dorsal stream have been associated with worse visual search performance in conjunction search tasks (Müller-Oehring, Schulte, Rohlfing, Pfefferbaum, & Sullivan, 2013).

COMPENSATION AND DEDIFFERENTIATION ACCOUNTS OF FRONTOPARIETAL NETWORK CHANGES

Traditional frameworks of age-related changes in the brain can be used to conceptualize underlying changes in the frontoparietal network. Compensation and dedifferentiation theories are two main hypotheses about age-related changes in the brain, and they apply to both brain structures and functional networks.

Dedifferentiation refers to a process when neural processors lose their functional specificity or selectivity (see Park et al., 2004). If neural representations are no longer as specific as they used to be, dedifferentiation would make it harder to select target stimuli among distractors. Evidence of age-related dedifferentiation has been observed in individual brain structures and for particular functional networks and connectivity (Geerligs et al., 2015; Goh, 2011; Park et al., 2004), including network connectivity and functionality of the frontoparietal network (Geerligs et al., 2015). Altogether, the lessened distinctiveness and modularity of regions responsible for particular processing in younger adulthood may make distinguishing task-relevant targets from task-irrelevant distractors more difficult in older age—and make it harder to direct goal-directed attentional inhibition.

Compensation theories also apply to the frontoparietal network. Despite deficits in performance, older adults often show more activity in related brain areas compared with younger adults (C. L. Grady & Craik, 2000; Reuter-Lorenz, 2002; Reuter-Lorenz & Cappell, 2008). This has been interpreted as a "compensation" for underlying deficits (Reuter-Lorenz & Cappell, 2008). Compensation theories of aging suggest that greater activity reflects greater task-related effort (Reuter-Lorenz & Cappell, 2008). However, when task demands are too great, frontoparietal activation in older adults decreases and is less active than for younger adults; a decrease that coincides with impaired task performance compared with younger adults (Campbell et al., 2012; Reuter-Lorenz & Cappell, 2008). Accordingly, compared with younger adults, older adults often demonstrate greater brain activation during cognitive tasks to achieve a similar level of performance, particularly in frontoparietal areas (Cabeza, 2002; Campbell et al., 2012; Madden, 2007).

Traditional dedifferentiation and compensation theories thus may help explain age-related changes in frontoparietal network activity. Furthermore, specific underlying functional and chemical changes have been identified that relate to the ability to ignore distraction. For example, the frontoparietal network's involvement in attentional selectivity has been linked with both alpha rhythms (e.g., Capotosto, Babiloni, Romani, & Corbetta, 2009) and with GABAergic action (Womelsdorf & Everling, 2015; Zhang et al., 2014). Both of these processes involved in implementing frontoparietal network function decline with aging, as reviewed in the following two sections.

ALPHA ELECTROENCEPHALOGRAM, SELECTIVE ATTENTION, AND THE FRONTOPARIETAL NETWORK

Oscillatory waveforms measured with electroencephalogram (EEG) are associated with mental processing and are correlated with performance on attentional tasks (for reviews, see Kahana, 2006; Klimesch, 1999; Ward, 2003). These waveforms are believed to represent synchronous activity in the brain, and unique waveforms can be distinguished on the basis of their individual frequency and power bands (Klimesch, 1999). Alpha EEG, with frequency ranges between 7.5 and 12.5 Hz, is the most dominant waveform in humans (Klimesch, 1999). It is also a waveform believed to reflect attention: Alpha EEG changes amplitude with task-related stimuli presentation or increased task demands in attentional tasks.

Furthermore, there is much evidence indicating that alpha oscillations reflect inhibitory and selective aspects of attention (Foxe & Snyder, 2011; Händel, Haarmeier, & Jensen, 2011; Klimesch, 1999, 2012). Alpha amplitude is typically suppressed when people process events, but it increases in situations when participants must exert top-down control over responses (for a review, see Klimesch, Sauseng, & Hanslmayr, 2007). The ability to perceive external stimuli oscillates in tandem with alpha oscillations, suggesting that alpha oscillations may provide rhythmic pulses that inhibit attentional processes (Mathewson et al., 2011). The causal role of alpha band rhythms in blocking stimuli processing was demonstrated in a study that applied rhythmic transmagnetic stimulation at a frequency within the alpha range (10 Hz) to parietal and occipital sites (Romei, Gross, & Thut, 2010). This alpha stimulation impaired visual detection contralateral to the stimulation site more than stimulation at higher or lower frequencies, while improving detection at an ipsilateral site.

Alpha EEG and activity in frontoparietal regions appear to be linked (Laufs et al., 2003). For example, in a study combining continuous EEG with fMRI, alpha rhythms were negatively correlated with activity specifically in frontal and parietal areas (Laufs et al., 2003). Attentional activity in the frontoparietal regions thus seems to be reflected through alpha rhythms. Frontoparietal brain regions also play a key role in modulating alpha activity (Mathewson et al., 2014). For instance, a transcranial magnetic stimulation study showed that interfering with activity in the intraparietal sulcus or frontal eye field (two nodes of the dorsal frontoparietal network) disrupted anticipatory alpha desynchronization and impaired identification of targets appearing a couple of seconds later (Capotosto et al., 2009).

AGE-RELATED CHANGES IN ALPHA EEG

Age-related slowing in alpha band oscillatory activity is a pronounced effect that is among the first documented observations of age differences in brain activity (e.g., Davis, 1941; Harvald, 1958) and has been replicated many times (e.g., Clark et al., 2004; McEvoy, Pellouchoud, Smith, & Gevins, 2001; Vlahou, Thurm, Kolassa, & Schlee, 2014; Woodruff & Kramer, 1979). Such slowing has been particularly observed in frontal areas of the brain (Clark et al., 2004) and has been linked with lowered reaction times on attentional tasks (Woodruff & Kramer, 1979) and decreased working memory performance (Clark et al., 2004; Sander, Werkle-Bergner, & Lindenberger, 2012).

Alpha-band activity is high during rest, and increases further when eyes are closed. In response to stimuli or task demands, it typically decreases in amplitude (showing an *alpha band desynchronization*). However, it can also increase in amplitude when stimuli are task irrelevant or potentially interfering with current goals. Thus, alpha band synchronization in response to stimuli appears to reflect inhibition (Klimesch, 2012). For instance, when performing the inhibition-intensive Stroop task that requires inhibition, younger adults showed a trade-off pattern between alpha and theta bands during a Stroop task, such that alpha was suppressed when participants resolved Stroop conflicts, and theta (theta band amplitude tends to increase with engaged attention; Klimesch, 1999) increased during these trials—but the trade-off was less pronounced in older adults compared with younger adults (Nombela et al., 2014). Furthermore, aging is associated with delays in the latency of alpha synchronization responses to task-irrelevant stimuli but not in the alpha band desynchronization responses to attended stimuli (Deiber et al., 2010). In other words, alpha band responses associated with inhibition show age-related decline, whereas alpha band responses associated with focused attention do not.

Alpha EEG is also believed to act as an anticipatory signal for information, and the frontoparietal network modulates these anticipatory alpha rhythms (Capotosto et al., 2009). For instance, the anticipatory change in alpha rhythms can be seen when participants are presented with a short sequence of stimuli in which the second item should be ignored on some trials but remembered on other trials (Vaden, Hutcheson, McCollum, Kentros, & Visscher, 2012). Younger adults show more alpha power from parietal electrodes in the 400 ms before that second stimulus when it should be ignored than when it should be remembered, indicating they increase alpha when anticipating the need to ignore something. In contrast, older adults did not show greater alpha power in the to-be-ignored than the to-be-remembered condition.

In younger adults, anticipatory shifts in alpha tend to be lateralized if cues indicate they should shift spatial attention to a left or right visual location (Sauseng et al., 2005). However, these spatially specific anticipatory shifts in alpha power are not seen in older adults even though older adults showed clear indications of spatial orienting and good task performance (Hong, Sun, Bengson, Mangun, & Tong, 2015; van der Waal, Farquhar, Fasotti, & Desain, 2017). The selective impairment of alpha was evident from classifier analyses that could decode the cue direction (left or right) on each trial from either ERPs or alpha lateralization in younger adults but only from ERPs in older adults (van der Waal et al., 2017).

Thus, in the context of attentional suppression in older adults, increased age correlates with a decrease in alpha EEG frequency (particularly decreased in frontal areas), which often correlates with decreased performance on attentional tasks. Nevertheless, the mechanisms underlying alpha EEG remain unknown. The slowing of alpha EEG with age may represent changes in the higher and lower bands of the alpha frequency, such that age reduces upper band power or decreases lower band power of the alpha EEG (or both; Clark et al., 2004). Altogether, while the underlying brain areas associated with age-related decreases in alpha EEG remain relatively unknown, the frontally specific, attention-related decline suggests that frontoparietal regions are involved in its age-related change.

Although it is not known what generates the alpha rhythms in the brain, they have been linked to thalamic oscillatory activity (e.g., Hughes & Crunelli, 2005) and rhythmic GABAergic activity (Lőrincz, Kékesi, Juhász, Crunelli, & Hughes, 2009). Gamma-aminobutyric acid (GABA) is a neurotransmitter that is widely distributed in the brain and is known to be involved in inhibition. Diazepam, a drug that increases GABAergic neurotransmission, increases alpha frequency, the inverse of the alpha slowing that occurs with aging (Hall, Barnes, Furlong, Seri, & Hillebrand, 2010). However, the mechanism does not seem to be as simple as "GABAergic processing increases alpha oscillations" in general. For instance, lorazepam, a drug enhancing GABAergic conductance, reduces alpha EEG power (Ahveninen et al., 2007; Lozano-Soldevilla, ter Huurne, Cools, & Jensen, 2014; Schreckenberger et al., 2004). In the next section, we review how GABAergic neurotransmission decreases in aging and how this might contribute to age-related impairments in attentional selection.

AGE-RELATED DECLINES IN GABA

GABA is the primary neurotransmitter driving inhibition in the brain. Compared with excitatory neurons, inhibitory neurons are less prevalent in the brain, making up only 10% to 20% of all neurons (Caputi, Melzer, Michael, & Monyer, 2013), but they are critical for maintaining effective brain function. In particular, GABA is associated with perceptual and attentional selectivity (Clark, 1996; Sumner, Edden, Bompas, Evans, & Singh, 2010); for example, greater concentrations of GABA are associated with increased inhibitory function in visual receptive fields (Wolf, Hicks, & Albus, 1986), increased working memory performance (Yoon, Grandelis, & Maddock, 2016), and faster eye-gaze movement toward task-relevant stimuli over task-irrelevant stimuli (Sumner et al., 2010). Moreover, inhibition in cognitive performance has been correlated specifically with GABA concentrations in frontal regions (Sumner et al., 2010; Yoon et al., 2016).

GABAergic interneurons are highly metabolically demanding (Bazzigaluppi, Ebrahim Amini, Weisspapir, Stefanovic, & Carlen, 2017), which may help explain why inhibitory GABA function seems to decline more in aging than excitatory glutamatergic function (Rozycka & Liguz-Lecznar, 2017). With age in human prefrontal cortex, the ratio of excitatory pyramidal neurons to nonpyramidal neurons (a category including GABAergic neurons) shifts as the proportion of nonpyramidal neurons decreases, whereas pyramidal neuron counts remain more constant (Braak & Braak, 1986). Likewise, in cat visual cortex, the ratio of GABAergic neurons to total neurons decreases with age (Hua, Kao, Sun, Li, & Zhou, 2008). In rats, aging reduces GABA, but not glutamate, efflux within the hippocampus and leads to significant loss of GABAergic interneurons (Stanley, Fadel, & Mott, 2012). Furthermore, in older mice somatosensory cortex, the overall responses of neurons and astrocytes is unchanged, but fast-spiking GABAergic parvalbumin-positive interneuron shows reduced activity (Jessen, Mathiesen, Lind, & Lauritzen, 2017).

In humans, GABA concentrations quantified noninvasively using magnetic resonance spectroscopy confirm that GABA concentrations decrease with age (Gao et al., 2013; Porges et al., 2017), and decreased GABA concentrations in frontal regions of the brain are associated with age-related cognitive functioning (Porges et al., 2017).

Reductions in GABA are likely to have significant effects in the aging brain. In particular, fast-spiking GABAergic parvalbumin-positive inter-neurons serve as pacemakers that help generate high-frequency gamma oscillations in local circuits associated with focused attention (Uhlhaas & Singer, 2012). Optogenetic techniques indicate that inhibiting parvalbumin interneurons suppresses gamma oscillations but increases oscillations in the alpha frequency range (Sohal, Zhang, Yizhar, & Deisseroth, 2009). Further, as already mentioned, pharmacological manipulations also link GABA to modulation of alpha EEG rhythms (Ahveninen et al., 2007; Hall et al., 2010; Lozano-Soldevilla et al., 2014; Schreckenberger et al., 2004).

Reductions in GABA are also likely to impair frontoparietal network function. The frontoparietal network relies on long-range communication across its subcomponent regions as well as with target regions (Womelsdorf & Everling, 2015). Although most inhibitory neurons make only local connec-tions, recent research indicates that a small number of cortical GABAergic neurons have long-range connections to other cortical regions or to sub-cortical regions (Higo, Udaka, & Tamamaki, 2007; Tomioka et al., 2005), with the basal ganglia a frequent target (Tomioka, Sakimura, & Yanagawa, 2015). In addition, prefrontal GABAergic interneurons regulate the out-put of long-range excitatory pyramidal cells (Giustino & Maren, 2017; Lu et al., 2017) and long-range excitatory connections from frontal regions acti-vate local GABAergic activity in visual cortex (Zhang et al., 2014). Thus, impaired GABA processing is likely to reduce the efficacy of frontoparietal network to coordinate attentional selectivity across the brain. Consistent with this potential link between GABA and frontoparietal function, in humans GABA levels in frontal and parietal regions are associated with selective attention effects such as the attentional blink (Kihara, Kondo, & Kawahara, 2016). Given its primary role in inhibition and its change in fron-tal regions with age, GABA is a strong candidate as a contributor for age-related inhibitory changes.

AGE-RELATED DECLINES IN DOPAMINE

Another neurotransmitter potentially involved in attentional selec-tivity changes in aging is dopamine. Dopamine is a neurotransmitter that is involved in motor processing and higher level cognitive processing (Bäckman, Nyberg, Lindenberger, Li, & Farde, 2006; Braver & Barch, 2002). This neurotransmitter is believed to play a role in cognitive control and also for gating information to further processing, such that dopaminergic phasic activity helps bias task-relevant information over task-irrelevant information (Braver & Barch, 2002).

Dopamine has been implicated in traditional models of age-related cognitive impairments of dedifferentiation (Abdulrahman, Fletcher, Bullmore, & Morcom, 2017; Li & Lindenberger, 1999). Moreover, connections have been drawn between dopamine and the integrity of the frontoparietal network. Dopamine appears to modulate the communication between the frontoparietal network and other attentional networks (Dang, O'Neil, & Jagust, 2012) and has been shown to play a role in synchronizing oscillations in prefrontal activity (Bäckman et al., 2006). Moreover, in a study of individual differences in caudate dopamine density, dopamine density was found to be predictive of connectivity between frontal and parietal brain areas, but not between areas of the default mode network or between bilateral prefrontal areas (Rieckmann, Karlsson, Fischer, & Bäckman, 2011). Thus, dopamine appears to play a modulatory role during attention, particularly to enhance communication within the frontoparietal network.

The density of dopamine, including both dopamine subtypes D_1, D_2, and the dopamine transporter (DAT), decreases with age, and the rate of decrease seems to be relatively similar throughout areas of the brain (Bäckman et al., 2006). These decreases in dopamine density have been associated with poorer cognitive function with age (Bäckman et al., 2006; Braver & Barch, 2002), in a proposed theoretical "correlative triad" between aging, cognition, and dopamine (Bäckman et al., 2011, 2006). Although increasing dopamine levels in older adults pharmacologically has failed to yield significant behavioral performance improvements, brain activation patterns under dopaminergic drugs have shown shifts in the right direction (Abdulrahman et al., 2017; Chowdhury et al., 2013; Morcom et al., 2010). Altogether, because of its role in the connectivity of the frontoparietal network, and the decrease of dopamine density with age, dopamine may well play a role in the decreased attentional inhibition in older adults.

AGE-RELATED CHANGES IN THE LOCUS COERULEUS–NOREPINEPHRINE SYSTEM AND ATTENTIONAL SELECTIVITY

The locus coeruleus (LC) is the brain's primary source of norepinephrine and activates with arousal. The role of the LC–norepinephrine (LC–NE) system in attentional selectivity is outlined in the GANE (glutamate amplifies noradrenergic effects) model (Mather, Clewett, Sakaki, & Harley, 2016). In this framework, glutamate spills over from active synapses in neural networks that are currently "high priority." This spillover glutamate from highly active synapses reaches N-methyl-D-aspartate (NMDA) receptors on nearby axons from LC neurons. Glutamate activates these NMDA receptors if the associated LC neuron is simultaneously depolarized (activated), stimulating local norepinephrine release. This can allow norepinephrine levels to get high enough in that local area to stimulate high-threshold β-adrenergic receptors via both presynaptic and postsynaptic mechanisms (e.g., Ji et al., 2008) that stimulate even more glutamate release at the excited synapse. This feedback loop can ignite "hot spots" of prioritized representation when arousal is high and therefore the LC is active. In areas with lower priority, norepinephrine release will be limited to the relatively low levels induced by LC activation alone. This should lead to insufficient release to activate β-adrenergic receptors but enough to stimulate lower threshold α2a inhibitory receptors (for more details, see Mather et al., 2016).

A recent study used fMRI to examine age differences in the dynamics of LC interactions with cortical representations of salient high-priority stimuli and with the frontoparietal network (Lee et al., 2018). On each trial in this study, participants were shown a place and an object image next to each other and had to indicate which one was more salient. On half of the trials, the place image was made more salient by highlighting it with a yellow border and by reducing the perceptual contrast on the other image. On the other trials, the object image was more salient. In addition, immediately before each trial, participants heard either a tone that had been previously conditioned to predict shock (CS+) or a tone conditioned to predict no shock (CS−). The GANE model predicts that high activation of stimuli representations should be further amplified when LC is activated at the same time. Consistent with this hypothesis, functional connectivity between the LC and the parahippocampal place area showed an arousal-by-salience interaction, such that the greatest functional connectivity was seen when both the place image was salient on that trial and it was an arousing (CS+) trial. This significant interaction in functional connectivity between the LC and a cortical brain area representing current stimuli was seen for both younger and older adults, suggesting that the GANE hot spot mechanisms are still intact in later life.

In contrast, the ability of the LC and arousal to modulate frontoparietal network activity was significantly diminished among the older adults in this study. Younger adults showed stronger functional connectivity between the frontoparietal network regions and the LC on high than on low arousal trials. In addition, for younger adults, functional connectivity between the parahippocampal place area and frontoparietal network regions was modulated both by the salience of the place stimulus and by arousal. These modulations of frontoparietal connectivity to the LC and to the brain region representing

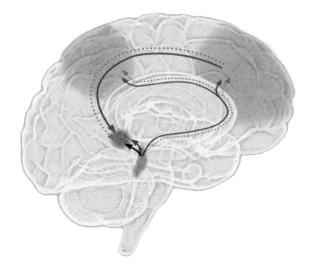

Figure 2.2. A depiction of the theorized network connectivity among the locus coeruleus, frontoparietal network, and parahippocampal place area in the Lee et al. (2018) study. Younger adults (pathway depicted with a solid gray line) demonstrated intact network connectivity among the locus coeruleus, parahippocampal place area, and frontoparietal network. Older adults (pathway depicted with a black line) demonstrated an intact connectivity between the locus coeruleus and parahippocampal place area, but disrupted connectivity with the frontoparietal network. From "Arousal Increases Neural Gain via the Locus Coeruleus–Norepinephrine System in Younger Adults but Not in Older Adults," by T. H. Lee, S. G. Greening, T. Ueno, D. Clewett, A. Ponzio, M. Sakaki, and M. Mather, 2018, *Nature Human Behaviour, 2*, p. 363. Copyright 2018 by SpringerNature. Adapted with permission.

a current salient stimulus were significantly diminished among older adults (see Figure 2.2). Thus, for younger adults, arousal increased the coordination of LC and frontoparietal activity, which in turn may have modulated how the frontoparietal network amplified or suppressed representations.

These findings suggest that even among older adults with intact ability of LC to differentially amplify cortical representations based on salience, the influence of the LC over frontoparietal selectivity processes is diminished. This may be due to decreases in the sensitivity of noradrenergic receptors in frontoparietal regions. Interestingly, in a sample aged 18 to 47, functional connectivity between the LC and the frontoparietal network during a resting state scan was positively correlated with age (Zhang, Hu, Chao, & Li, 2016). Higher circulating levels of norepinephrine among older adults at rest (e.g., Gannon & Wang, 2019) may lead to high levels of frontoparietal network stimulation at baseline with little capacity to increase frontoparietal resources when attentional demands (and arousal) increase. Furthermore, age-related decline in the LC itself may contribute to decreases in attentional selectivity under arousal. In general, recent findings indicate that age-related decreases in LC integrity are associated with decline in cognitive function (Clewett et al., 2016; Dahl et al., 2018; Hämmerer et al., 2018; Mather & Harley, 2016; Wilson et al., 2013). The Lee et al. (2018) findings suggest that changes in the LC–NE system in aging may target some aspects of cognition more than others. In particular, older adults may get the benefits of arousal for amplifying activation of salient stimuli but lose the benefits of arousal for inhibition of competing stimuli.

ALTERNATIVE MECHANISMS AND DIRECTIONS FOR FUTURE RESEARCH

We have outlined several mechanisms that may contribute to age-related differences in goal-related inhibition of distracting information. In particular, we have focused on changes that occur within the frontoparietal network, a likely candidate for age-related decline in attentional selectivity. However, further work needs to examine how these mechanisms interact, whether their contributions are specifically related to attentional selectivity, and how other brain areas or networks may also play a role.

Default Mode Network

Although the frontoparietal network is a strong candidate for attentional selectivity changes with age, other candidates have been put forward. For example, changes within the default mode network have been proposed as contributors to age-related decline in attentional selectivity (e.g., Chadick, Zanto, & Gazzaley, 2014; Stevens, Hasher, Chiew, & Grady, 2008).

The default mode network tends to be active when people are not engaged in a particular task, and decreases activity—a pattern termed *deactivation*—with increased task demands (Anticevic et al., 2012; Mevel, Chételat, Eustache, & Desgranges, 2011). The network includes areas of the posterior cingulate cortex, precuneus, anterior cingulate cortex, dorsal and ventral medial prefrontal cortex, lateral parietal cortices, and medial temporal lobes (Hafkemeijer, van der Grond, & Rombouts, 2012; Mevel et al., 2011). Older adults tend to show lessened deactivation between rest and during cognitive tasks, suggesting that they are less able to transition between a task-free state and one that requires cognitive task demands (Hafkemeijer et al., 2012; Mevel et al., 2011). The functional connectivity of the default mode network also appears to decrease in older age (Hafkemeijer et al., 2012; Ng, Lo, Lim, Chee, & Zhou, 2016; Vidal-Piñeiro et al., 2014), and even more in individuals with mild cognitive impairment (Hafkemeijer et al., 2012; Zanchi et al., 2017) or Alzheimer's disease (Hafkemeijer et al., 2012).

In a task that required attentional selection for faces over scenes or vice versa, older adults demonstrated decreased deactivation in default network areas compared with younger adults—particularly in the medial prefrontal cortex—and older adult's lowered suppression of the medial prefrontal cortex was related to greater distraction in behavioral performance on the task (Chadick et al., 2014; see also Stevens et al., 2008). Moreover, connectivity between the medial prefrontal cortex and visual areas were associated with less suppression of distracting information in older adults compared to younger adults (Chadick et al., 2014). Thus, areas identified as within the default mode network in the medial prefrontal cortex were especially indicative of attentional selection with age.

Both the frontoparietal network and default network include areas of the prefrontal cortex, are related to attentional demands, and demonstrate decreased connectivity with age (Chadick et al., 2014; Sala-Llonch et al., 2015). Moreover, emerging evidence suggests that age-related changes in both networks can be predictive of performance (e.g., Zanchi et al., 2017), suggesting that underlying impairments in both networks should be considered for age-related changes. However, the default mode network is typically measured during nontask situations, and its coupling with other networks, such as the frontoparietal network, may vary by task demands (Avelar-Pereira et al., 2017). Although still in its infancy, more research exploring age-related connectivity changes seems a fruitful avenue for explaining complex age-related changes like attentional selectivity—whether it be a particular network or a combination of networks (see Amer, Anderson, Campbell, Hasher, & Grady, 2016; Avelar-Pereira et al., 2017; Ng et al., 2016; Zhao, Lu, Metmer, Li, & Lu, 2018).

Defining Inhibition

We also discussed several functional and chemical mechanisms that change with age and likely contribute to impairments in the functions of the frontoparietal network. Nevertheless, it remains unclear which of these mechanisms and their interactions are most potent in the underlying impairments in attentional selectivity. In this chapter so far, we have discussed *inhibition* as a general concept, which may not be representative of the complex mechanistic underpinnings involved in different attentional, inhibitory situations (see Kramer, Humphrey, Larish, Logan, & Strayer, 1994). That is, just because inhibitory differences have been observed across many tasks does not mean that their underlying mechanisms are the same (e.g., Eich, Razlighi, & Stern, 2017); for example, the mechanisms through which arousal amplifies inhibition of stimuli that are not perceptually salient (e.g., Lee, Sakaki, Cheng, Velasco, & Mather, 2014) may work differently from inhibition of goal-irrelevant stimuli (e.g., Sutherland, McQuiggan, Ryan, & Mather, 2017). Specifying differences between such inhibitory effects will help identify mechanisms responsible for specific aspects of attentional inhibition.

Mechanistic Influences on Individual Stages of Cognition

Inhibition may also rely on separable underlying mechanisms during different cognitive processing stages. In an fMRI study to compare activation related to older adults' inhibition during early versus late memory processing, activation patterns reflected separable regions for inhibition during different memory processes (Eich et al., 2017). Different stages of attentional processing may thus involve different contributory mechanisms in inhibitory functionality (see also Turner & Spreng, 2012). Future research exploring the mechanisms underlying age-related inhibition changes should thus consider the specific contributory processing stages.

CONCLUSION

Goal-directed attentional selection requires selecting task-relevant information while simultaneously inhibiting task-irrelevant information. Across many studies and task designs, older adults demonstrate impaired attentional inhibition. We reviewed literature suggesting the frontoparietal network may play a key role in age-related changes in inhibitory processing and discussed mechanisms that may contribute to alterations in the integrity of the network, including alpha band activity, GABAergic processing, dopaminergic decreases, and noradrenergic influences via the LC–NE system under arousal. We also discussed the potential role of the default mode network. Future research will inform which of these mechanisms—or their interactions—play the largest role in driving age-related changes in attentional inhibition.

REFERENCES

Abdulrahman, H., Fletcher, P. C., Bullmore, E., & Morcom, A. M. (2017). Dopamine and memory dedifferentiation in aging. *NeuroImage, 153,* 211–220. http://dx.doi.org/10.1016/j.neuroimage.2015.03.031

Ahveninen, J., Lin, F. H., Kivisaari, R., Autti, T., Hämäläinen, M., Stufflebeam, S., . . . Kähkönen, S. (2007). MRI-constrained spectral imaging of benzodiazepine modulation of spontaneous neuromagnetic activity in human cortex. *NeuroImage, 35*, 577–582. http://dx.doi.org/10.1016/j.neuroimage.2006.12.033

Allen, J. S., Bruss, J., Brown, C. K., & Damasio, H. (2005). Normal neuroanatomical variation due to age: The major lobes and a parcellation of the temporal region. *Neurobiology of Aging, 26*, 1245–1260. http://dx.doi.org/10.1016/j.neurobiolaging.2005.05.023

Amer, T., Anderson, J. A. E., Campbell, K. L., Hasher, L., & Grady, C. L. (2016). Age differences in the neural correlates of distraction regulation: A network interaction approach. *NeuroImage, 139*, 231–239. http://dx.doi.org/10.1016/j.neuroimage.2016.06.036

Andrés, P., Guerrini, C., Phillips, L. H., & Perfect, T. J. (2008). Differential effects of aging on executive and automatic inhibition. *Developmental Neuropsychology, 33*, 101–123. http://dx.doi.org/10.1080/87565640701884212

Andrés, P., Parmentier, F. B. R., & Escera, C. (2006). The effect of age on involuntary capture of attention by irrelevant sounds: A test of the frontal hypothesis of aging. *Neuropsychologia, 44*, 2564–2568. http://dx.doi.org/10.1016/j.neuropsychologia.2006.05.005

Anticevic, A., Cole, M. W., Murray, J. D., Corlett, P. R., Wang, X.-J., & Krystal, J. H. (2012). The role of default network deactivation in cognition and disease. *Trends in Cognitive Sciences, 16*, 584–592. http://dx.doi.org/10.1016/j.tics.2012.10.008

Avelar-Pereira, B., Bäckman, L., Wåhlin, A., Nyberg, L., & Salami, A. (2017). Age-related differences in dynamic interactions among default mode, frontoparietal control, and dorsal attention networks during resting-state and interference resolution. *Frontiers in Aging Neuroscience, 9*, 152. Advance online publication. http://dx.doi.org/10.3389/fnagi.2017.00152

Bäckman, L., Karlsson, S., Fischer, H., Karlsson, P., Brehmer, Y., Rieckmann, A., . . . Nyberg, L. (2011). Dopamine D(1) receptors and age differences in brain activation during working memory. *Neurobiology of Aging, 32*, 1849–1856. http://dx.doi.org/10.1016/j.neurobiolaging.2009.10.018

Bäckman, L., Nyberg, L., Lindenberger, U., Li, S.-C., & Farde, L. (2006). The correlative triad among aging, dopamine, and cognition: Current status and future prospects. *Neuroscience & Biobehavioral Reviews, 30*, 791–807. http://dx.doi.org/10.1016/j.neubiorev.2006.06.005

Bazzigaluppi, P., Ebrahim Amini, A., Weisspapir, I., Stefanovic, B., & Carlen, P. L. (2017). Hungry neurons: Metabolic insights on seizure dynamics. *International Journal of Molecular Sciences, 18*, 2269. http://dx.doi.org/10.3390/ijms18112269

Braak, H., & Braak, E. (1986). Ratio of pyramidal cells versus non-pyramidal cells in the human frontal isocortex and changes in ratio with ageing and Alzheimer's disease. *Progress in Brain Research, 70*, 185–212. http://dx.doi.org/10.1016/S0079-6123(08)64305-8

Braver, T. S., & Barch, D. M. (2002). A theory of cognitive control, aging cognition, and neuromodulation. *Neuroscience and Biobehavioral Reviews, 26*, 809–817. http://dx.doi.org/10.1016/S0149-7634(02)00067-2

Cabeza, R. (2002). Hemispheric asymmetry reduction in older adults: The HAROLD model. *Psychology and Aging, 17*, 85–100. http://dx.doi.org/10.1037/0882-7974.17.1.85

Campbell, K. L., Grady, C. L., Ng, C., & Hasher, L. (2012). Age differences in the frontoparietal cognitive control network: Implications for distractibility. *Neuropsychologia, 50*, 2212–2223. http://dx.doi.org/10.1016/j.neuropsychologia.2012.05.025

Capotosto, P., Babiloni, C., Romani, G. L., & Corbetta, M. (2009). Frontoparietal cortex controls spatial attention through modulation of anticipatory alpha rhythms. *The Journal of Neuroscience, 29*, 5863–5872. http://dx.doi.org/10.1523/JNEUROSCI.0539-09.2009

Caputi, A., Melzer, S., Michael, M., & Monyer, H. (2013). The long and short of GABAergic neurons. *Current Opinion in Neurobiology, 23*, 179–186. http://dx.doi.org/10.1016/j.conb.2013.01.021

Chadick, J. Z., Zanto, T. P., & Gazzaley, A. (2014). Structural and functional differences in medial prefrontal cortex underlie distractibility and suppression deficits in ageing. *Nature Communications, 5*, 4223. http://dx.doi.org/10.1038/ncomms5223

Chang, L. H., Shibata, K., Andersen, G. J., Sasaki, Y., & Watanabe, T. (2014). Age-related declines of stability in visual perceptual learning. *Current Biology, 24*, 2926–2929. http://dx.doi.org/10.1016/j.cub.2014.10.041

Chee, M. W. L., Goh, J. O. S., Venkatraman, V., Tan, J. C., Gutchess, A., Sutton, B., . . . Park, D. (2006). Age-related changes in object processing and contextual binding revealed using fMR adaptation. *Journal of Cognitive Neuroscience, 18*, 495–507. http://dx.doi.org/10.1162/jocn.2006.18.4.495

Chowdhury, R., Guitart-Masip, M., Lambert, C., Dayan, P., Huys, Q., Düzel, E., & Dolan, R. J. (2013). Dopamine restores reward prediction errors in old age. *Nature Neuroscience, 16*, 648–653. http://dx.doi.org/10.1038/nn.3364

Clark, C. R., Veltmeyer, M. D., Hamilton, R. J., Simms, E., Paul, R., Hermens, D., & Gordon, E. (2004). Spontaneous alpha peak frequency predicts working memory performance across the age span. *International Journal of Psychophysiology, 53*, 1–9. http://dx.doi.org/10.1016/j.ijpsycho.2003.12.011

Clark, J. M. (1996). Contributions of inhibitory mechanisms to unified theory in neuroscience and psychology. *Brain and Cognition, 30*, 127–152. http://dx.doi.org/10.1006/brcg.1996.0008

Clewett, D. V., Lee, T. H., Greening, S., Ponzio, A., Margalit, E., & Mather, M. (2016). Neuromelanin marks the spot: Identifying a locus coeruleus biomarker of cognitive reserve in healthy aging. *Neurobiology of Aging, 37*, 117–126.

Colcombe, A. M., Kramer, A. F., Irwin, D. E., Peterson, M. S., Colcombe, S., & Hahn, S. (2003). Age-related effects of attentional and oculomotor capture by onsets and color singletons as a function of experience. *Acta Psychologica, 113*, 205–225. http://dx.doi.org/10.1016/S0001-6918(03)00019-2

Commodari, E., & Guarnera, M. (2008). Attention and aging. *Aging Clinical and Experimental Research, 20*, 578–584. http://dx.doi.org/10.1007/BF03324887

Dahl, M. J., Mather, M., Duezel, S., Bodammer, N. C., Lindenberger, U., Kuehn, S., & Werkle-Bergner, M. (2018). Locus coeruleus integrity preserves memory performance across the adult life span. *bioRxiv*, 332098. Retrieved from https://www.biorxiv.org/content/early/2018/05/28/332098.article-metrics

Dang, L. C., O'Neil, J. P., & Jagust, W. J. (2012). Dopamine supports coupling of attention-related networks. *The Journal of Neuroscience, 32*, 9582–9587. http://dx.doi.org/10.1523/JNEUROSCI.0909-12.2012

Davis, P. A. (1941). The electroencephalogram in old age. *Diseases of the Nervous System, 2*, 77.

Deiber, M. P., Rodriguez, C., Jaques, D., Missonnier, P., Emch, J., Millet, P., . . . Ibañez, V. (2010). Aging effects on selective attention-related electro-encephalographic patterns during face encoding. *Neuroscience, 171*, 173–186. http://dx.doi.org/10.1016/j.neuroscience.2010.08.051

DuPre, E., & Spreng, R. N. (2017). Structural covariance networks across the life span, from 6 to 94 years of age. *Network Neuroscience, 1*, 302–323. http://dx.doi.org/10.1162/NETN_a_00016

Eich, T. S., Razlighi, Q. R., & Stern, Y. (2017). Perceptual and memory inhibition deficits in clinically healthy older adults are associated with region-specific, doubly dissociable patterns of cortical thinning. *Behavioral Neuroscience, 131*, 220–225. http://dx.doi.org/10.1037/bne0000194

Foster, J. K., Behrmann, M., & Stuss, D. T. (1995). Aging and visual search: Generalized cognitive slowing or selective deficit in attention? *Aging, Neuropsychology and Cognition, 2*, 279–299. http://dx.doi.org/10.1080/13825589508256604

Foxe, J. J., & Snyder, A. C. (2011). The role of alpha-band brain oscillations as a sensory suppression mechanism during selective attention. *Frontiers in Psychology, 2*, 154. Advance online publication. http://dx.doi.org/10.3389/fpsyg.2011.00154

Gannon, M., & Wang, Q. (2019). Complex noradrenergic dysfunction in Alzheimer's disease: Low norepinephrine input is not always to blame. *Brain Research, 1702*, 12–16.

Gao, F., Edden, R. A. E., Li, M., Puts, N. A. J., Wang, G., & Liu, C., . . . Barker, P. B. (2013). Edited magnetic resonance spectroscopy detects an age-related decline in brain GABA levels. *NeuroImage, 78*, 75–82. http://dx.doi.org/10.1016/j.neuroimage.2013.04.012

Gazzaley, A., Cooney, J. W., Rissman, J., & D'Esposito, M. (2005). Top-down suppression deficit underlies working memory impairment in normal aging [erratum at http://dx.doi.org/10.1038/nn1205-1791c]. *Nature Neuroscience, 8*, 1298–1300. http://dx.doi.org/10.1038/nn1543

Gazzaley, A., & D'Esposito, M. (2007). Top-down modulation and normal aging. *Annals of the New York Academy of Sciences, 1097*, 67–83. http://dx.doi.org/10.1196/annals.1379.010

Geerligs, L., Renken, R. J., Saliasi, E., Maurits, N. M., & Lorist, M. M. (2015). A brain-wide study of age-related changes in functional connectivity. *Cerebral Cortex, 25,* 1987–1999. http://dx.doi.org/10.1093/cercor/bhu012

Giustino, T. F., & Maren, S. (2017). Chandelier cells illuminate inhibitory control of prefrontal–amygdala outputs. *Trends in Neurosciences, 40,* 640–642. http://dx.doi.org/10.1016/j.tins.2017.09.005

Goh, J. O. S. (2011). Functional dedifferentiation and altered connectivity in older adults: Neural accounts of cognitive aging. *Aging and Disease, 2,* 30–48. Retrieved from http://www.pubmedcentral.nih.gov/articlerender.fcgi?artid=3066008&tool=pmcentrez&rendertype=abstract

Grady, C. L., & Craik, F. I. M. (2000). Changes in memory processing with age. *Current Opinion in Neurobiology, 10,* 224–231. http://dx.doi.org/10.1016/S0959-4388(00)00073-8

Grady, C. L., Sarraf, S., Saverino, C., & Campbell, K. (2016). Age differences in the functional interactions among the default, frontoparietal control, and dorsal attention networks. *Neurobiology of Aging, 41,* 159–172. http://dx.doi.org/10.1016/j.neurobiolaging.2016.02.020

Hafkemeijer, A., van der Grond, J., & Rombouts, S. A. R. B. (2012). Imaging the default mode network in aging and dementia. *Biochimica et Biophysica Acta, 1822,* 431–441. http://dx.doi.org/10.1016/j.bbadis.2011.07.008

Hall, S. D., Barnes, G. R., Furlong, P. L., Seri, S., & Hillebrand, A. (2010). Neuronal network pharmacodynamics of GABAergic modulation in the human cortex determined using pharmaco-magnetoencephalography. *Human Brain Mapping, 31,* 581–594.

Hämmerer, D., Callaghan, M. F., Hopkins, A., Kosciessa, J., Betts, M., Cardenas-Blanco, A., . . . Düzel, E. (2018). Locus coeruleus integrity in old age is selectively related to memories linked with salient negative events. *Proceedings of the National Academy of Sciences of the United States of America, 115,* 2228–2233. http://dx.doi.org/10.1073/pnas.1712268115

Händel, B. F., Haarmeier, T., & Jensen, O. (2011). Alpha oscillations correlate with the successful inhibition of unattended stimuli. *Journal of Cognitive Neuroscience, 23,* 2494–2502. http://dx.doi.org/10.1162/jocn.2010.21557

Harvald, B. (1958). EEG in old age. *Acta Psychiatrica Scandinavica, 33,* 193–196. http://dx.doi.org/10.1111/j.1600-0447.1958.tb03512.x

Hasher, L., Stoltzfus, E. R., Zacks, R. T., & Rypma, B. (1991). Age and inhibition. *Journal of Experimental Psychology: Learning, Memory, and Cognition, 17,* 163–169. http://dx.doi.org/10.1037/0278-7393.17.1.163

Hasher, L., & Zacks, R. T. (1988). Working memory, comprehension, and aging: A review and a new view. *Psychology of Learning and Motivation, 22,* 193–225. http://dx.doi.org/10.1016/S0079-7421(08)60041-9

Hasher, L., Zacks, R. T., & May, C. P. (1999). Inhibitory control, circadian arousal, and age. *Attention and Performance XVII, Cognitive Regulation of Performance:*

Interaction of Theory and Application. Cambridge, MA: MIT Press. Retrieved from http://search.ebscohost.com/login.aspx?direct=true&db=psyh&AN=1999-02468-022&lang=fr&site=ehost-live

Healey, M. K., Campbell, K. L., & Hasher, L. (2008). Cognitive aging and increased distractibility: Costs and potential benefits. *Progress in Brain Research, 169,* 353–363. http://dx.doi.org/10.1016/S0079-6123(07)00022-2

Higo, S., Udaka, N., & Tamamaki, N. (2007). Long-range GABAergic projection neurons in the cat neocortex. *The Journal of Comparative Neurology, 503,* 421–431. http://dx.doi.org/10.1002/cne.21395

Hong, X., Sun, J., Bengson, J. J., Mangun, G. R., & Tong, S. (2015). Normal aging selectively diminishes alpha lateralization in visual spatial attention. *Neuro-Image, 106,* 353–363. http://dx.doi.org/10.1016/j.neuroimage.2014.11.019

Hua, T., Kao, C., Sun, Q., Li, X., & Zhou, Y. (2008). Decreased proportion of GABA neurons accompanies age-related degradation of neuronal function in cat striate cortex. *Brain Research Bulletin, 75,* 119–125. http://dx.doi.org/10.1016/j.brainresbull.2007.08.001

Hughes, S. W., & Crunelli, V. (2005). Thalamic mechanisms of EEG alpha rhythms and their pathological implications. *The Neuroscientist, 11,* 357–372. http://dx.doi.org/10.1177/1073858405277450

Hwang, K., Shine, J. M., & D'Esposito, M. (2018). Frontoparietal activity interacts with task-evoked changes in functional connectivity. *Cerebral Cortex.* Advance online publication. http://dx.doi.org/10.1093/cercor/bhy011

Jerde, T. A., Merriam, E. P., Riggall, A. C., Hedges, J. H., & Curtis, C. E. (2012). Prioritized maps of space in human frontoparietal cortex. *The Journal of Neuroscience, 32,* 17382–17390. http://dx.doi.org/10.1523/JNEUROSCI.3810-12.2012

Jessen, S. B., Mathiesen, C., Lind, B. L., & Lauritzen, M. (2017). Interneuron deficit associates attenuated network synchronization to mismatch of energy supply and demand in aging mouse brains. *Cerebral Cortex, 27,* 646–659. http://dx.doi.org/10.1093/cercor/bhv261

Ji, X.-H., Cao, X.-H., Zhang, C.-L., Feng, Z.-J., Zhang, X.-H., Ma, L., & Li, B.-M. (2008). Pre- and postsynaptic β-adrenergic activation enhances excitatory synaptic transmission in layer V/VI pyramidal neurons of the medial prefrontal cortex of rats. *Cerebral Cortex, 18,* 1506–1520. http://dx.doi.org/10.1093/cercor/bhm177

Kahana, M. J. (2006). The cognitive correlates of human brain oscillations. *The Journal of Neuroscience, 26,* 1669–1672. http://dx.doi.org/10.1523/JNEUROSCI.3737-05c.2006

Kihara, K., Kondo, H. M., & Kawahara, J. I. (2016). Differential contributions of GABA concentration in frontal and parietal regions to individual differences in attentional blink. *The Journal of Neuroscience, 36,* 8895–8901. http://dx.doi.org/10.1523/JNEUROSCI.0764-16.2016

Klimesch, W. (1999). EEG alpha and theta oscillations reflect cognitive and memory performance: A review and analysis. *Brain Research Reviews, 29,* 169–195. http://dx.doi.org/10.1016/S0165-0173(98)00056-3

Klimesch, W. (2012). α-band oscillations, attention, and controlled access to stored information. *Trends in Cognitive Sciences, 16*, 606–617. http://dx.doi.org/10.1016/j.tics.2012.10.007

Klimesch, W., Sauseng, P., & Hanslmayr, S. (2007). EEG alpha oscillations: The inhibition-timing hypothesis. *Brain Research Reviews, 53*, 63–88. http://dx.doi.org/10.1016/j.brainresrev.2006.06.003

Kramer, A. F., Hahn, S., Irwin, D. E., & Theeuwes, J. (2000). Age differences in the control of looking behavior: Do you know where your eyes have been? *Psychological Science, 11*, 210–217. http://dx.doi.org/10.1111/1467-9280.00243

Kramer, A. F., Humphrey, D. G., Larish, J. F., Logan, G. D., & Strayer, D. L. (1994). Aging and inhibition: Beyond a unitary view of inhibitory processing in attention. *Psychology and Aging, 9*, 491–512. http://dx.doi.org/10.1037/0882-7974.9.4.491

Kubo-Kawai, N., & Kawai, N. (2010). Elimination of the enhanced Simon effect for older adults in a three-choice situation: Ageing and the Simon effect in a go/no-go Simon task. *Quarterly Journal of Experimental Psychology, 63*, 452–64. http://dx.doi.org/10.1080/17470210902990829

Laird, A. R., Fox, P. M., Eickhoff, S. B., Turner, J. A., Ray, K. L., McKay, D. R., . . . Fox, P. T. (2011). Behavioral interpretations of intrinsic connectivity networks. *Journal of Cognitive Neuroscience, 23*, 4022–4037. http://dx.doi.org/10.1162/jocn_a_00077

Laufs, H., Kleinschmidt, A., Beyerle, A., Eger, E., Salek-Haddadi, A., Preibisch, C., & Krakow, K. (2003). EEG-correlated fMRI of human alpha activity. *NeuroImage, 19*, 1463–1476. http://dx.doi.org/10.1016/S1053-8119(03)00286-6

Lee, T. H., Greening, S. G., Ueno, T., Clewett, D., Ponzio, A., Sakaki, M., & Mather, M. (2018). Arousal increases neural gain via the locus coeruleus–norepinephrine system in younger adults but not in older adults. *Nature Human Behaviour, 2*, 356–366. http://dx.doi.org/10.1038/s41562-018-0344-1

Lee, T. H., Sakaki, M., Cheng, R., Velasco, R., & Mather, M. (2014). Emotional arousal amplifies the effects of biased competition in the brain. *Social Cognitive and Affective Neuroscience, 9*, 2067–2077. http://dx.doi.org/10.1093/scan/nsu015

Li, S.-C., & Lindenberger, U. (1999). Cross-level unification: A computational exploration of the link between deterioration of neurotransmitter systems and dedifferentiation of cognitive abilities in old age. In L.-G. Nilsson & H. J. Markowitsch (Eds.), *Cognitive neuroscience of memory* (pp. 103–146). Ashland, OH: Hogrefe & Huber.

Lőrincz, M. L., Kékesi, K. A., Juhász, G., Crunelli, V., & Hughes, S. W. (2009). Temporal framing of thalamic relay-mode firing by phasic inhibition during the alpha rhythm. *Neuron, 63*, 683–696. http://dx.doi.org/10.1016/j.neuron.2009.08.012

Lozano-Soldevilla, D., ter Huurne, N., Cools, R., & Jensen, O. (2014). GABAergic modulation of visual gamma and alpha oscillations and its consequences for working memory performance. *Current Biology, 24*, 2878–2887. http://dx.doi.org/10.1016/j.cub.2014.10.017

Lu, J., Tucciarone, J., Padilla-Coreano, N., He, M., Gordon, J. A., & Huang, Z. J. (2017). Selective inhibitory control of pyramidal neuron ensembles and cortical subnetworks by chandelier cells. *Nature Neuroscience, 20*, 1377–1383. http://dx.doi.org/10.1038/nn.4624

Lustig, C., Hasher, L., & Zacks, R. T. (2007). Inhibitory deficit theory: Recent developments in a new view. In D. S. Gorfein & C. M. MacLeod (Eds.), *Inhibition in cognition* (pp. 145–162). Washington, DC: American Psychological Association. http://dx.doi.org/10.1037/11587-008

Madden, D. J. (2007). Aging and visual attention. *Current Directions in Psychological Science, 16*, 70–74. http://dx.doi.org/10.1111/j.1467-8721.2007.00478.x

Mather, M., Clewett, D., Sakaki, M., & Harley, C. W. (2016). Norepinephrine ignites local hot spots of neuronal excitation: How arousal amplifies selectivity in perception and memory. *Behavioral and Brain Sciences, 39*, e200. Advance online publication. http://dx.doi.org/10.1017/S0140525X15000667

Mather, M., & Harley, C. W. (2016). The locus coeruleus: Essential for maintaining cognitive function and the aging brain. *Trends in Cognitive Sciences, 20*, 214–226. http://dx.doi.org/10.1016/j.tics.2016.01.001

Mathewson, K. E., Beck, D. M., Ro, T., Maclin, E. L., Low, K. A., Fabiani, M., & Gratton, G. (2014). Dynamics of alpha control: Preparatory suppression of posterior alpha oscillations by frontal modulators revealed with combined EEG and event-related optical signal. *Journal of Cognitive Neuroscience, 26*, 2400–2415. http://dx.doi.org/10.1162/jocn_a_00637

Mathewson, K. E., Lleras, A., Beck, D. M., Fabiani, M., Ro, T., & Gratton, G. (2011). Pulsed out of awareness: EEG alpha oscillations represent a pulsed-inhibition of ongoing cortical processing. *Frontiers in Psychology, 2*, 99. Advance online publication. http://dx.doi.org/10.3389/fpsyg.2011.00099

McEvoy, L. K., Pellouchoud, E., Smith, M. E., & Gevins, A. (2001). Neurophysiological signals of working memory in normal aging. *Cognitive Brain Research, 11*, 363–376. http://dx.doi.org/10.1016/S0926-6410(01)00009-X

Mevel, K., Chételat, G., Eustache, F., & Desgranges, B. (2011). The default mode network in healthy aging and Alzheimer's disease. *International Journal of Alzheimer's Disease, 2011*, 535816. http://dx.doi.org/10.4061/2011/535816

Mitchell, K. J., Ankudowich, E., Durbin, K. A., Greene, E. J., & Johnson, M. K. (2013). Age-related differences in agenda-driven monitoring of format and task information. *Neuropsychologia, 51*, 2427–2441. http://dx.doi.org/10.1016/j.neuropsychologia.2013.01.012

Morcom, A. M., Bullmore, E. T., Huppert, F. A., Lennox, B., Praseedom, A., Linnington, H., & Fletcher, P. C. (2010). Memory encoding and dopamine in the aging brain: A psychopharmacological neuroimaging study. *Cerebral Cortex, 20*, 743–757. http://dx.doi.org/10.1093/cercor/bhp139

Müller-Oehring, E. M., Schulte, T., Rohlfing, T., Pfefferbaum, A., & Sullivan, E. V. (2013). Visual search and the aging brain: Discerning the effects of age-related brain volume shrinkage on alertness, feature binding, and attentional control. *Neuropsychology, 27*, 48–59. http://dx.doi.org/10.1037/a0030921

Nashiro, K., Sakaki, M., Braskie, M. N., & Mather, M. (2017). Resting-state networks associated with cognitive processing show more age-related decline than those associated with emotional processing. *Neurobiology of Aging, 54*, 152–162. http://dx.doi.org/10.1016/j.neurobiolaging.2017.03.003

Ng, K. K., Lo, J. C., Lim, J. K. W., Chee, M. W. L., & Zhou, J. (2016). Reduced functional segregation between the default mode network and the executive control network in healthy older adults: A longitudinal study. *NeuroImage, 133*, 321–330. http://dx.doi.org/10.1016/j.neuroimage.2016.03.029

Nombela, C., Nombela, M., Castell, P., García, T., López-Coronado, J., & Herrero, M. T. (2014). Alpha-theta effects associated with ageing during the Stroop test. *PLoS One, 9*, e95657. Advance online publication. http://dx.doi.org/10.1371/journal.pone.0095657

Park, D. C., Polk, T. A., Park, R., Minear, M., Savage, A., & Smith, M. R. (2004). Aging reduces neural specialization in ventral visual cortex. *Proceedings of the National Academy of Sciences of the United States of America, 101*, 13091–13095. http://dx.doi.org/10.1073/pnas.0405148101

Porges, E. C., Woods, A. J., Edden, R. A. E., Puts, N. A. J., Harris, A. D., Chen, H., . . . Cohen, R. A. (2017). Frontal gamma-aminobutyric acid concentrations are associated with cognitive performance in older adults. *Biological Psychiatry: Cognitive Neuroscience and Neuroimaging, 2*, 38–44.

Ptak, R. (2012). The frontoparietal attention network of the human brain: Action, saliency, and a priority map of the environment. *The Neuroscientist, 18*, 502–515. http://dx.doi.org/10.1177/1073858411409051

Reuter-Lorenz, P. A. (2002). New visions of the aging mind and brain. *Trends in Cognitive Sciences, 6*, 394–400. http://dx.doi.org/10.1016/S1364-6613(02)01957-5

Reuter-Lorenz, P. A., & Cappell, K. A. (2008). Neurocognitive ageing and the Compensation Hypothesis. *Current Directions in Psychological Science, 17*, 177–182. http://dx.doi.org/10.1111/j.1467-8721.2008.00570.x

Rieckmann, A., Karlsson, S., Fischer, H., & Bäckman, L. (2011). Caudate dopamine D1 receptor density is associated with individual differences in frontoparietal connectivity during working memory. *The Journal of Neuroscience, 31*, 14284–14290. http://dx.doi.org/10.1523/JNEUROSCI.3114-11.2011

Romei, V., Gross, J., & Thut, G. (2010). On the role of prestimulus alpha rhythms over occipito-parietal areas in visual input regulation: Correlation or causation? *The Journal of Neuroscience, 30*, 8692–8697. http://dx.doi.org/10.1523/JNEUROSCI.0160-10.2010

Rowe, G., Valderrama, S., Hasher, L., & Lenartowicz, A. (2006). Attentional disregulation: A benefit for implicit memory. *Psychology and Aging, 21*, 826–830. http://dx.doi.org/10.1037/0882-7974.21.4.826

Rozycka, A., & Liguz-Lecznar, M. (2017). The space where aging acts: Focus on the GABAergic synapse. *Aging Cell, 16*, 634–643. http://dx.doi.org/10.1111/acel.12605

Sala-Llonch, R., Bartrés-Faz, D., & Junqué, C. (2015). Reorganization of brain networks in aging: A review of functional connectivity studies. *Frontiers in Psychology, 6*, 663. http://dx.doi.org/10.3389/fpsyg.2015.00663

Sander, M. C., Werkle-Bergner, M., & Lindenberger, U. (2012). Amplitude modulations and inter-trial phase stability of alpha-oscillations differentially reflect working memory constraints across the lifespan. *NeuroImage, 59*, 646–654. http://dx.doi.org/10.1016/j.neuroimage.2011.06.092

Sauseng, P., Klimesch, W., Stadler, W., Schabus, M., Doppelmayr, M., Hanslmayr, S., . . . Birbaumer, N. (2005). A shift of visual spatial attention is selectively associated with human EEG alpha activity. *European Journal of Neuroscience, 22*, 2917–2926. http://dx.doi.org/10.1111/j.1460-9568.2005.04482.x

Schreckenberger, M., Lange-Asschenfeldt, C., Lochmann, M., Mann, K., Siessmeier, T., Buchholz, H. G., . . . Gründer, G. (2004). The thalamus as the generator and modulator of EEG alpha rhythm: A combined PET/EEG study with lorazepam challenge in humans. *NeuroImage, 22*, 637–644. http://dx.doi.org/10.1016/j.neuroimage.2004.01.047

Scolari, M., Seidl-Rathkopf, K. N., & Kastner, S. (2015). Functions of the human frontoparietal attention network: Evidence from neuroimaging. *Current Opinion in Behavioral Sciences, 1*, 32–39. http://dx.doi.org/10.1016/j.cobeha.2014.08.003

Siman-Tov, T., Bosak, N., Sprecher, E., Paz, R., Eran, A., Aharon-Peretz, J., & Kahn, I. (2017). Early age-related functional connectivity decline in high-order cognitive networks. *Frontiers in Aging Neuroscience, 8*, 330. Advance online publication. http://dx.doi.org/10.3389/fnagi.2016.00330

Sohal, V. S., Zhang, F., Yizhar, O., & Deisseroth, K. (2009). Parvalbumin neurons and gamma rhythms enhance cortical circuit performance. *Nature, 459*, 698–702. http://dx.doi.org/10.1038/nature07991

Stanley, E. M., Fadel, J. R., & Mott, D. D. (2012). Interneuron loss reduces dendritic inhibition and GABA release in hippocampus of aged rats. *Neurobiology of Aging, 33*, 431.e1–431.e13. http://dx.doi.org/10.1016/j.neurobiolaging.2010.12.014

Stevens, W. D., Hasher, L., Chiew, K. S., & Grady, C. L. (2008). A neural mechanism underlying memory failure in older adults. *The Journal of Neuroscience, 28*, 12820–12824. http://dx.doi.org/10.1523/JNEUROSCI.2622-08.2008

Sumner, P., Edden, R. A. E., Bompas, A., Evans, C. J., & Singh, K. D. (2010). More GABA, less distraction: A neurochemical predictor of motor decision speed. *Nature Neuroscience, 13*, 825–827. http://dx.doi.org/10.1038/nn.2559

Sutherland, M. R., McQuiggan, D. A., Ryan, J. D., & Mather, M. (2017). Perceptual salience does not influence emotional arousal's impairing effects on top-down attention. *Emotion, 17*, 700–706. http://dx.doi.org/10.1037/emo0000245

Tomioka, R., Okamoto, K., Furuta, T., Fujiyama, F., Iwasato, T., Yanagawa, Y., . . . Tamamaki, N. (2005). Demonstration of long-range GABAergic connections distributed throughout the mouse neocortex. *The European Journal of Neuroscience, 21*, 1587–1600. http://dx.doi.org/10.1111/j.1460-9568.2005.03989.x

Tomioka, R., Sakimura, K., & Yanagawa, Y. (2015). Corticofugal GABAergic projection neurons in the mouse frontal cortex. *Frontiers in Neuroanatomy, 9,* 133. Advance online publication. http://dx.doi.org/10.3389/fnana.2015.00133

Treisman, A. (1998). Feature binding, attention and object perception. *Philosophical Transactions of the Royal Society of London: Series B. Biological Sciences, 353,* 1295–1306. http://dx.doi.org/10.1098/rstb.1998.0284

Turner, G. R., & Spreng, R. N. (2012). Executive functions and neurocognitive aging: Dissociable patterns of brain activity. *Neurobiology of Aging, 33,* 826.e1–826.e13. Advance online publication. http://dx.doi.org/10.1016/j.neurobiolaging.2011.06.005

Uhlhaas, P. J., & Singer, W. (2012). Neuronal dynamics and neuropsychiatric disorders: Toward a translational paradigm for dysfunctional large-scale networks. *Neuron, 75,* 963–980. http://dx.doi.org/10.1016/j.neuron.2012.09.004

Vaden, R. J., Hutcheson, N. L., McCollum, L. A., Kentros, J., & Visscher, K. M. (2012). Older adults, unlike younger adults, do not modulate alpha power to suppress irrelevant information. *NeuroImage, 63,* 1127–1133. http://dx.doi.org/10.1016/j.neuroimage.2012.07.050

van der Waal, M., Farquhar, J., Fasotti, L., & Desain, P. (2017). Preserved and attenuated electrophysiological correlates of visual spatial attention in elderly subjects. *Behavioural Brain Research, 317,* 415–423. http://dx.doi.org/10.1016/j.bbr.2016.09.052

Vidal-Piñeiro, D., Valls-Pedret, C., Fernández-Cabello, S., Arenaza-Urquijo, E. M., Sala-Llonch, R., Solana, E., . . . Bartrés-Faz, D. (2014). Decreased default mode network connectivity correlates with age-associated structural and cognitive changes. *Frontiers in Aging Neuroscience, 6,* 256.

Vlahou, E. L., Thurm, F., Kolassa, I.-T., & Schlee, W. (2014). Resting-state slow wave power, healthy aging and cognitive performance. *Scientific Reports, 4,* 5101. http://dx.doi.org/10.1038/srep05101

Ward, L. M. (2003). Synchronous neural oscillations and cognitive processes. *Trends in Cognitive Sciences, 7,* 553–559. http://dx.doi.org/10.1016/j.tics.2003.10.012

Weeks, J. C., & Hasher, L. (2014). The disruptive—and beneficial—effects of distraction on older adults' cognitive performance. *Frontiers in Psychology, 5,* 133. Advance online publication. http://dx.doi.org/10.3389/fpsyg.2014.00133

West, R., & Alain, C. (2000). Age-related decline in inhibitory control contributes to the increased Stroop effect observed in older adults. *Psychophysiology, 37,* 179–189. http://dx.doi.org/10.1111/1469-8986.3720179

Whiting, W. L., Madden, D. J., Pierce, T. W., & Allen, P. A. (2005). Searching from the top down: Ageing and attentional guidance during singleton detection. *The Quarterly Journal of Experimental Psychology, 58,* 72–97. http://dx.doi.org/10.1080/02724980443000205

Wilson, R. S., Nag, S., Boyle, P. A., Hizel, L. P., Yu, L., Buchman, A. S., . . . Bennett, D. A. (2013). Neural reserve, neuronal density in the locus ceruleus, and cognitive decline. *Neurology, 80,* 1202–1208. http://dx.doi.org/10.1212/WNL.0b013e3182897103

Wolf, W., Hicks, T. P., & Albus, K. (1986). The contribution of GABA-mediated inhibitory mechanisms to visual response properties of neurons in the kitten's striate cortex [Abstract]. *The Journal of Neuroscience, 6,* 2779–2795. http://www.jneurosci.org/content/6/10/2779. http://dx.doi.org/10.1523/JNEUROSCI.06-10-02779.1986

Wolfe, J. M., & Horowitz, T. S. (2017). Five factors that guide attention in visual search. *Nature Human Behaviour, 1,* 0058. http://dx.doi.org/10.1038/s41562-017-0058

Womelsdorf, T., & Everling, S. (2015). Long-range attention networks: Circuit motifs underlying endogenously controlled stimulus selection. *Trends in Neurosciences, 38,* 682–700. http://dx.doi.org/10.1016/j.tins.2015.08.009

Woodruff, D. S., & Kramer, D. A. (1979). EEG alpha slowing, refractory period, and reaction time in aging. *Experimental Aging Research, 5,* 279–292. http://dx.doi.org/10.1080/03610737908257205

Yoon, J. H., Grandelis, A., & Maddock, R. J. (2016). Dorsolateral prefrontal cortex GABA concentration in humans predicts working memory load processing capacity. *The Journal of Neuroscience, 36,* 11788–11794. http://dx.doi.org/10.1523/JNEUROSCI.1970-16.2016

Zanchi, D., Montandon, M. L., Sinanaj, I., Rodriguez, C., Depoorter, A., Herrmann, F. R., . . . Haller, S. (2017). Decreased fronto-parietal and increased default mode network activation is associated with subtle cognitive deficits in elderly controls. *Neuro-Signals, 25,* 127–138. http://dx.doi.org/10.1159/000486152

Zanto, T. P., & Gazzaley, A. (2017). Selective attention and inhibitory control in the aging brain. In R. Cabeza, L. Nyberg, & D. C. Park (Eds.), *Cognitive neuroscience of aging: Linking cognitive and cerebral aging* (2nd ed., pp. 207–234). New York, NY: Oxford University Press. http://dx.doi.org/10.1093/acprof:oso/9780199372935.003.0009

Zeef, E. J., Sonke, C. J., Kok, A., Buiten, M. M., & Kenemans, J. L. (1996). Perceptual factors affecting age-related differences in focused attention: Performance and psychophysiological analyses. *Psychophysiology, 33,* 555–565. http://dx.doi.org/10.1111/j.1469-8986.1996.tb02432.x

Zhang, S., Hu, S., Chao, H. H., & Li, C. S. R. (2016). Resting-state functional connectivity of the locus coeruleus in humans: In comparison with the ventral tegmental area/substantia nigra pars compacta and the effects of age. *Cerebral Cortex, 26,* 3413–3427. http://dx.doi.org/10.1093/cercor/bhv172

Zhang, S., Xu, M., Kamigaki, T., Hoang Do, J. P., Chang, W. C., Jenvay, S., . . . Dan, Y. (2014). Selective attention. Long-range and local circuits for top-down modulation of visual cortex processing. *Science, 345,* 660–665. http://dx.doi.org/10.1126/science.1254126

Zhao, Q., Lu, H., Metmer, H., Li, W. X. Y., & Lu, J. (2018). Evaluating functional connectivity of executive control network and frontoparietal network in Alzheimer's disease. *Brain Research, 1678,* 262–272. http://dx.doi.org/10.1016/j.brainres.2017.10.025

3

LEARNING AND MEMORY IN THE AGING BRAIN: THE FUNCTION OF DECLARATIVE AND NONDECLARATIVE MEMORY OVER THE LIFESPAN

NICHOLE R. LIGHTHALL, LINDSAY B. CONNER, AND KELLY S. GIOVANELLO

Human memory is not a unitary faculty. Rather, it consists of distinct learning and memory systems, each contributing in unique ways to the acquisition, retention, and subsequent retrieval of information. This chapter focuses on age-related changes to long-term learning and memory systems defined as the acquisition and retention of information over long intervals of time (i.e., beyond working memory capacity). Long-term memory is often subdivided into declarative memory (the acquisition and retention of knowledge) and nondeclarative memory (experience-induced changes in performance). In this chapter, we draw on behavioral and neuroimaging studies of young adults and older adults to describe the functional-anatomic architecture of multiple memory systems including declarative and nondeclarative memory. First, we present the neural correlates of the declarative memory system, followed by a discussion of how age-related changes to declarative memory mechanisms affect episodic memory while leaving semantic memory relatively intact. We then present the neural correlates of the nondeclarative memory system,

http://dx.doi.org/10.1037/0000143-004

The Aging Brain: Functional Adaptation Across Adulthood, G. R. Samanez-Larkin (Editor)

followed by a discussion of how age-related changes to mechanisms of priming, classical conditioning, procedural, and reinforcement learning affect associated learning and memory performance with age. Finally, we discuss interactions across and between memory systems with age, and potential future directions in research on learning and memory function in the aging brain.

NEURAL CORRELATES OF THE DECLARATIVE SYSTEM

Declarative memory encompasses the acquisition, long-term retention, and retrieval of events, facts, and concepts (Squire, 2009). Such knowledge can be retrieved at will and used in a variety of contexts. Declarative memory is typically subdivided based on whether memories are concerned with personally relevant events (i.e., episodic memory) or impersonal information (i.e., semantic memory). Broadly speaking, declarative learning and memory processes depend predominantly on the prefrontal cortex (PFC), medial temporal lobe (MTL), and lateral temporal cortex (see Figure 3.1). Research suggests that the PFC plays a supervisory role over other brain regions, including the MTL (Miller & Cohen, 2001; Norman & Shallice, 1986), via consciously controlled bias mechanisms (Buckner, 2003). During encoding, the PFC implements the processes that organize input to the MTL and during retrieval, the PFC mediates search and postretrieval monitoring processes (Cabeza, 2006; Moscovitch, 1992). In contrast, the MTL, particularly the hippocampus, serves to bind the conceptual, perceptual, and affective components of an episodic event into an integrated memory trace (Eichenbaum, Yonelinas, & Ranganath, 2007; Moscovitch, 1992). These binding processes operate both during the initial registration of novel events and when subjects retrieve recently acquired information (Gabrieli, Brewer, Desmond, & Glover, 1997; Nyberg, McIntosh, Houle, Nilsson, & Tulving, 1996), particularly during the encoding of experiences that are later remembered versus later forgotten. (Brewer, Zhao, Desmond, Glover, & Gabrieli, 1998; Wagner et al., 1998). Finally, neuroimaging studies investigating the brain basis of semantic memory have observed neural activity in the inferior frontal gyri, left superior temporal gyrus, and bilateral supramarginal gyri—specifically during the production of semantic exemplars and judgments of semantic similarity (Dapretto & Bookheimer, 1999; Friederici, Meyer, & von Cramon, 2000; Poldrack et al., 1999; Tyler et al., 2010, 2011; Wierenga et al., 2008; Zhuang, Johnson, Madden, Burke, & Diaz, 2016).

Functional neuroimaging studies of declarative memory in healthy older adults have demonstrated age-related alterations in neural activity (for general discussions of relevant issues, see Cabeza, 2006; Giovanello & Dew, 2015; Grady, 2008; Maillet & Rajah, 2014; Park & Reuter-Lorenz, 2009).

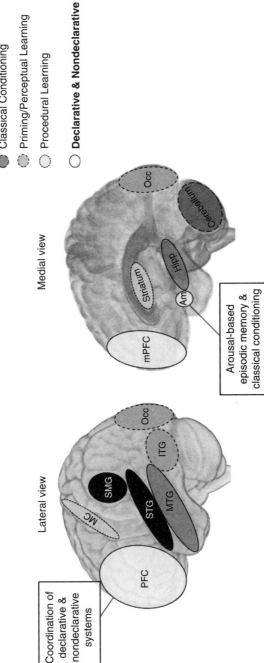

Figure 3.1. Primary brain structures associated with declarative and nondeclarative memory and learning. Generally, the declarative system relies on the prefrontal cortex (PFC) and temporal lobe, including the superior temporal (STG) and supramarginal (SMG) gyri for semantic memory and the middle temporal gyrus (MTG)—including the amygdala (Am) and hippocampus (Hipp)—for episodic memory. The nondeclarative system includes the striatum and motor cortex (MC) for procedural learning, stimulus-relevant neocortical areas for priming and perceptual learning (occipital [Occ] and inferior temporal gyrus [ITG]), and the amygdala and cerebellum for classical conditioning. Importantly, areas of the prefrontal cortex (PFC) are involved in coordination of both memory and learning systems (e.g., ventromedial PFC inhibition of the amygdala in fear conditioning; orbitofrontal and ventromedial PFC for reward and value processing) and undergoes the greatest amount of structural atrophy with age. The amygdala is involved in both fear conditioning in classical conditioning paradigms and the encoding and retrieval of emotional components of episodic memories.

Such alterations have taken the form of *underrecruitment* (i.e., failures to recruit specific brain regions to the same extent as young adults) or *nonselective recruitment* (i.e., recruitment of brain regions beyond those of young adults). Age-related functional alterations in declarative memory likely arise from age-dependent structural atrophy differences across distinct brain regions, including regions within the PFC (Gunning-Dixon & Raz, 2003; Maillet & Rajah, 2013; Pfefferbaum, Sullivan, Rosenbloom, Mathalon, & Lim, 1998; Raz et al., 2005; Resnick, Pham, Kraut, Zonderman, & Davatzikos, 2003) and MTL (Persson et al., 2006; Raz et al., 2005; Rodrigue & Raz, 2004). In what follows, we define the declarative memory subsystems, specifically episodic and semantic memory, and then describe experimental behavioral studies and neuroimaging investigations of aging.

EPISODIC MEMORY

Episodic memory enables individuals to recollect conscious experiences from their personal past (e.g., remembering what you ate for lunch yesterday). According to Tulving (1983), episodic memories are characterized by a sense of subjective awareness of having experienced remembered events in the past. To tap this *recollective experience*, Tulving developed the widely used remember–know paradigm, in which participants are initially presented with stimulus material and then asked to indicate whether the information is remembered (i.e., recollected with specific information) or known (i.e., retrieved with a sense of knowing something, yet void of any event details). This approach led to the proposal that two distinct mnemonic processes mediate episodic memory: recollection, as assessed with remember judgments, and familiarity, as indexed by know judgments (Yonelinas, 2002). However, such dual-process models of episodic memory have been consistently challenged by the view that episodic memory does not inherently rely on recollection and familiarity processes, but rather that episodic memories may be strong or weak (Wais, Squire, & Wixted, 2010).

Cognitive aging studies, including those that have used the remember–know paradigm or assessed the status of recollection and familiarity in aging (Anderson et al., 2008; Bastin & Van der Linden, 2003; Davidson & Glisky, 2002; Jacoby, 1999; Jennings & Jacoby, 1993; Naveh-Benjamin et al., 2009; Spencer & Raz, 1995; Yonelinas, 2002), have shown that older adults do not perform as well as young adults on tests of episodic memory. Several prominent theories have been proposed to account for age-related episodic memory declines, including general slowing (Salthouse, 1996), reductions in attentional resources (Craik & Byrd, 1982), dysfunction of inhibitory processes (Hasher, Lustig, & Zacks, 2007), and changes in sensory and perceptual abilities (Lindenberger & Baltes, 1994). Although these influential theories attempt to explain the range of cognitive changes observed in adulthood, two theoretical views have been proposed to explicitly account for age-related changes in episodic memory (for a review, see Giovanello & Dew, 2015). More specifically, the binding deficit view asserts that older adults have a fundamental deficit in linking or integrating the separate elements of an episode (Bayen, Phelps, & Spaniol, 2000; Burke & Light, 1981; Chalfonte & Johnson, 1996; Lyle, Bloise, & Johnson, 2006; Mitchell, Johnson, Raye, & D'Esposito, 2000; Naveh-Benjamin, 2000; Ryan, Leung, Turk-Browne, & Hasher, 2007), whereas the control deficit view suggests that older adults experience more generalized declines in cognitive control processes (Anderson & Craik, 2000; Craik, 1986; Craik & Byrd, 1982; Jennings & Jacoby, 1993; Light, Prull, LaVoie, & Healy, 2000; Moscovitch & Winocur, 1995; A. D. Smith, Park, Earles, Shaw, & Whiting, 1998), such as the strategic manipulation, organization, or evaluation of contextual attributes and the intentional retrieval of associative or relational information (Dew & Giovanello, 2010).

Accumulating evidence suggests that age-related declines in episodic memory are linked to structural and functional changes in the PFC. The frontal aging hypothesis proposes that age-related episodic memory changes are primarily due to PFC dysfunction (Moscovitch & Winocur, 1995; West, 1996). In support of this view, structural magnetic resonance imaging (MRI) studies of the aging brain consistently demonstrate frontal atrophy (Coffey et al., 1998; Convit et al., 2001; Cowell et al., 1994; Gur, Gunning-Dixon, Bilker, & Gur, 2002; Raz et al., 1997). The frontal lobes show the steepest rate of age-related atrophy (Pfefferbaum et al., 1998; Raz et al., 2005; Resnick et al., 2003), and, critically, this atrophy has been shown to correspond to cognitive changes (Gunning-Dixon & Raz, 2003; Maillet & Rajah, 2013). Additional evidence linking age-related episodic deficits with PFC dysfunction comes from functional neuroimaging studies showing age-related decreases in PFC activity during tasks of episodic memory. Age-related decreases in PFC activity have been observed during both encoding (Dennis, Hayes, et al., 2008; Iidaka et al., 2001; Kim & Giovanello, 2011; Mitchell et al., 2000) and retrieval (Cabeza, Anderson, Locantore, & McIntosh, 2002; Giovanello & Schacter, 2012) of episodic information.

There is also evidence suggesting that age-related episodic memory declines are linked to MTL structure and function. The MTL has a hierarchical organization, whereby information from sensory association cortices are channeled through the parahippocampal region (e.g., perirhinal and parahippocampal cortices), to the entorhinal cortex, and on to the hippocampus (Squire & Zola-Morgan, 1991). These memory structures undergo age-related atrophic changes, with significant atrophy observed in the hippocampus and minimal change in the entorhinal cortex (Raz et al., 2005), although shrinkage of the entorhinal cortex has been shown to correlate with poorer memory performance, whereas changes in the PFC and hippocampus have not (Rodrigue & Raz, 2004). Persson and colleagues (2006) reported reduced hippocampal volume in a group of older adults whose episodic memory performance declined over time compared with that of a group whose memory performance remained stable. Relatedly, Yonelinas and colleagues (2007) showed that reductions in hippocampal volume resulted in decreased recollection of episodic memories. More recently, Braskie, Small, and Bookheimer (2009) examined the relationship between entorhinal cortex thickness and functional MRI (fMRI) activity during an associative verbal (word pair) memory task. The results showed that participants with a thicker left entorhinal cortex had greater activation in anterior cingulate and medial frontal regions during memory retrieval, but not encoding. This result was independent of hippocampal volume. Finally, de Chastelaine and colleagues (2011) investigated the effects of age, memory performance, and callosal integrity on the neural correlates of successful episodic encoding. Participants in the study were scanned while making judgments about word pairs. A relationship was found between encoding trials that were subsequently remembered and activity in left inferior frontal gyrus, as well as bilateral hippocampus. Negative effects (i.e., greater activity for forgotten than remembered trials) were observed in default mode network regions (e.g., medial brain regions) for young adults but were reversed in the old—and that reversal correlated negatively with memory performance.

The relationship between age-related episodic memory deficits and MTL atrophy is also supported by fMRI studies demonstrating age-related reductions in MTL activity during encoding (Daselaar, Veltman, Rombouts, Raaijmakers, & Jonker, 2003; Dennis, Hayes, et al., 2008; Mitchell et al., 2000) and retrieval (Daselaar, Fleck, Dobbins, Madden, & Cabeza, 2006; Giovanello & Schacter, 2012; Tsukiura & Cabeza, 2008) of episodic information, particularly in the hippocampus. For example, Giovanello and Schacter (2012) hypothesized that healthy older adults would show age-related changes in MTL recruitment when the experimental task required the retrieval of specific, detailed, relational information. In young adults, left posterior ventrolateral PFC and bilateral hippocampal activity was modulated by the extent to which the retrieval task depended on relational processing (i.e., activity was greater during retrieval of relation, relative to item, information). For older adults, in contrast, activity in these regions was equivalent for item memory and relational (associative) memory conditions, suggesting an age-related change in the recruitment of ventrolateral PFC and hippocampal regions during retrieval of episodic information. In line with these findings, fMRI evidence has shown that aging reduces recollection-related hippocampal activity (Dennis, Kim, & Cabeza, 2008; Morcom, Li, &

Rugg, 2007; but see Persson, Kalpouzos, Nilsson, Ryberg, & Nyberg, 2011), yet enhances familiarity-related activity in the perirhinal cortex (Daselaar, Fleck, Dobbins, Madden, & Cabeza, 2006).

SEMANTIC MEMORY

Semantic memory encompasses a wide range of information, including facts about the world, the meanings of words and concepts, and the names attached to people and objects. Both cross-sectional and longitudinal studies indicate less age-related decline in semantic memory compared with episodic memory (e.g., Rönnlund, Nyberg, Bäckman, & Nilsson, 2005; see Figure 3.2). At a processing level, semantic memories differ from episodic memories in that they may be retrieved without associated information about the context

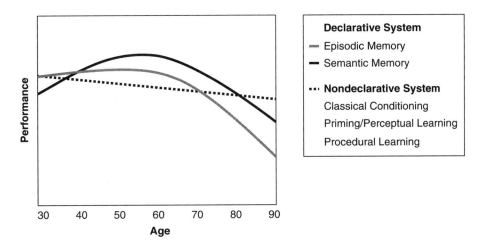

Figure 3.2. Estimated aging trajectory of declarative and nondeclarative memory and learning systems. Although explicit memory and learning tasks have been able to successfully estimate the relative rates of maintenance and decline of declarative episodic and semantic memory performance in later life, implicit learning and memory tasks have not fully informed separate trajectories of the nondeclarative system with age. While components such as name recall, value processing, and task maintenance that rely on the prefrontal cortex undergo decline with age, processes dependent on the accumulation of world knowledge and slow, implicit procedural learning are generally maintained and strengthened throughout the lifetime, allowing for individual differences in successful compensation on memory and learning tasks (e.g., the use of explicit strategies). Adapted from "Stability, Growth, and Decline in Adult Life Span Development of Declarative Memory: Cross-Sectional and Longitudinal Data From a Population-Based Study," by M. Rönnlund, L. Nyberg, L. Bäckman, and L.-G. Nilsson, 2005, *Psychology and Aging, 20,* p. 14. Copyright 2005 by the American Psychological Association.

in which they were learned. Importantly, not all forms of semantic knowledge share the same properties. Some forms of knowledge may be acquired after a single exposure (e.g., knowledge that Boston is the capital of Massachusetts), whereas other forms may be gradually acquired across multiple repetitions (e.g., understanding the concept *website*). Additionally, semantic learning may involve establishing new associations between preexisting representations in memory (e.g., learning that William Shakespeare wrote *Romeo and Juliet*) or acquiring a new label for information already represented in memory (e.g., learning a foreign language). Finally, a new label and a novel set of properties may be linked to each other (e.g., learning the concept of a *microbrew*).

Given the varied nature of semantic information and its accrual over the lifetime, behavioral aging studies have primarily focused on retrieval of semantic information using tests of picture naming, vocabulary, and text comprehension (Burke & Shafto, 2008). Studies investigating age-related changes in vocabulary knowledge and text comprehension have consistently reported that these measures are well preserved in aging and, in the case of vocabulary knowledge, improve over the adult lifespan (Alwin & McCammon, 2001; Verhaeghen, 2003). Additionally, preserved semantic function in older adults has also been reported during semantic judgments (Little, Prentice, & Wingfield, 2004) and semantic priming (Madden, Pierce, & Allen, 1993). In contrast, one of the most frequent cognitive complaints among older adults is difficulty with finding words (Albert et al., 2009; Clark-Cotton, Williams, Goral, & Obler, 2007; Mortensen, Meyer, & Humphreys, 2006; Neumann, Obler, Gomes, & Shafer, 2009). These naming difficulties have been confirmed in both cross-sectional (MacKay, Connor, Albert, & Obler, 2002; Mariën, Mampaey, Vervaet, Saerens, & de Deyn, 1998) and longitudinal (Au et al., 1995; Barresi, Nicholas, Connor, Obler, & Albert, 2000; Connor, Spiro, Obler, & Albert, 2004; Goral, Spiro, Albert, Obler, & Connor, 2007) studies. Although older adults complain of word-finding difficulties, not all studies have found age-related declines in naming. Moreover, determining when such age-related decreases in naming performance arise during the adult lifespan has been controversial. To investigate this issue, Verhaegen and Poncelet (2013) assessed picture-naming performance in participants at the ages of 25 to 35, 50 to 59, 60 to 69, and older than 70 years. In addition to naming accuracy, naming latencies were assessed to reveal subtle naming difficulties. Importantly, to control for general slowing (as opposed to slowing specific to the naming task), participants were also given an odd–even judgment task to assess cognitive processing speed. The researchers reported that participants in their 50s showed decline in naming performance, reflected by an increase in naming latencies, while adults in their 60s and their 70s showed both a decrease in accuracy and an increase in latency. The increase in naming latencies remained significant even after controlling for odd–even judgment latencies, suggesting a specific decline in picture naming. Finally, to further assess the degradation of semantic knowledge, participants were tested with a synonym judgment task and the Pyramids and Palm Trees test (the latter task requires participants to identify pairings of conceptually related words or pictures). The results revealed semantic degradation in the group older than 70 years.

Neuroimaging studies have consistently shown activation in left prefrontal and temporal cortices during semantic retrieval. However, disagreement exists about the specific nature of the processes mediated by subregions within the PFC. One theoretical view proposes that the left inferior frontal gyrus (IFG), particularly the ventral region (Brodmann's area 47), is involved in semantic processing (Dapretto & Bookheimer, 1999; Friederici, Meyer, & von Cramon, 2000; Poldrack et al., 1999), while another theoretical views asserts that the left IFG has a domain-general role in selecting among competing candidates (Humphreys & Gennari, 2014; January, Trueswell, & Thompson-Schill, 2009; Moss et al., 2005; Schnur et al., 2009; Thompson-Schill, Bedny, & Goldberg, 2005; Thompson-Schill, D'Esposito, Aguirre, & Farah, 1997). The role of the left temporal cortex in semantic memory has been informed by patient-based and functional neuroimaging studies investigating the continuum of general semantic knowledge to knowledge of specific exemplars or items. For example, Tyler and colleagues (2011) suggested that naming at the specific level requires retrieval and integration of more detailed semantic information than at the domain-general level. That is, naming a picture at the domain-general level requires activation of item features only, whereas naming a picture at the specific level entails retrieval and integration of additional, more precise features. Tyler and colleagues observed that patients with lesions to the anterior temporal lobes cannot reliably name exemplars (e.g., tiger) at the specific level, indicating that retrieval and integration of more detailed semantic information is impaired. Moreover, convergent evidence comes from fMRI studies in young adults in which greater activation in the anterior temporal lobes is observed with specific level naming than with domain level naming.

As with episodic memory, age-related functional activity changes during semantic memory tasks have taken the form of nonselective recruitment (i.e., recruitment of brain regions engaged beyond those of young adults) resulting in reduced laterality, such that young adults may engage only the left PFC, whereas older adults activate the PFC bilaterally. Although debate exists about whether such age-related increase in right PFC activation reflect compensatory processes (Cabeza, Anderson, Locantore, & McIntosh, 2002; Park & Reuter-Lorenz, 2009; Peelle, Troiani, Wingfield, & Grossman, 2010; Wierenga et al., 2008) or less efficient neural responses (Li, Lindenberger, & Sikström, 2001; Park et al., 2004), both patterns have been observed in neural investigations of semantic memory and aging. Consistent with the compensation view, Wierenga et al. (2008) reported age-related increased functional activation of the right IFG associated with higher accuracy during picture naming, and Tyler and colleagues (2010) observed age-related increased activation in right inferior frontal cortex during a comprehension task, under conditions in which performance was matched between young and older adults. In contrast, age-related increases right IFG activity have also been observed during poor performance. For example, during a semantic fluency task, Meinzer et al. (2009) found negative correlations between neural activity in the right IFG in older adults and the production of semantic exemplars. Likewise, Diaz et al. (2014) showed that older adults produced more errors than young adults on a phonological judgment task that required covert production of picture names and, although older adults exhibited greater activation than younger adults, this activity was not related to behavioral performance.

More recently, Zhuang and colleagues (2016) investigated the neural underpinnings of phonological and semantic retrieval in young and older adults using rhyme and semantic similarity judgment tasks. Although all participants responded faster and more accurately during the rhyme task compared to the semantic task, older adults demonstrated higher accuracy than young adults during semantic similarity judgments. Analysis of the fMRI data revealed no overall age-related differences, with bilateral IFG, bilateral supramarginal gyri, cingulate, and left superior temporal gyrus supporting performance. However, an interaction of age (young, old) and task (phonological, semantic) was observed during the semantic judgment task, with older adults showing greater activation than younger adults in left inferior frontal, bilateral posterior cingulate, and left fusiform regions. Taken together, these results indicate that at lower levels of task difficulty, older and younger adults engaged similar neural networks that benefited behavioral performance. However, as task difficulty increased during the semantic task, older adults relied more heavily on left hemisphere regions, as well as regions involved in perception and strategic monitoring. Zhuang et al. suggested that these results are consistent with the stability of language comprehension across the adult lifespan and illustrate how the preservation of semantic representations with age may influence performance during high task difficulty.

NEURAL CORRELATES OF THE NONDECLARATIVE SYSTEM

Brain regions most commonly associated with the nondeclarative system include the striatum for procedural and reinforcement learning, stimulus-relevant neocortical areas for priming and perceptual learning, and the amygdala and cerebellum for conditioning (see Figure 3.1; Squire, 2004; Squire

& Dede, 2015). More specifically, skill and reward-based learning depend on dopamine projections of value signals from the midbrain (e.g., substantia nigra and ventral tegmental area) to the striatum (Schultz, 2013), which is divided into functionally distinct subregions (K. S. Smith & Graybiel, 2013; Yin et al., 2009). The ventral striatum (e.g., nucleus accumbens, ventral caudate nucleus, and putamen) is associated with early learning and valuation processing in conjunction with medial PFC regions, while the dorsal striatum (e.g., dorsal caudate nucleus and putamen) supports overlearned behaviors through coordination with the dorsal PFC and motor regions (Haber & Knutson, 2010; Haruno & Kawato, 2006; Hiebert et al., 2014). Neural mechanisms of priming and perceptual learning involve attenuated cortical activity upon repetition of previously experienced stimuli and their associates (Schacter, Wig, & Stevens, 2007). Facilitated processing has been attributed to stimulus-specific neural assemblies "sharpening" their responses for more efficient processing (Wiggs & Martin, 1998), whereas the PFC appears to drive the efficiency of communication across regions (Schacter et al., 2007). Finally, with respect to classical conditioning, motor conditioning and emotion-based conditioning are distinct in their neural correlates. Motor conditioning relies on the cerebellum (e.g., delayed eyeblink task; Thompson & Steinmetz, 2009), including simultaneous activation of the cerebellar cortex and its nuclei during learning acquisition (Thürling et al., 2015). In contrast, the amygdala is critically involved in classical conditioning involving arousal states such as threat (Bechara et al., 1995; LaBar, LeDoux, Spencer, & Phelps, 1995; Morris, DeGelder, Weiskrantz, & Dolan, 2001). The prefrontal cortex also plays a role in classical conditioning—for example, through inhibition of the amygdala when automatic defensive behaviors do not allow for escape from threat (Moscarello & LeDoux, 2013).

Cross-sectional and longitudinal structural neuroimaging evidence shows age-related volume loss in all of the aforementioned brain regions, with considerable heterogeneity in the nature of change and some notable similarities to aging in the declarative memory system. For example, comparable age effects are observed for the amygdala and hippocampus (Fjell & Walhovd, 2010). In an analysis of 883 adults from ages 18 to 93, Walhovd and colleagues (2011) found that the striatum and hippocampus age at approximately the same rate—but within the striatum some structures age faster (e.g., putamen, pallidum, accumbens) relative to others (e.g., caudate). The hippocampus and caudate are also associated with nonlinear changes, but whereas shrinkage of the hippocampus appears to accelerate in late life, shrinkage of the caudate seems to decelerate (Fjell & Walhovd, 2010; Raz, Ghisletta, Rodrigue, Kennedy, & Lindenberger, 2010; Raz et al., 2005; Walhovd et al., 2011). Across brain regions, the cerebral cortex exhibits the greatest gray matter loss across adulthood and accelerating white matter loss in later life (Walhovd et al.,

2011). However, gray matter volume in the occipital lobe (implicated in perceptual priming) appears to be relatively stable with age (Driscoll et al., 2009; Fjell & Walhovd, 2010; Raz et al., 2010). Thus, age-related changes to macrostructure suggest that all forms of learning and memory are subject to age effects, and processing changes may be driven by the subregions within memory systems that are most vulnerable to age-related decline.

PROCEDURAL AND REINFORCEMENT LEARNING

The literature on age-related changes to procedure and reinforcement learning mechanisms has expanded greatly in recent years. Indeed, prior reviews of learning and memory in aging dedicated only small sections to the topic (Craik, 1994; Hoyer & Verhaeghen, 2006; Lustig & Flegal, 2008; Nilsson, 2003). This lack of attention reflected the low number of human studies and the general conclusion, based on limited findings, that these forms of procedural learning showed little age-related change. This seems odd in retrospect because it had been known since the 1980s that the striatum played a critical role in feedback-based learning (Packard, Hirsh, & White, 1989), and normal aging was associated with significant decline in striatal dopamine receptors (Severson, Marcusson, Winblad, & Finch, 1982; Wong et al., 1984). Renewed interest in this topic coincided with the birth of neuroeconomics as a field of study, as researchers tried to understand whether and how brain aging affects our ability to make value-based decisions (Eppinger, Hämmerer, & Li, 2011).

Reinforcement learning yields habit-based behaviors that make up a significant part of our everyday decision-making. Such behaviors arise from the slow building of associations between actions and their likely consequences through trial and error (Thorndike, 1911). Typical tasks involve stimuli with probabilistic associations to immediate choice outcomes (e.g., rewards, punishments). Learning results in higher selection rates for reward-predicting stimuli and/or lower selection rates of punishment-predicting stimuli over time. Most behavioral findings indicate that older adults maintain the ability to acquire adaptive behaviors through trial-and-error learning with probabilistic outcomes but typically find declines in learning performance for older adults relative to young (Eppinger, Schuck, Nystrom, & Cohen, 2013; Hämmerer, Li, Müller, & Lindenberger, 2011; Lighthall, Gorlick, Schoeke, Frank, & Mather, 2013; Wood, Busemeyer, Koling, Cox, & Davis, 2005), although age effects often depend on the precise metrics of performance or specific task conditions. Recent advances in cognitive neuroscience research have shed light on both the likely mechanisms of age-related change in procedural learning and sources of heterogeneity in the learning behavior of older adults. Much progress in this area of study is attributable to computational learning models, which allow for the examination of discrete learning components and their neural correlates. Functional imaging studies using these approaches can investigate how the brain processes action-based outcomes (e.g., rewards) according to valence and magnitude, integrates past reward histories into accurate expected values for states or situations, and then generates prediction errors when actual rewards differ from expected rewards (Niv, 2009; Schultz, Dayan, & Montague, 1997; Sutton & Barto, 1998).

In considering mechanisms of change to learning, one possibility is that aging has a negative impact on the ability to respond to the positive and negative outcomes of our choices. Within the cortex, delivery of reward is consistently associated with activation in the orbitofrontal, ventromedial prefrontal, and anterior cingulate regions (Haber & Knutson, 2010; Schultz, 2000). Extant research indicates that both simple reward detection and the representation of reward magnitude are preserved in healthy older adults. Responses to positive outcomes (e.g., rewards, gains) are generally maintained or may even increase with age in regions such as the medial PFC, anterior cingulate, and striatum in healthy aging (e.g., Dreher, Meyer-Lindenberg, Kohn, & Berman, 2008; Samanez-Larkin et al., 2007; Schott et al., 2007). Neural mechanisms of responses to negative outcomes (e.g., punishments, losses) are less established (Schultz, 2017), but similar response patterns have been observed across younger and older adults in the anterior cingulate, inferior parietal cortex, dorsolateral PFC, insula, and putamen (Eppinger et al., 2013). Eppinger et al. (2013) also found age differences based on outcome valence, such that older adults showed reduced neural responses to gains but not losses in the ventromedial PFC. However, other studies have specifically tested for age-by-valence effects in this region and found no significant interaction (Samanez-Larkin et al., 2007; Samanez-Larkin, Worthy, Mata, McClure, & Knutson, 2014). Notably, Samanez-Larkin and associates (2007) observed the maintenance of neural responses to positive and negative outcomes across and within different levels of magnitude and, in another investigation (Samanez-Larkin et al., 2014), observed increased response to gains in the anterior cingulate for older versus younger adults. These mixed results highlight the need for future research to further examine potential age-by-outcome valence interactions. However, consistencies across studies suggest that age-related change to simple outcome response is not the primary driver of age differences in reinforcement learning.

In contrast, age-related changes to the behavioral and neural correlates of value updating are frequently observed. When stimulus-outcome likelihoods are stable or explicitly stated, older adults' performance is often similar to that of younger adults, but relatively poorer when outcome likelihoods are probabilistic or involve reversal learning (Eppinger, Heekeren, & Li, 2015;

Eppinger, Kray, Mock, & Mecklinger, 2008; Hämmerer et al., 2011; Lighthall et al., 2013; Mata, Josef, Samanez-Larkin, & Hertwig, 2011; Mell et al., 2005; Pietschmann, Endrass, Czerwon, & Kathmann, 2011; Samanez-Larkin et al., 2014; van de Vijver, Ridderinkhof, & de Wit, 2015; Weiler, Bellebaum, & Daum, 2008). It is important to note that providing outcome contingencies, or making them easy to learn, can effectively diminish or altogether eliminate the need for implicit learning and its neural mechanisms. As such, an environment where outcome likelihoods are uncertain or changing will increase the reliance on truly implicit procedural learning. Under such conditions, the representation of accurate expected values critically depends on predictor error signals for value updating (Chase, Kumar, Eickhoff, & Dombrovski, 2015). These signals correspond to discrepancies between actual and expected rewards, with positive prediction errors (i.e., actual > expected) enhancing phasic dopamine neuron firing (Schultz, 2017). Further, functional imaging studies in humans, along with electrophysiological and lesion studies in animals, have shown that reward prediction error signals act on subject behavior via mesostriatal dopamine projections and the synaptic modification of cortical–striatal–midbrain networks (Chase et al., 2015; Eppinger et al., 2011).

Evidence that older adults are specifically impaired in value updating led to the hypothesis that age-related alterations to striatal prediction error signals cause deficits in reinforcement-based learning among older adults (Eppinger et al., 2011; Samanez-Larkin & Knutson, 2015). Consistent with this hypothesis, fMRI studies of reinforcement learning have observed age-related reductions in activation of the medial PFC and nucleus accumbens, corresponding to learning model-based reward prediction errors among older adults (Eppinger et al., 2013; Samanez-Larkin et al., 2014). Others have manipulated dopamine levels using L-DOPA in older adults to determine if increasing available dopamine can improve older adults' learning performance and restore their neural prediction error signal to the canonical form observed in young adults (Chowdhury et al., 2013). Chowdhury and colleagues (2013) found that L-DOPA had different effects on subgroups of older adults. Whereas one subgroup performed at the level of younger adults on placebo and experienced a decrease in performance on L-DOPA ($n = 17$), the other subgroup experienced a boost in learning performance, bringing them up to the level of young adults when on the drug ($n = 15$). Critically, within the group that benefitted from L-DOPA, fMRI results revealed that the drug restored their reward prediction error signal in the ventral striatum. The impact of L-DOPA was specific to the expected value component of the prediction error (vs. the reward response). In contrast, the subgroup of older adults who performed worse on L-DOPA appeared to have greater noise in their neural prediction error components when on the drug. Consistent with results in the former subgroup of older adults (worse performance on L-DOPA), a recent fMRI study demonstrated that older adults with reinforcement learning performance equal to younger adults had no age-related decline in striatal prediction error response to immediate feedback (Lighthall, Pearson, Huettel, & Cabeza, 2018). Critically, however, the same group of older adults exhibited relatively diminished hippocampal prediction error signals that support learning from delayed feedback. Thus, striatally mediated learning functions appear to be relatively well preserved in at least a subpopulation of high-functioning older adults who nonetheless exhibit decline in hippocampally mediated learning functions.

The preceding findings are consistent with earlier studies suggesting that trial-and-error learning from immediate feedback is well preserved in a large percentage of healthy older adults (Denburg et al., 2005, 2006) and studies finding no impact of aging on basic reward outcome responses (Dreher et al., 2008; Samanez-Larkin et al., 2007; Schott et al., 2007). They also provide convincing evidence that age effects on habit development are driven by dopamine-mediated alterations to expected value representations in the striatum. In addition, a current hypothesis proposes that age effects on reward learning stem from declines in the structural integrity of frontostriatal white matter connections that support corrections to reward predictions (Samanez-Larkin & Knutson, 2015). Consistent with this proposal, a study of age effects on reward learning using diffusion tensor imaging found that age was associated with declines in the coherence of frontostriatal pathways (i.e., connections from thalamus to medial PFC and medial PFC to nucleus accumbens; Samanez-Larkin, Levens, Perry, Dougherty, & Knutson, 2012). Furthermore, age differences in reward learning were fully explained by white matter coherence within these specific tracts.

Given that reinforcement learning and procedural skill learning share both neural mechanisms (e.g., striatum) and process features (e.g., effects of outcome probabilities, magnitudes, variabilities, and delays; Fu & Anderson, 2006), one may expect similar trajectories of age-related changes as behaviors go from processing recurrent choices to developing complex skills. Indeed, as with reinforcement learning, the overall ability to learn new skills is maintained into old age (Ren, Wu, Chan, & Yan, 2013), while learning rates and skill performance levels are typically lower in older adults compared with younger and middle-aged adults (Durkina, Prescott, Furchtgott, Cantor, & Powell, 1995; King, Fogel, Albouy, & Doyon, 2013; Rodrigue, Kennedy, & Raz, 2005; Voelcker-Rehage, 2008).

Like simple reward learning, individual differences and task-related factors can affect both the existence and magnitude of age differences in procedural skill learning, as well as the specific performance measure on which age effects are observed. Motor sequence learning tasks (e.g., serial reaction time) are commonly used in laboratory studies to index skill learning and performance. Motor sequence learning tasks involve the development of smooth, effortless movements from repeated sequence training. For instance, in the classic serial reaction time task, button-response sequences are implicitly learned by following a pattern of visual cues over many trials. A key finding from motor sequence learning studies is that the initial sequence learning abilities are relatively intact in healthy older adults (King et al., 2013), as well as in patients with damage to the medial temporal lobes (van Halteren-van Tilborg, Scherder, & Hulstijn, 2007). Importantly, similar age-related changes to skill learning and performance are also observed for motor tasks that do not involve sequences (e.g., force production, simple tracking; Voelcker-Rehage, 2008) as well as skill learning tasks that do not require a motor response (e.g., mirror-reversed reading; Durkina et al., 1995).

For simple skills, older adults may exhibit performance levels similar to those of younger adults; however, as task complexity increases, initial learning rates are reduced in older adults (King et al., 2013). For example, one study found that older adults performed worse under dual-task versus single-task conditions during sequence learning (Gamble, Howard, & Howard, 2014). Yet, in the same study, postlearning probes indicated equivalent performance among older adults for sequences learned across conditions. Thus, executive demands during motor sequence learning may sometimes suppress the expression of learning in older adults, rather than impairing learning itself. Another factor mediating age effects is whether explicit knowledge is involved in the motor sequence-learning task. For example, when older adults are told that a motor sequence learning task has an embedded sequence and that learning the sequence can help them respond more quickly, they show poorer learning relative to older adults without this explicit knowledge (Howard & Howard, 2001). Notably, younger adults' sequence learning is unaffected or enhanced by explicit knowledge (Howard & Howard, 2001; Willingham & Goedert-Eschmann, 1999; Willingham, Salidis, & Gabrieli, 2002). With respect to postlearning performance, age is associated with poorer consolidation of motor memories (e.g., during sleep; Spencer, Gouw, & Ivry, 2007; Wilson, Baran, Pace-Schott, Ivry, & Spencer, 2012) and poorer adaptation to sensorimotor perturbations. Older adults' difficulty in adapting to changes in required motor patterns (i.e., motor adaptation) appears to be most pronounced immediately at the change initiation (King et al., 2013), and this deficit has been linked to reduced explicit awareness of pattern changes among older adults (Heuer & Hegele, 2008). Thus, again, aging is associated with a reduced ability to use explicit knowledge to benefit procedural learning.

Among the most direct evidence linking age-related changes to the brain and changes to skill learning are findings showing decreased putamen activation among older adults during the late phase of learning in serial reaction tasks and altered patterns of PFC activation during learning (Aizenstein et al., 2006). Correspondingly, while reduced reaction time from early to late learning has been associated with decreasing MTL activation and increasing caudate activation in young adults, older adults exhibit associated increasing activation in both regions (Rieckmann, Fischer, & Bäckman, 2010). Such findings may reflect age-related compensation in the MTL; however, more conclusive support for this interpretation requires age comparisons of MTL activation with trial-level performance measures (e.g., slow vs. fast reaction-time trials within subjects; Cabeza & Dennis, 2013). Other critical findings include that lateral PFC and caudate volumes predict skill learning performance, but lateral PFC volumes change more with aging and are more predictive of skill learning in older compared with younger adults (Kennedy & Raz, 2005). Together, these findings suggest that age-related changes to the basal ganglia and its connections to the PFC may be responsible for decline in simple habit and skill learning with age. Large-scale age differences observed in motor adaptation, more complex learning tasks, and procedural learning with "contamination" from explicit processing are likely due to age-related changes in the MTL and PFC.

PRIMING AND PERCEPTUAL LEARNING

Repetition priming, also known simply as *priming*, involves facilitated processing of previously experienced items or associates of those items (Squire & Dede, 2015). Experienced information may be perceptual or conceptual, and individuals need not be aware that the stimulus previously occurred, although processing may be affected by conscious awareness (Roediger & McDermott, 1993). Typical priming tasks involve the presentation of words or pictures followed by a delay and then a second "unrelated" task. The second task includes primed material or associates as potential response options and such responses are more readily produced, as indicated by speed, accuracy, and response bias. Priming has been linked to *repetition suppression* effects, such that brain activation is reduced upon repetition of a stimulus in the neocortical regions initially involved in processing the stimulus or its associates (Wiggs & Martin, 1998). The prevailing theory of repetition-related reductions in activation is that stimuli-associated neurons become more precise in their response with repeated exposure (Grill-Spector, Henson, & Martin, 2006).

Although a lack of age differences has been reported in numerous priming studies, careful reviews and meta-analyses indicate a decline in priming effects on perceptual and conceptual information in normal aging (Fleischman & Gabrieli, 1998; La Voie & Light, 1994; Ward, Berry, & Shanks, 2013). Earlier research indicated that age differences in priming may be small or negligible depending on the specific task; however, a more recent report suggests that small but reliable age effects may have been obscured by low power and reliability in many priming studies (Ward et al., 2013). Correspondingly, event-related potentials and oscillatory responses to priming indicate attenuated repetition suppression effects in older compared with younger adults, even in the absence of behavioral differences (Sebastián & Ballesteros, 2012).

Well-designed behavioral studies have revealed that age differences in the neural correlates of priming may relate to greater use of controlled encoding among younger adults. Gopie, Craik, and Hasher (2011) found that when individuals are told to ignore presented words and only respond to their text color, older adults show relatively greater *implicit* memory for primed words, but younger adults showed relatively greater *explicit* memory for primed words. The young adults' advantage for explicit memory disappeared when their attention was divided at encoding. This suggests that some age differences in priming and repetition suppression can be explained by deeper processing of "incidental" details by younger adults. With that said, the effectiveness of priming in older populations suggests cortical plasticity that may be leveraged to ameliorate declines in sensory processing via perceptual learning. Indeed, research shows that healthy older adults who engage in brief training sessions to improve visual discrimination (e.g., texture, motion) can retain benefits for at least several months (Andersen, Ni, Bower, & Watanabe, 2010; Bower, Watanabe, & Andersen, 2013). These findings suggest that neural plasticity in early and later visual processing regions (Schwartz, Maquet, & Frith, 2002) is maintained in late life.

CLASSICAL CONDITIONING

Classical conditioning represents one of the most basic forms of learning—its functions and related mechanisms are conserved within mammals and are similar between vertebrates. In such tasks, a neutral stimulus (CS) is repeatedly paired with an unconditioned stimulus (US), the latter eliciting arousal and/or behavioral states prior to training. Learning is said to have occurred when the CS in isolation can elicit responses previously only attributed to the US. Across a range of studies, eyeblink conditioning (anticipatory blink from a CS) is more pronounced in younger versus older adults (Bellebaum & Daum, 2004; Cheng, Faulkner, Disterhoft, & Desmond, 2010; Knuttinen, Power, Preston, & Disterhoft, 2001; Solomon, Pomerleau, Bennett, James, & Morse, 1989). In contrast, aging impairs extinguishing of conditioned responses (Thürling et al., 2014). Cerebellar volume predicts eyeblink conditioned responses (Woodruff-Pak, Goldenberg, Downey-Lamb, Boyko, & Lemieux, 2000), as well as the change in storage of conditioned responses with advancing age (Thürling et al., 2014). The hippocampus also plays a role in eyeblink conditioning, particularly when the CS and US are separated in time (e.g., *trace conditioning*; Cheng, Disterhoft, Power, Ellis, & Desmond, 2008), but further work must be conducted to determine if age-related change to the hippocampus drives trace-conditioning deficits.

Age-related decline has also been observed for arousal-based conditioning. Contributing factors appear to include declines in autonomic responses to conditioned stimuli from middle age to late adulthood, along with lower levels of contingency awareness (LaBar, Cook, Torpey, & Welsh-Bohmer, 2004). In fact, simultaneously controlling for these two factors eliminated age differences in fear learning. Critically, middle aged and older adults exhibited lower autonomic response to the US during learning acquisition and lower orienting response to the CS. This age effect mirrors impaired older adults' reduced anticipatory physiological signal to losses in the Iowa Gambling Task (Denburg, Recknor, Bechara, & Tranel, 2006; Denburg, Tranel, & Bechara, 2005). The Iowa Gambling Task, developed by Bechara, Damasio, Damasio, and Anderson (1994), requires feedback-based learning about card deck outcome probabilities over time and is commonly used to examine ventromedial PFC function and the integrated role of cognition and emotion in risky decision-making. Thus, despite the fact that aging is associated with more "pure" implicit learning during classical conditioning, this is not enough to overcome learning deficits associated with age-related decline in autonomic signaling.

CONCLUSIONS AND FUTURE DIRECTIONS

Taken together, the reviewed literature suggests unique trajectories of age-related change for different memory systems. Behavioral research indicates relatively greater stability in nondeclarative versus declarative forms of learning and memory, with a midlife peak in declarative memory and more accelerated decline in episodic versus semantic memory (see Figure 3.2). Age-related changes in the neural mechanisms of these memory systems likewise suggests generally greater decline in episodic relative to semantic and nondeclarative memory. Notably, however, there is currently a dearth of research comparing trajectories of age-related changes to different forms of nondeclarative memory and their neural correlates. Additional research is required to determine the precise rate and nature of change to different types of nondeclarative memory in aging.

Before closing, it is important to note that focal lesion studies strongly suggest independence of declarative and nondeclarative memory (Knowlton, Mangels, & Squire, 1996; Packard et al., 1989), but accumulating evidence points to interactions between systems (e.g., Lee, Shimojo, & O'Doherty, 2014; Poldrack et al., 2001; Shohamy & Wagner, 2008; Wimmer, Braun, Daw,

& Shohamy, 2014). The latter studies involve innovative designs and analytic methods that allow for examination of memory mechanism interactions across systems and have not yet been applied to investigate age-related changes. Indeed, few studies to date have directly compared age-related changes to the neural mechanisms of declarative and nondeclarative memory systems in the same participants (e.g., Dennis & Cabeza, 2011; Lighthall et al., 2018). The available findings suggest that uncontrolled crossover between memory systems may be more common in older adults due to age-related dedifferentiation of neural networks (Park & Reuter-Lorenz, 2009), but these conclusions require additional evidence.

Further, the degree to which classic nondeclarative tasks represent "pure" unconscious processing has been called into question (LeDoux, 2014; Nilsson, 2003). This chapter included several examples of porous boundaries between systems. Thus, although age differences generally decrease as limitations on explicit processing increase, younger adults can use structures and functions of the declarative system to their advantage in many classic nondeclarative tasks. Situations that allow for crossover from explicit to implicit processing are likely to increase observed age differences in learning and memory performance and benefit only the most cognitively fit older adults. As such, although this chapter largely highlighted age effects on learning and memory within traditional memory-system boundaries, a frontier in the cognitive neuroscience of aging is emerging at their intersections.

REFERENCES

Aizenstein, H. J., Butters, M. A., Clark, K. A., Figurski, J. L., Andrew Stenger, V., Nebes, R. D., . . . Carter, C. S. (2006). Prefrontal and striatal activation in elderly subjects during concurrent implicit and explicit sequence learning. *Neurobiology of Aging, 27,* 741–751. http://dx.doi.org/10.1016/j.neurobiolaging. 2005.03.017

Albert, M. L., Spiro, A., III, Sayers, K. J., Cohen, J. A., Brady, C. B., Goral, M., & Obler, L. K. (2009). Effects of health status on word finding in aging. *Journal of the American Geriatrics Society, 57,* 2300–2305. http://dx.doi.org/10.1111/ j.1532-5415.2009.02559.x

Alwin, D. F., & McCammon, R. J. (2001). Aging, cohorts, and verbal ability. *Journal of Gerontology: Series B. Psychological Sciences and Social Sciences, 56,* S151–S161. http://dx.doi.org/10.1093/geronb/56.3.S151

Andersen, G. J., Ni, R., Bower, J. D., & Watanabe, T. (2010). Perceptual learning, aging, and improved visual performance in early stages of visual processing. *Journal of Vision, 10,* 4–4. http://dx.doi.org/10.1167/10.13.4

Anderson, N. D., & Craik, F. I. M. (2000). Memory in the aging brain. In E. Tulving & F. I. M. Craik (Eds.), *The Oxford handbook of memory* (pp. 411–425). New York, NY: Oxford University Press.

Anderson, N. D., Ebert, P. L., Jennings, J. M., Grady, C. L., Cabeza, R., & Graham, S. J. (2008). Recollection- and familiarity-based memory in healthy aging and amnestic mild cognitive impairment. *Neuropsychology, 22,* 177–187. http://dx.doi.org/10.1037/0894-4105.22.2.177

Au, R., Joung, P., Nicholas, M., Obler, L. K., Kass, R., & Albert, M. L. (1995). Naming ability across the adult life span. *Aging and Cognition, 2,* 300–311. http://dx.doi.org/10.1080/13825589508256605

Barresi, B., Nicholas, M., Connor, L. T., Obler, L. K., & Albert, M. L. (2000). Semantic degradation and lexical access in age-related naming failures. *Aging, Neuropsychology and Cognition, 7,* 169–178. http://dx.doi.org/10.1076/1382-5585(200009)7:3;1-Q;FT169

Bastin, C., & Van der Linden, M. (2003). The contribution of recollection and familiarity to recognition memory: A study of the effects of test format and aging. *Neuropsychology, 17,* 14–24. http://dx.doi.org/10.1037/0894-4105.17.1.14

Bayen, U. J., Phelps, M. P., & Spaniol, J. (2000). Age-related differences in the use of contextual information in recognition memory: A global matching approach. *Journals of Gerontology: Series B. Psychological Sciences and Social Sciences, 55,* 131–141. http://dx.doi.org/10.1093/geronb/55.3.P131

Bechara, A., Damasio, A. R., Damasio, H., & Anderson, S. W. (1994). Insensitivity to future consequences following damage to human prefrontal cortex. *Cognition, 50,* 7–15. http://dx.doi.org/10.1016/0010-0277(94)90018-3

Bechara, A., Tranel, D., Damasio, H., Adolphs, R., Rockland, C., & Damasio, A. R. (1995). Double dissociation of conditioning and declarative knowledge relative to the amygdala and hippocampus in humans. *Science, 269,* 1115–1118. http://dx.doi.org/10.1126/science.7652558

Bellebaum, C., & Daum, I. (2004). Effects of age and awareness on eyeblink conditional discrimination learning. *Behavioral Neuroscience, 118,* 1157–1165. http://dx.doi.org/10.1037/0735-7044.118.6.1157

Bower, J. D., Watanabe, T., & Andersen, G. J. (2013). Perceptual learning and aging: Improved performance for low-contrast motion discrimination. *Frontiers in Psychology, 4,* 66. http://dx.doi.org/10.3389/fpsyg.2013.00066

Braskie, M. N., Small, G. W., & Bookheimer, S. Y. (2009). Entorhinal cortex structure and functional MRI response during an associative verbal memory task. *Human Brain Mapping, 30,* 3981–3992. http://dx.doi.org/10.1002/hbm.20823

Brewer, J. B., Zhao, Z., Desmond, J. E., Glover, G. H., & Gabrieli, J. D. E. (1998). Making memories: Brain activity that predicts how well visual experience will be remembered. *Science, 281,* 1185–1187. http://dx.doi.org/10.1126/science.281.5380.1185

Buckner, R. L. (2003). Functional-anatomic correlates of control processes in memory. *The Journal of Neuroscience, 23,* 3999–4004. http://dx.doi.org/10.1523/JNEUROSCI.23-10-03999.2003

Burke, D. M., & Light, L. L. (1981). Memory and aging: The role of retrieval processes. *Psychological Bulletin, 90,* 513–546. http://dx.doi.org/10.1037/0033-2909.90.3.513

Burke, D. M., & Shafto, M. A. (2008). Language and aging. In F. I. M. Craik & T. A. Salthouse (Eds.), *The handbook of aging and cognition* (3rd ed., pp. 373–443). New York, NY: Psychology Press.

Cabeza, R. (2006). Prefrontal and medial temporal contributions to relational memory in young and older adults. In D. Zimmer, A. Mecklinger, & U. Lindenberger (Eds.), *Binding in human memory: A neurocognitive approach* (pp. 595–626). New York, NY: Oxford University Press. http://dx.doi.org/10.1093/acprof:oso/9780198529675.003.0024

Cabeza, R., Anderson, N. D., Locantore, J. K., & McIntosh, A. R. (2002). Aging gracefully: Compensatory brain activity in high-performing older adults. *NeuroImage, 17,* 1394–1402. http://dx.doi.org/10.1006/nimg.2002.1280

Cabeza, R., & Dennis, N. A. (2013). Frontal lobes and aging: Deterioration and compensation. In D. T. Stuss & R. T. Knight (Eds.), *Principles of frontal lobe function* (2nd ed., pp. 628–652). New York, NY: Oxford University Press.

Chalfonte, B. L., & Johnson, M. K. (1996). Feature memory and binding in young and older adults. *Memory & Cognition, 24,* 403–416. http://dx.doi.org/10.3758/BF03200930

Chase, H. W., Kumar, P., Eickhoff, S. B., & Dombrovski, A. Y. (2015). Reinforcement learning models and their neural correlates: An activation likelihood estimation meta-analysis. *Cognitive, Affective & Behavioral Neuroscience, 15,* 435–459. http://dx.doi.org/10.3758/s13415-015-0338-7

Cheng, D. T., Disterhoft, J. F., Power, J. M., Ellis, D. A., & Desmond, J. E. (2008). Neural substrates underlying human delay and trace eyeblink conditioning. *Proceedings of the National Academy of Sciences of the United States of America, 105,* 8108–8113. http://dx.doi.org/10.1073/pnas.0800374105

Cheng, D. T., Faulkner, M. L., Disterhoft, J. F., & Desmond, J. E. (2010). The effects of aging in delay and trace human eyeblink conditioning. *Psychology and Aging, 25,* 684–690. http://dx.doi.org/10.1037/a0017978

Chowdhury, R., Guitart-Masip, M., Lambert, C., Dayan, P., Huys, Q., Düzel, E., & Dolan, R. J. (2013). Dopamine restores reward prediction errors in old age. *Nature Neuroscience, 16,* 648–653. http://dx.doi.org/10.1038/nn.3364

Clark-Cotton, M. R., Williams, R. K., Goral, M., & Obler, L. K. (2007). Language and communication in aging. In J. E. Birren (Ed.), *Encyclopedia of gerontology: Age, aging, and the aged* (2nd ed., pp. 1–8). London, England: Elsevier. http://dx.doi.org/10.1016/B0-12-370870-2/00103-7

Coffey, J. F., Lucke, J. A., Saxton, G., Ratcliff, L. J., Unitas, B., Billig, B., & Byran, R. N. (1998). Sex differences in brain imaging. *Archives of Neurology, 55,* 169–179. http://dx.doi.org/10.1001/archneur.55.2.169

Connor, L. T., Spiro, A., Obler, L. K., & Albert, M. L. (2004). Change in object naming ability during adulthood. *The Journals of Gerontology: Series B. Psychological Sciences and Social Sciences, 59,* 203–209. http://dx.doi.org/10.1093/geronb/59.5.P203

Convit, A., Wolf, O. T., de Leon, M. J., Patalinjug, M., Kandil, E., Caraos, C., . . . Cancro, R. (2001). Volumetric analysis of the pre-frontal regions: Findings in aging and schizophrenia. *Psychiatry Research: Neuroimaging, 107,* 61–73. http://dx.doi.org/10.1016/S0925-4927(01)00097-X

Cowell, P. E., Turetsky, B. I., Gur, R. C., Grossman, R. I., Shtasel, D. L., & Gur, R. E. (1994). Sex differences in aging of the human frontal and temporal lobes. *The Journal of Neuroscience, 14,* 4748–4755. http://dx.doi.org/10.1523/JNEUROSCI.14-08-04748.1994

Craik, F. I. M. (1986). A functional account of age differences in memory. In F. Klix & H. Hagendorf (Eds.), *Human memory and cognitive capabilities, mechanisms, and performances* (pp. 409–422). North Holland, Netherlands: Elsevier.

Craik, F. I. M. (1994). Memory changes in normal aging. *Current Directions in Psychological Science, 3,* 155–158. http://dx.doi.org/10.1111/1467-8721.ep10770653

Craik, F. I. M., & Byrd, M. (1982). Aging and cognitive deficits: The role of attentional resources. In F. I. M. Craik & S. Trehub (Eds.), *Aging and cognitive processes* (pp. 191–211). New York, NY: Plenum Press.

Dapretto, M., & Bookheimer, S. Y. (1999). Form and content: Dissociating syntax and semantics in sentence comprehension. *Neuron, 24,* 427–432. http://dx.doi.org/10.1016/S0896-6273(00)80855-7

Daselaar, S. M., Fleck, M. S., Dobbins, I. G., Madden, D. J., & Cabeza, R. (2006). Effects of healthy aging on hippocampal and rhinal memory functions: An event-related fMRI study. *Cerebral Cortex, 16,* 1771–1782. http://dx.doi.org/10.1093/cercor/bhj112

Daselaar, S. M., Veltman, D. J., Rombouts, S. A., Raaijmakers, J. G., & Jonker, C. (2003). Deep processing activates the medial temporal lobe in young but not in old adults. *Neurobiology of Aging, 24,* 1005–1011. http://dx.doi.org/10.1016/S0197-4580(03)00032-0

Davidson, P. S., & Glisky, E. L. (2002). Neuropsychological correlates of recollection and familiarity in normal aging. *Cognitive, Affective & Behavioral Neuroscience, 2,* 174–186. http://dx.doi.org/10.3758/CABN.2.2.174

de Chastelaine, M., Wang, T. H., Minton, B., Muftuler, L. T., & Rugg, M. D. (2011). The effects of age, memory performance, and callosal integrity on the neural correlates of successful associative encoding. *Cerebral Cortex, 21,* 2166–2176. http://dx.doi.org/10.1093/cercor/bhq294

Denburg, N. L., Recknor, E. C., Bechara, A., & Tranel, D. (2006). Psychophysiological anticipation of positive outcomes promotes advantageous decision-making in normal older persons. *International Journal of Psychophysiology, 61,* 19–25. http://dx.doi.org/10.1016/j.ijpsycho.2005.10.021

Denburg, N. L., Tranel, D., & Bechara, A. (2005). The ability to decide advantageously declines prematurely in some normal older persons. *Neuropsychologia, 43,* 1099–1106. http://dx.doi.org/10.1016/j.neuropsychologia.2004.09.012

Dennis, N. A., & Cabeza, R. (2011). Age-related dedifferentiation of learning systems: An fMRI study of implicit and explicit learning. *Neurobiology of Aging, 32,* 2318.e17–2318.e30. http://dx.doi.org/10.1016/j.neurobiolaging.2010.04.004

Dennis, N. A., Hayes, S. M., Prince, S. E., Madden, D. J., Huettel, S. A., & Cabeza, R. (2008). Effects of aging on the neural correlates of successful item and source memory encoding. *Journal of Experimental Psychology: Learning, Memory, and Cognition, 34,* 791–808. http://dx.doi.org/10.1037/0278-7393.34.4.791

Dennis, N. A., Kim, H., & Cabeza, R. (2008). Age-related differences in brain activity during true and false memory retrieval. *Journal of Cognitive Neuroscience, 20,* 1390–1402. http://dx.doi.org/10.1162/jocn.2008.20096

Dew, I. T. Z., & Giovanello, K. S. (2010). Differential age effects for implicit and explicit conceptual associative memory. *Psychology and Aging, 25,* 911–921. http://dx.doi.org/10.1037/a0019940

Diaz, M. T., Johnson, M. A., Burke, D. M., & Madden, D. J. (2014). Age-related differences in the neural bases of phonological and semantic processes. *Journal of Cognitive Neuroscience, 26,* 2798–2811. http://dx.doi.org/10.1162/jocn_a_00665

Dreher, J. C., Meyer-Lindenberg, A., Kohn, P., & Berman, K. F. (2008). Age-related changes in midbrain dopaminergic regulation of the human reward system. *Proceedings of the National Academy of Sciences of the United States of America, 105,* 15106–15111. http://dx.doi.org/10.1073/pnas.0802127105

Driscoll, I., Davatzikos, C., An, Y., Wu, X., Shen, D., Kraut, M., & Resnick, S. M. (2009). Longitudinal pattern of regional brain volume change differentiates normal aging from MCI. *Neurology, 72,* 1906–1913. http://dx.doi.org/10.1212/WNL.0b013e3181a82634

Durkina, M., Prescott, L., Furchtgott, E., Cantor, J., & Powell, D. A. (1995). Performance but not acquisition of skill learning is severely impaired in the elderly. *Archives of Gerontology and Geriatrics, 20,* 167–183. http://dx.doi.org/10.1016/0167-4943(94)00594-W

Eichenbaum, H., Yonelinas, A. P., & Ranganath, C. (2007). The medial temporal lobe and recognition memory. *Annual Review of Neuroscience, 30,* 123–152. http://dx.doi.org/10.1146/annurev.neuro.30.051606.094328

Eppinger, B., Hämmerer, D., & Li, S. C. (2011). Neuromodulation of reward-based learning and decision making in human aging. *Annals of the New York Academy of Sciences, 1235,* 1–17. http://dx.doi.org/10.1111/j.1749-6632.2011.06230.x

Eppinger, B., Heekeren, H. R., & Li, S. C. (2015). Age-related prefrontal impairments implicate deficient prediction of future reward in older adults. *Neurobiology of Aging, 36*, 2380–2390. http://dx.doi.org/10.1016/j.neurobiolaging.2015.04.010

Eppinger, B., Kray, J., Mock, B., & Mecklinger, A. (2008). Better or worse than expected? Aging, learning, and the ERN. *Neuropsychologia, 46*, 521–539. http://dx.doi.org/10.1016/j.neuropsychologia.2007.09.001

Eppinger, B., Schuck, N. W., Nystrom, L. E., & Cohen, J. D. (2013). Reduced striatal responses to reward prediction errors in older compared with younger adults. *The Journal of Neuroscience, 33*, 9905–9912. http://dx.doi.org/10.1523/JNEUROSCI.2942-12.2013

Fjell, A. M., & Walhovd, K. B. (2010). Structural brain changes in aging: Courses, causes and cognitive consequences. *Reviews in the Neurosciences, 21*, 187–221. http://dx.doi.org/10.1515/REVNEURO.2010.21.3.187

Fleischman, D. A., & Gabrieli, J. D. (1998). Repetition priming in normal aging and Alzheimer's disease: A review of findings and theories. *Psychology and Aging, 13*, 88–119. http://dx.doi.org/10.1037/0882-7974.13.1.88

Friederici, A. D., Meyer, M., & von Cramon, D. Y. (2000). Auditory language comprehension: An event-related fMRI study on the processing of syntactic and lexical information. *Brain and Language, 74*, 289–300. http://dx.doi.org/10.1006/brln.2000.2313

Fu, W. T., & Anderson, J. R. (2006). From recurrent choice to skill learning: A reinforcement-learning model. *Journal of Experimental Psychology: General, 135*, 184–206. http://dx.doi.org/10.1037/0096-3445.135.2.184

Gabrieli, J. D. E., Brewer, J. B., Desmond, J. E., & Glover, G. H. (1997). Separate neural bases of two fundamental memory processes in the human medial temporal lobe. *Science, 276*, 264–266. http://dx.doi.org/10.1126/science.276.5310.264

Gamble, K. R., Howard, J. H., Jr., & Howard, D. V. (2014). Does a simultaneous memory load affect older and younger adults' implicit associative learning? *Aging, Neuropsychology and Cognition, 21*, 52–67. http://dx.doi.org/10.1080/13825585.2013.782998

Giovanello, K. S., & Dew, I. T. Z. (2015). Relational memory and its relevance to aging. In D. R. Addis, M. Barense, & A. Duarte (Eds.), *The Wiley handbook on the cognitive neuroscience of human memory* (pp. 371–392). Hoboken, NJ: Wiley. http://dx.doi.org/10.1002/9781118332634.ch18

Giovanello, K. S., & Schacter, D. L. (2012). Reduced specificity of hippocampal and posterior ventrolateral prefrontal activity during relational retrieval in normal aging. *Journal of Cognitive Neuroscience, 24*, 159–170. http://dx.doi.org/10.1162/jocn_a_00113

Gopie, N., Craik, F. I., & Hasher, L. (2011). A double dissociation of implicit and explicit memory in younger and older adults. *Psychological Science, 22*, 634–640. http://dx.doi.org/10.1177/0956797611403321

Goral, M., Spiro, A. I., Albert, M. L., Obler, L. K., & Connor, L. T. (2007). Change in lexical skills in adulthood: Not a uniform decline. *The Mental Lexicon, 2*, 215–238. http://dx.doi.org/10.1075/ml.2.2.05gor

Grady, C. L. (2008). Cognitive neuroscience of aging. *Annual Review of the New York Academy of Sciences, 1124*, 127–144. http://dx.doi.org/10.1196/annals.1440.009

Grill-Spector, K., Henson, R., & Martin, A. (2006). Repetition and the brain: Neural models of stimulus-specific effects. *Trends in Cognitive Sciences, 10*, 14–23. http://dx.doi.org/10.1016/j.tics.2005.11.006

Gunning-Dixon, F. M., & Raz, N. (2003). Neuroanatomical correlates of selected executive functions in middle-aged and older adults: A prospective MRI study. *Neuropsychologia, 41*, 1929–1941. http://dx.doi.org/10.1016/S0028-3932(03)00129-5

Gur, R. C., Gunning-Dixon, F., Bilker, W. B., & Gur, R. E. (2002). Sex differences in temporo-limbic and frontal brain volumes of healthy adults. *Cerebral Cortex, 12*, 998–1003. http://dx.doi.org/10.1093/cercor/12.9.998

Haber, S. N., & Knutson, B. (2010). The reward circuit: Linking primate anatomy and human imaging. *Neuropsychopharmacology, 35*, 4–26. http://dx.doi.org/10.1038/npp.2009.129

Hämmerer, D., Li, S.-C., Müller, V., & Lindenberger, U. (2011). Life span differences in electrophysiological correlates of monitoring gains and losses during probabilistic reinforcement learning. *Journal of Cognitive Neuroscience, 23*, 579–592. http://dx.doi.org/10.1162/jocn.2010.21475

Haruno, M., & Kawato, M. (2006). Heterarchical reinforcement-learning model for integration of multiple cortico-striatal loops: fMRI examination in stimulus-action-reward association learning. *Neural Networks, 19*, 1242–1254. http://dx.doi.org/10.1016/j.neunet.2006.06.007

Hasher, L., Lustig, C., & Zacks, R. T. (2007). Inhibitory mechanisms and the control of attention. In A. R. A. Conway, C. Jarrold, M. J. Kane, A. Miyake, & J. N. Towes (Eds.), *Variation in working memory* (pp. 227–249). New York, NY: Oxford University Press.

Heuer, H., & Hegele, M. (2008). Adaptation to visuomotor rotations in younger and older adults. *Psychology and Aging, 23*, 190–202. http://dx.doi.org/10.1037/0882-7974.23.1.190

Hiebert, N. M., Vo, A., Hampshire, A., Owen, A. M., Seergobin, K. N., & MacDonald, P. A. (2014). Striatum in stimulus-response learning via feedback and in decision making. *NeuroImage, 101*, 448–457. http://dx.doi.org/10.1016/j.neuroimage.2014.07.013

Howard, D. V., & Howard, J. H., Jr. (2001). When it does hurt to try: Adult age differences in the effects of instructions on implicit pattern learning. *Psychonomic Bulletin & Review, 8*, 798–805. http://dx.doi.org/10.3758/BF03196220

Hoyer, W. J., & Verhaeghen, P. (2006). Memory aging. In J. E. Birren & K. W. Schaire (Eds.), *Handbook of the psychology of aging* (pp. 209–232). Amsterdam, Netherlands: Elsevier. http://dx.doi.org/10.1016/B978-012101264-9/50013-6

Humphreys, G. F., & Gennari, S. P. (2014). Competitive mechanisms in sentence processing: Common and distinct production and reading comprehension networks linked to the prefrontal cortex. *NeuroImage, 84,* 354–366. http://dx.doi.org/10.1016/j.neuroimage.2013.08.059

Iidaka, T., Sadato, N., Yamada, H., Murata, T., Omori, M., & Yonekura, Y. (2001). An fMRI study of the functional neuroanatomy of picture encoding in younger and older adults. *Cognitive Brain Research, 11,* 1–11. http://dx.doi.org/10.1016/S0926-6410(00)00058-6

Jacoby, L. L. (1999). Ironic effects of repetition: Measuring age-related differences in memory. *Journal of Experimental Psychology: Learning, Memory, and Cognition, 25,* 3–22. http://dx.doi.org/10.1037/0278-7393.25.1.3

January, D., Trueswell, J. C., & Thompson-Schill, S. L. (2009). Co-localization of Stroop and syntactic ambiguity resolution in Broca's area: Implications for the neural basis of sentence processing. *Journal of Cognitive Neuroscience, 21,* 2434–2444. http://dx.doi.org/10.1162/jocn.2008.21179

Jennings, J. M., & Jacoby, L. L. (1993). Automatic versus intentional uses of memory: Aging, attention, and control. *Psychology and Aging, 8,* 283–293. http://dx.doi.org/10.1037/0882-7974.8.2.283

Kennedy, K. M., & Raz, N. (2005). Age, sex and regional brain volumes predict perceptual-motor skill acquisition. *Cortex, 41,* 560–569. http://dx.doi.org/10.1016/S0010-9452(08)70196-5

Kim, S. Y., & Giovanello, K. S. (2011). The effects of attention on age-related relational memory deficits: fMRI evidence from a novel attentional manipulation. *Journal of Cognitive Neuroscience, 23,* 3637–3656. http://dx.doi.org/10.1162/jocn_a_00058

King, B. R., Fogel, S. M., Albouy, G., & Doyon, J. (2013). Neural correlates of the age-related changes in motor sequence learning and motor adaptation in older adults. *Frontiers in Human Neuroscience, 7,* 142. http://dx.doi.org/10.3389/fnhum.2013.00142

Knowlton, B. J., Mangels, J. A., & Squire, L. R. (1996). A neostriatal habit learning system in humans. *Science, 273,* 1399–1402. http://dx.doi.org/10.1126/science.273.5280.1399

Knuttinen, M. G., Power, J. M., Preston, A. R., & Disterhoft, J. F. (2001). Awareness in classical differential eyeblink conditioning in young and aging humans. *Behavioral Neuroscience, 115,* 747–757. http://dx.doi.org/10.1037/0735-7044.115.4.747

LaBar, K. S., Cook, C. A., Torpey, D. C., & Welsh-Bohmer, K. A. (2004). Impact of healthy aging on awareness and fear conditioning. *Behavioral Neuroscience, 118,* 905–915. http://dx.doi.org/10.1037/0735-7044.118.5.905

LaBar, K. S., LeDoux, J. E., Spencer, D. D., & Phelps, E. A. (1995). Impaired fear conditioning following unilateral temporal lobectomy in humans. *The Journal of Neuroscience, 15,* 6846–6855. http://dx.doi.org/10.1523/JNEUROSCI.15-10-06846.1995

La Voie, D., & Light, L. L. (1994). Adult age differences in repetition priming: A meta-analysis. *Psychology and Aging, 9,* 539–553. http://dx.doi.org/10.1037/0882-7974.9.4.539

LeDoux, J. E. (2014). Coming to terms with fear. *Proceedings of the National Academy of Sciences of the United States of America, 111,* 2871–2878. http://dx.doi.org/10.1073/pnas.1400335111

Lee, S. W., Shimojo, S., & O'Doherty, J. P. (2014). Neural computations underlying arbitration between model-based and model-free learning. *Neuron, 81,* 687–699. http://dx.doi.org/10.1016/j.neuron.2013.11.028

Li, S. C., Lindenberger, U., & Sikström, S. (2001). Aging cognition: From neuromodulation to representation. *Trends in Cognitive Sciences, 5,* 479–486. http://dx.doi.org/10.1016/S1364-6613(00)01769-1

Light, L. L., Prull, M. W., LaVoie, D. J., & Healy, M. R. (2000). Dual-process theories of memory in old age. In T. J. Perfect & E. A. Maylor (Eds.), *Models of cognitive aging* (pp. 238–300). New York, NY: Oxford University Press.

Lighthall, N. R., Gorlick, M. A., Schoeke, A., Frank, M. J., & Mather, M. (2013). Stress modulates reinforcement learning in younger and older adults. *Psychology and Aging, 28,* 35–46. http://dx.doi.org/10.1037/a0029823

Lighthall, N. R., Pearson, J. M., Huettel, S. A., & Cabeza, R. (2018). Feedback-based learning in aging: Contributions and trajectories of change in striatal and hippocampal systems. *The Journal of Neuroscience, 38,* 8453–8462. http://dx.doi.org/10.1523/JNEUROSCI.0769-18.2018

Lindenberger, U., & Baltes, P. B. (1994). Sensory functioning and intelligence in old age: A strong connection. *Psychology and Aging, 9,* 339–355. http://dx.doi.org/10.1037/0882-7974.9.3.339

Little, D. M., Prentice, K. J., & Wingfield, A. (2004). Adult age differences in judgments of semantic fit. *Applied Psycholinguistics, 25,* 135–143. http://dx.doi.org/10.1017/S0142716404001079

Lustig, C., & Flegal, K. (2008). Age differences in memory: Demands on cognitive control and association processes. *Advances in Psychology, 139,* 137–149. http://dx.doi.org/10.1016/S0166-4115(08)10012-7

Lyle, K. B., Bloise, S. M., & Johnson, M. K. (2006). Age-related binding deficits and the content of false memories. *Psychology and Aging, 21,* 86–95. http://dx.doi.org/10.1037/0882-7974.21.1.86

MacKay, A. I., Connor, L. T., Albert, M. L., & Obler, L. K. (2002). Noun and verb retrieval in healthy aging. *Journal of the International Neuropsychological Society, 8,* 764–770. http://dx.doi.org/10.1017/S1355617702860040

Madden, D. J., Pierce, T. W., & Allen, P. A. (1993). Age-related slowing and the time course of semantic priming in visual word identification. *Psychology and Aging, 8,* 490–507. http://dx.doi.org/10.1037/0882-7974.8.4.490

Maillet, D., & Rajah, M. N. (2013). Association between prefrontal activity and volume change in prefrontal and medial temporal lobes in aging and dementia: A review. *Ageing Research Reviews, 12*, 479–489. http://dx.doi.org/10.1016/j.arr.2012.11.001

Maillet, D., & Rajah, M. N. (2014). Age-related differences in brain activity in the subsequent memory paradigm: A meta-analysis. *Neuroscience and Biobehavioral Reviews, 45*, 246–257. http://dx.doi.org/10.1016/j.neubiorev.2014.06.006

Mariën, P., Mampaey, E., Vervaet, A., Saerens, J., & De Deyn, P. P. (1998). Normative data for the Boston naming test in native Dutch-speaking Belgian elderly. *Brain and Language, 65*, 447–467. http://dx.doi.org/10.1006/brln.1998.2000

Mata, R., Josef, A. K., Samanez-Larkin, G. R., & Hertwig, R. (2011). Age differences in risky choice: A meta-analysis. *Annals of the New York Academy of Sciences, 1235*, 18–29. http://dx.doi.org/10.1111/j.1749-6632.2011.06200.x

Meinzer, M., Flaisch, T., Wilser, L., Eulitz, C., Rockstroh, B., Conway, T., . . . Crosson, B. (2009). Neural signatures of semantic and phonemic fluency in young and old adults. *Journal of Cognitive Neuroscience, 21*, 2007–2018. http://dx.doi.org/10.1162/jocn.2009.21219

Mell, T., Heekeren, H. R., Marschner, A., Wartenburger, I., Villringer, A., & Reischies, F. M. (2005). Effect of aging on stimulus-reward association learning. *Neuropsychologia, 43*, 554–563. http://dx.doi.org/10.1016/j.neuropsychologia.2004.07.010

Miller, E. K., & Cohen, J. D. (2001). An integrative theory of prefrontal cortex function. *Annual Review of Neuroscience, 24*, 167–202. http://dx.doi.org/10.1146/annurev.neuro.24.1.167

Mitchell, K. J., Johnson, M. K., Raye, C. L., & D'Esposito, M. (2000). fMRI evidence of age-related hippocampal dysfunction in feature binding in working memory. *Cognitive Brain Research, 10*, 197–206. http://dx.doi.org/10.1016/S0926-6410(00)00029-X

Morcom, A. M., Li, J., & Rugg, M. D. (2007). Age effects on the neural correlates of episodic retrieval: Increased cortical recruitment with matched performance. *Cerebral Cortex, 17*, 2491–2506. http://dx.doi.org/10.1093/cercor/bhl155

Morris, J. S., DeGelder, B., Weiskrantz, L., & Dolan, R. J. (2001). Differential extrageniculostriate and amygdala responses to presentation of emotional faces in a cortically blind field. *Brain, 124*, 1241–1252. http://dx.doi.org/10.1093/brain/124.6.1241

Mortensen, L., Meyer, A. S., & Humphreys, G. W. (2006). Age-related effects on speech production: A review. *Language and Cognitive Processes, 21*, 238–290. http://dx.doi.org/10.1080/01690960444000278

Moscarello, J. M., & LeDoux, J. E. (2013). Active avoidance learning requires prefrontal suppression of amygdala-mediated defensive reactions. *The Journal of Neuroscience, 33*, 3815–3823. http://dx.doi.org/10.1523/JNEUROSCI.2596-12.2013

Moscovitch, M. (1992). Memory and working-with-memory: A component process model based on modules and central systems. *Journal of Cognitive Neuroscience, 4*, 257–267. http://dx.doi.org/10.1162/jocn.1992.4.3.257

Moscovitch, M., & Winocur, G. (1995). Frontal lobes, memory, and aging. In J. Grafman, K. J. Holyoak, & F. Boller (Eds.), *Structure and functions of the human prefrontal cortex* (pp. 119–150). New York, NY: New York Academy of Sciences.

Moss, H. E., Abdallah, S., Fletcher, P., Bright, P., Pilgrim, L., Acres, K., & Tyler, L. K. (2005). Selecting among competing alternatives: Selection and retrieval in the left inferior frontal gyrus. *Cerebral Cortex, 15,* 1723–1735. http://dx.doi.org/10.1093/cercor/bhi049

Naveh-Benjamin, M. (2000). Adult age differences in memory performance: Tests of an associative deficit hypothesis. *Journal of Experimental Psychology: Learning, Memory, and Cognition, 26,* 1170–1187. http://dx.doi.org/10.1037/0278-7393.26.5.1170

Naveh-Benjamin, M., Shing, Y. L., Kilb, A., Werkle-Bergner, M., Lindenberger, U., & Li, S. C. (2009). Adult age differences in memory for name-face associations: The effects of intentional and incidental learning. *Memory, 17,* 220–232. http://dx.doi.org/10.1080/09658210802222183

Neumann, Y., Obler, L. K., Gomes, H., & Shafer, V. (2009). Phonological vs sensory contributions to age effects in naming: An electrophysiological study. *Aphasiology, 23*(7–8), 1028–1039. http://dx.doi.org/10.1080/02687030802661630

Nilsson, L. G. (2003). Memory function in normal aging. *Acta Neurologica Scandinavica, 179,* 7–13. http://dx.doi.org/10.1034/j.1600-0404.107.s179.5.x

Niv, Y. (2009). Reinforcement learning in the brain. *Journal of Mathematical Psychology, 53,* 139–154. http://dx.doi.org/10.1016/j.jmp.2008.12.005

Norman, D. A., & Shallice, T. (1986). Attention to action: Willed and automatic control of behavior. In R. J. Davidson, G. E. Schwartz, & D. Shapiro (Eds.), *Consciousness and self-regulation: Advances in research and theory* (pp. 1–18). New York, NY: Plenum. http://dx.doi.org/10.1007/978-1-4757-0629-1_1

Nyberg, L., McIntosh, A. R., Houle, S., Nilsson, L. G., & Tulving, E. (1996). Activation of medial temporal structures during episodic memory retrieval. *Nature, 380,* 715–717. http://dx.doi.org/10.1038/380715a0

Packard, M. G., Hirsh, R., & White, N. M. (1989). Differential effects of fornix and caudate nucleus lesions on two radial maze tasks: Evidence for multiple memory systems. *The Journal of Neuroscience, 9,* 1465–1472. http://dx.doi.org/10.1523/JNEUROSCI.09-05-01465.1989

Park, D. C., Polk, T. A., Park, R., Minear, M., Savage, A., & Smith, M. R. (2004). Aging reduces neural specialization in ventral visual cortex. *Proceedings of the National Academy of Sciences of the United States of America, 101,* 13091–13095. http://dx.doi.org/10.1073/pnas.0405148101

Park, D. C., & Reuter-Lorenz, P. (2009). The adaptive brain: Aging and neurocognitive scaffolding. *Annual Review of Psychology, 60,* 173–196. http://dx.doi.org/10.1146/annurev.psych.59.103006.093656

Peelle, J. E., Troiani, V., Wingfield, A., & Grossman, M. (2010). Neural processing during older adults' comprehension of spoken sentences: Age differences in resource allocation and connectivity. *Cerebral Cortex, 20,* 773–782. http://dx.doi.org/10.1093/cercor/bhp142

Persson, J., Kalpouzos, G., Nilsson, L. G., Ryberg, M., & Nyberg, L. (2011). Preserved hippocampus activation in normal aging as revealed by fMRI. *Hippocampus, 21,* 753–766. http://dx.doi.org/10.1002/hipo.20794

Persson, J., Nyberg, L., Lind, J., Larsson, A., Nilsson, L. G., Ingvar, M., & Buckner, R. L. (2006). Structure-function correlates of cognitive decline in aging. *Cerebral Cortex, 16,* 907–915. http://dx.doi.org/10.1093/cercor/bhj036

Pfefferbaum, A., Sullivan, E. V., Rosenbloom, M. J., Mathalon, D. H., & Lim, K. O. (1998). A controlled study of cortical gray matter and ventricular changes in alcoholic men over a 5-year interval. *Archives of General Psychiatry, 55,* 905–912. http://dx.doi.org/10.1001/archpsyc.55.10.905

Pietschmann, M., Endrass, T., Czerwon, B., & Kathmann, N. (2011). Aging, probabilistic learning and performance monitoring. *Biological Psychology, 86,* 74–82. http://dx.doi.org/10.1016/j.biopsycho.2010.10.009

Poldrack, R. A., Clark, J., Paré-Blagoev, E. J., Shohamy, D., Creso Moyano, J., Myers, C., & Gluck, M. A. (2001). Interactive memory systems in the human brain. *Nature, 414,* 546–550. http://dx.doi.org/10.1038/35107080

Poldrack, R. A., Wagner, A. D., Prull, M. W., Desmond, J. E., Glover, G. H., & Gabrieli, J. D. E. (1999). Functional specialization for semantic and phonological processing in the left inferior prefrontal cortex. *NeuroImage, 10,* 15–35. http://dx.doi.org/10.1006/nimg.1999.0441

Raz, N., Ghisletta, P., Rodrigue, K. M., Kennedy, K. M., & Lindenberger, U. (2010). Trajectories of brain aging in middle-aged and older adults: Regional and individual differences. *NeuroImage, 51,* 501–511. http://dx.doi.org/10.1016/j.neuroimage.2010.03.020

Raz, N., Gunning-Dixon, F. M., Head, D., Dupuis, J. H., McQuain, J., Briggs, S. D., . . . Acker, J. D. (1997). Selective aging of the human cerebral cortex observed in vivo: Differential vulnerability of the prefrontal gray matter. *Cerebral Cortex, 7,* 268–282.

Raz, N., Lindenberger, U., Rodrigue, K. M., Kennedy, K. M., Head, D., Williamson, A., . . . Acker, J. D. (2005). Regional brain changes in aging healthy adults: General trends, individual differences and modifiers. *Cerebral Cortex, 15,* 1676–1689. http://dx.doi.org/10.1093/cercor/bhi044

Ren, J., Wu, Y. D., Chan, J. S., & Yan, J. H. (2013). Cognitive aging affects motor performance and learning. *Geriatrics & Gerontology International, 13,* 19–27. http://dx.doi.org/10.1111/j.1447-0594.2012.00914.x

Resnick, S. M., Pham, D. L., Kraut, M. A., Zonderman, A. B., & Davatzikos, C. (2003). Longitudinal magnetic resonance imaging studies of older adults: A shrinking brain. *The Journal of Neuroscience, 23,* 3295–3301. http://dx.doi.org/10.1523/JNEUROSCI.23-08-03295.2003

Rieckmann, A., Fischer, H., & Bäckman, L. (2010). Activation in striatum and medial temporal lobe during sequence learning in younger and older adults:

Relations to performance. *NeuroImage, 50,* 1303–1312. http://dx.doi.org/10.1016/j.neuroimage.2010.01.015

Rodrigue, K. M., Kennedy, K. M., & Raz, N. (2005). Aging and longitudinal change in perceptual-motor skill acquisition in healthy adults. *The Journals of Gerontology: Series B. Psychological Sciences and Social Sciences, 60,* 174–181. http://dx.doi.org/10.1093/geronb/60.4.P174

Rodrigue, K. M., & Raz, N. (2004). Shrinkage of the entorhinal cortex over five years predicts memory performance in healthy adults. *The Journal of Neuroscience, 24,* 956–963. http://dx.doi.org/10.1523/JNEUROSCI.4166-03.2004

Roediger, H. L., & McDermott, K. B. (1993). Implicit memory in normal human subjects. In H. Spinnler & F. Boller (Eds.), *Handbook of neuropsychology* (pp. 63–131). Amsterdam, Netherlands: Elsevier.

Rönnlund, M., Nyberg, L., Bäckman, L., & Nilsson, L. G. (2005). Stability, growth, and decline in adult life span development of declarative memory: Cross-sectional and longitudinal data from a population-based study. *Psychology and Aging, 20,* 3–18. http://dx.doi.org/10.1037/0882-7974.20.1.3

Ryan, J. D., Leung, G., Turk-Browne, N. B., & Hasher, L. (2007). Assessment of age-related changes in inhibition and binding using eye movement monitoring. *Psychology and Aging, 22,* 239–250. http://dx.doi.org/10.1037/0882-7974.22.2.239

Salthouse, T. A. (1996). The processing-speed theory of adult age differences in cognition. *Psychological Review, 103,* 403–428. http://dx.doi.org/10.1037/0033-295X.103.3.403

Samanez-Larkin, G. R., Gibbs, S. E., Khanna, K., Nielsen, L., Carstensen, L. L., & Knutson, B. (2007). Anticipation of monetary gain but not loss in healthy older adults. *Nature Neuroscience, 10,* 787–791. http://dx.doi.org/10.1038/nn1894

Samanez-Larkin, G. R., & Knutson, B. (2015). Decision making in the ageing brain: Changes in affective and motivational circuits. *Nature Reviews Neuroscience, 16,* 278–289. http://dx.doi.org/10.1038/nrn3917

Samanez-Larkin, G. R., Levens, S. M., Perry, L. M., Dougherty, R. F., & Knutson, B. (2012). Frontostriatal white matter integrity mediates adult age differences in probabilistic reward learning. *The Journal of Neuroscience, 32,* 5333–5337. http://dx.doi.org/10.1523/JNEUROSCI.5756-11.2012

Samanez-Larkin, G. R., Worthy, D. A., Mata, R., McClure, S. M., & Knutson, B. (2014). Adult age differences in frontostriatal representation of prediction error but not reward outcome. *Cognitive, Affective & Behavioral Neuroscience, 14,* 672–682. http://dx.doi.org/10.3758/s13415-014-0297-4

Schacter, D. L., Wig, G. S., & Stevens, W. D. (2007). Reductions in cortical activity during priming. *Current Opinion in Neurobiology, 17,* 171–176. http://dx.doi.org/10.1016/j.conb.2007.02.001

Schnur, T. T., Schwartz, M. F., Kimberg, D. Y., Hirshorn, E., Coslett, H. B., & Thompson-Schill, S. L. (2009). Localizing interference during naming: Convergent neuroimaging and neuropsychological evidence for the function of

Broca's area. *Proceedings of the National Academy of Sciences of the United States of America, 106*, 322–327. http://dx.doi.org/10.1073/pnas.0805874106

Schott, B. H., Niehaus, L., Wittmann, B. C., Schütze, H., Seidenbecher, C. I., Heinze, H. J., & Düzel, E. (2007). Ageing and early-stage Parkinson's disease affect separable neural mechanisms of mesolimbic reward processing. *Brain, 130*, 2412–2424. http://dx.doi.org/10.1093/brain/awm147

Schultz, W. (2000). Multiple reward signals in the brain. *Nature Reviews Neuroscience, 1*, 199–207. http://dx.doi.org/10.1038/35044563

Schultz, W. (2013). Updating dopamine reward signals. *Current Opinion in Neurobiology, 23*, 229–238. http://dx.doi.org/10.1016/j.conb.2012.11.012

Schultz, W. (2017). Reward prediction error. *Current Biology, 27*, R369–R371. http://dx.doi.org/10.1016/j.cub.2017.02.064

Schultz, W., Dayan, P., & Montague, P. R. (1997). A neural substrate of prediction and reward. *Science, 275*, 1593–1599. http://dx.doi.org/10.1126/science.275.5306.1593

Schwartz, S., Maquet, P., & Frith, C. (2002). Neural correlates of perceptual learning: A functional MRI study of visual texture discrimination [erratum at http://dx.doi.org/10.1073/pnas.1030820100]. *Proceedings of the National Academy of Sciences of the United States of America, 99*, 17137–17142. http://dx.doi.org/10.1073/pnas.242414599

Sebastián, M., & Ballesteros, S. (2012). Effects of normal aging on event-related potentials and oscillatory brain activity during a haptic repetition priming task. *NeuroImage, 60*, 7–20. http://dx.doi.org/10.1016/j.neuroimage.2011.11.060

Severson, J. A., Marcusson, J., Winblad, B., & Finch, C. E. (1982). Age-correlated loss of dopaminergic binding sites in human basal ganglia. *Journal of Neurochemistry, 39*, 1623–1631. http://dx.doi.org/10.1111/j.1471-4159.1982.tb07996.x

Shohamy, D., & Wagner, A. D. (2008). Integrating memories in the human brain: Hippocampal-midbrain encoding of overlapping events. *Neuron, 60*, 378–389. http://dx.doi.org/10.1016/j.neuron.2008.09.023

Smith, A. D., Park, D. C., Earles, J. L. K., Shaw, R. J., & Whiting, W. L., IV. (1998). Age differences in context integration in memory. *Psychology and Aging, 13*, 21–28. http://dx.doi.org/10.1037/0882-7974.13.1.21

Smith, K. S., & Graybiel, A. M. (2013). A dual operator view of habitual behavior reflecting cortical and striatal dynamics [erratum at http://dx.doi.org/10.1016/j.neuron.2013.07.032]. *Neuron, 79*, 361–374. http://dx.doi.org/10.1016/j.neuron.2013.05.038

Solomon, P. R., Pomerleau, D., Bennett, L., James, J., & Morse, D. L. (1989). Acquisition of the classically conditioned eyeblink response in humans over the life span. *Psychology and Aging, 4*, 34–41. http://dx.doi.org/10.1037/0882-7974.4.1.34

Spencer, R. M., Gouw, A. M., & Ivry, R. B. (2007). Age-related decline of sleep-dependent consolidation. *Learning & Memory, 14*, 480–484. http://dx.doi.org/10.1101/lm.569407

Spencer, W. D., & Raz, N. (1995). Differential effects of aging on memory for content and context: A meta-analysis. *Psychology and Aging, 10*, 527–539. http://dx.doi.org/10.1037/0882-7974.10.4.527

Squire, L. R. (2004). Memory systems of the brain: A brief history and current perspective. *Neurobiology of Learning and Memory, 82*, 171–177. http://dx.doi.org/10.1016/j.nlm.2004.06.005

Squire, L. R. (2009). Memory and brain systems: 1969–2009. *The Journal of Neuroscience, 29*, 12711–12716. http://dx.doi.org/10.1523/JNEUROSCI.3575-09.2009

Squire, L. R., & Dede, A. J. O. (2015). Conscious and unconscious memory systems. *Cold Spring Harbor Perspectives in Biology, 7*, a021667. http://dx.doi.org/10.1101/cshperspect.a021667

Squire, L. R., & Zola-Morgan, S. (1991). The medial temporal lobe memory system. *Science, 253*, 1380–1386. http://dx.doi.org/10.1126/science.1896849

Sutton, R. S., & Barto, A. G. (1998). *Reinforcement learning: An introduction.* Cambridge, MA: The MIT Press.

Thompson, R. F., & Steinmetz, J. E. (2009). The role of the cerebellum in classical conditioning of discrete behavioral responses. *Neuroscience, 162*, 732–755. http://dx.doi.org/10.1016/j.neuroscience.2009.01.041

Thompson-Schill, S. L., Bedny, M., & Goldberg, R. F. (2005). The frontal lobes and the regulation of mental activity. *Current Opinion in Neurobiology, 15*, 219–224. http://dx.doi.org/10.1016/j.conb.2005.03.006

Thompson-Schill, S. L., D'Esposito, M., Aguirre, G. K., & Farah, M. J. (1997). Role of left inferior prefrontal cortex in retrieval of semantic knowledge: A reevaluation. *Proceedings of the National Academy of Sciences of the United States of America, 94*, 14792–14797. http://dx.doi.org/10.1073/pnas.94.26.14792

Thorndike, E. L. (1911). *Animal intelligence: Experimental studies.* New York, NY: Macmillan. http://dx.doi.org/10.5962/bhl.title.55072

Thürling, M., Galuba, J., Thieme, A., Burciu, R. G., Göricke, S., Beck, A., . . . Timmann, D. (2014). Age effects in storage and extinction of a naturally acquired conditioned eyeblink response. *Neurobiology of Learning and Memory, 109*, 104–112. http://dx.doi.org/10.1016/j.nlm.2013.12.007

Thürling, M., Kahl, F., Maderwald, S., Stefanescu, R. M., Schlamann, M., Boele, H. J., . . . Timmann, D. (2015). Cerebellar cortex and cerebellar nuclei are concomitantly activated during eyeblink conditioning: A 7T fMRI study in humans. *The Journal of Neuroscience, 35*, 1228–1239. http://dx.doi.org/10.1523/JNEUROSCI.2492-14.2015

Tsukiura, T., & Cabeza, R. (2008). Orbitofrontal and hippocampal contributions to memory for face-name associations: The rewarding power of a smile. *Neuropsychologia, 46*, 2310–2319. http://dx.doi.org/10.1016/j.neuropsychologia.2008.03.013

Tulving, E. (1983). *Elements of episodic memory.* Oxford, England: Oxford University Press.

Tyler, L. K., Marslen-Wilson, W. D., Randall, B., Wright, P., Devereux, B. J., Zhuang, J., . . . Stamatakis, E. A. (2011). Left inferior frontal cortex and syntax: Function, structure and behaviour in patients with left hemisphere damage. *Brain*, *134*, 415–431. http://dx.doi.org/10.1093/brain/awq369

Tyler, L. K., Shafto, M. A., Randall, B., Wright, P., Marslen-Wilson, W. D., & Stamatakis, E. A. (2010). Preserving syntactic processing across the adult life span: The modulation of the frontotemporal language system in the context of age-related atrophy. *Cerebral Cortex*, *20*, 352–364. http://dx.doi.org/10.1093/cercor/bhp105

van de Vijver, I., Ridderinkhof, K. R., & de Wit, S. (2015). Age-related changes in deterministic learning from positive versus negative performance feedback. *Aging, Neuropsychology and Cognition*, *22*, 595–619. http://dx.doi.org/10.1080/13825585.2015.1020917

van Halteren-van Tilborg, I. A., Scherder, E. J., & Hulstijn, W. (2007). Motor-skill learning in Alzheimer's disease: A review with an eye to the clinical practice. *Neuropsychology Review*, *17*, 203–212. http://dx.doi.org/10.1007/s11065-007-9030-1

Verhaegen, C., & Poncelet, M. (2013). Changes in naming and semantic abilities with aging from 50 to 90 years. *Journal of the International Neuropsychological Society*, *19*, 119–126. http://dx.doi.org/10.1017/S1355617712001178

Verhaeghen, P. (2003). Aging and vocabulary scores: A meta-analysis. *Psychology and Aging*, *18*, 332–339. http://dx.doi.org/10.1037/0882-7974.18.2.332

Voelcker-Rehage, C. (2008). Motor-skill learning in older adults: A review of studies on age-related differences. *European Review of Aging and Physical Activity*, *5*, 5–16. http://dx.doi.org/10.1007/s11556-008-0030-9

Wagner, A. D., Schacter, D. L., Rotte, M., Koutstaal, W., Maril, A., Dale, A. M., . . . Buckner, R. L. (1998). Building memories: Remembering and forgetting of verbal experiences as predicted by brain activity. *Science*, *281*, 1188–1191. http://dx.doi.org/10.1126/science.281.5380.1188

Wais, P. E., Squire, L. R., & Wixted, J. T. (2010). In search of recollection and familiarity signals in the hippocampus. *Journal of Cognitive Neuroscience*, *22*, 109–123. http://dx.doi.org/10.1162/jocn.2009.21190

Walhovd, K. B., Westlye, L. T., Amlien, I., Espeseth, T., Reinvang, I., Raz, N., . . . Fjell, A. M. (2011). Consistent neuroanatomical age-related volume differences across multiple samples. *Neurobiology of Aging*, *32*, 916–932. http://dx.doi.org/10.1016/j.neurobiolaging.2009.05.013

Ward, E. V., Berry, C. J., & Shanks, D. R. (2013). Age effects on explicit and implicit memory. *Frontiers in Psychology*, *4*, 639. http://dx.doi.org/10.3389/fpsyg.2013.00639

Weiler, J. A., Bellebaum, C., & Daum, I. (2008). Aging affects acquisition and reversal of reward-based associative learning. *Learning & Memory*, *15*, 190–197. http://dx.doi.org/10.1101/lm.890408

West, R. L. (1996). An application of prefrontal cortex function theory to cognitive aging. *Psychological Bulletin, 120,* 272–292. http://dx.doi.org/10.1037/0033-2909.120.2.272

Wierenga, C. E., Benjamin, M., Gopinath, K., Perlstein, W. M., Leonard, C. M., Rothi, L. J., . . . Crosson, B. (2008). Age-related changes in word retrieval: Role of bilateral frontal and subcortical networks. *Neurobiology of Aging, 29,* 436–451. http://dx.doi.org/10.1016/j.neurobiolaging.2006.10.024

Wiggs, C. L., & Martin, A. (1998). Properties and mechanisms of perceptual priming. *Current Opinion in Neurobiology, 8,* 227–233. http://dx.doi.org/10.1016/S0959-4388(98)80144-X

Willingham, D. B., & Goedert-Eschmann, K. (1999). The relation between implicit and explicit learning: Evidence for parallel development. *Psychological Science, 10,* 531–534. http://dx.doi.org/10.1111/1467-9280.00201

Willingham, D. B., Salidis, J., & Gabrieli, J. D. (2002). Direct comparison of neural systems mediating conscious and unconscious skill learning. *Journal of Neurophysiology, 88,* 1451–1460. http://dx.doi.org/10.1152/jn.2002.88.3.1451

Wilson, J. K., Baran, B., Pace-Schott, E. F., Ivry, R. B., & Spencer, R. M. (2012). Sleep modulates word-pair learning but not motor sequence learning in healthy older adults. *Neurobiology of Aging, 33,* 991–1000. http://dx.doi.org/10.1016/j.neurobiolaging.2011.06.029

Wimmer, G. E., Braun, E. K., Daw, N. D., & Shohamy, D. (2014). Episodic memory encoding interferes with reward learning and decreases striatal prediction errors. *The Journal of Neuroscience, 34,* 14901–14912. http://dx.doi.org/10.1523/JNEUROSCI.0204-14.2014

Wong, D. F., Wagner, H. N., Jr., Dannals, R. F., Links, J. M., Frost, J. J., Ravert, H. T., . . . Kuhar, M. J. (1984). Effects of age on dopamine and serotonin receptors measured by positron tomography in the living human brain. *Science, 226,* 1393–1396. http://dx.doi.org/10.1126/science.6334363

Wood, S., Busemeyer, J., Koling, A., Cox, C. R., & Davis, H. (2005). Older adults as adaptive decision makers: Evidence from the Iowa Gambling Task. *Psychology and Aging, 20,* 220–225. http://dx.doi.org/10.1037/0882-7974.20.2.220

Woodruff-Pak, D. S., Goldenberg, G., Downey-Lamb, M. M., Boyko, O. B., & Lemieux, S. K. (2000). Cerebellar volume in humans related to magnitude of classical conditioning. *NeuroReport, 11,* 609–615. http://dx.doi.org/10.1097/00001756-200002280-00035

Yin, H. H., Mulcare, S. P., Hilário, M. R., Clouse, E., Holloway, T., Davis, M. I., . . . Costa, R. M. (2009). Dynamic reorganization of striatal circuits during the acquisition and consolidation of a skill. *Nature Neuroscience, 12,* 333–341. http://dx.doi.org/10.1038/nn.2261

Yonelinas, A. P. (2002). The nature of recollection and familiarity: A review of 30 years of research. *Journal of Memory and Language, 46,* 441–517. http://dx.doi.org/10.1006/jmla.2002.2864

Yonelinas, A. P., Widaman, K., Mungas, D., Reed, B., Weiner, M. W., & Chui, H. C. (2007). Memory in the aging brain: Doubly dissociating the contribution of the hippocampus and entorhinal cortex. *Hippocampus, 17,* 1134–1140. http://dx.doi.org/10.1002/hipo.20341

Zhuang, J., Johnson, M. A., Madden, D. J., Burke, D. M., & Diaz, M. T. (2016). Age-related differences in resolving semantic and phonological competition during receptive language tasks. *Neuropsychologia, 93,* 189–199. http://dx.doi.org/10.1016/j.neuropsychologia.2016.10.016

4

AGE-RELATED CHANGES IN EPISODIC MEMORY

AUDREY DUARTE AND ELIZABETH KENSINGER

Memory changes are common in aging, even for older adults unaffected by dementia. Memory impairments are most notable within *episodic memory*, which is the ability to consciously encode and retrieve details and associations that allow us to distinguish one event from another. We discuss the neural factors that contribute to older adults' memory impairments in the first section. We then describe how these factors explain the relative preservation of older adults' emotional memories. In the third section, we discuss recent methods that should provide new insights into age-related memory changes. We conclude by noting the memory benefits to be gained by staying mentally and physically active in old age. Figure 4.1 depicts our conceptualization of age-related changes in episodic memory.

http://dx.doi.org/10.1037/0000143-005
The Aging Brain: Functional Adaptation Across Adulthood, G. R. Samanez-Larkin (Editor)

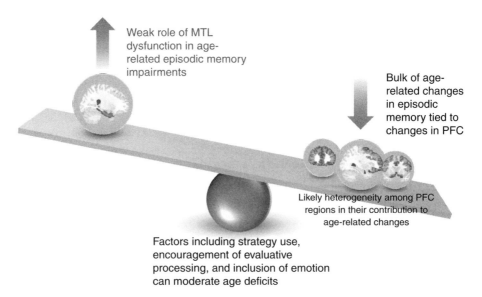

Weak role of MTL dysfunction in age-related episodic memory impairments

Bulk of age-related changes in episodic memory tied to changes in PFC

Likely heterogeneity among PFC regions in their contribution to age-related changes

Factors including strategy use, encouragement of evaluative processing, and inclusion of emotion can moderate age deficits

Figure 4.1. Factors including strategy use, encouragement of evaluative processing, and inclusion of emotion can moderate age deficits.

NEUROCOGNITIVE CONTRIBUTIONS TO OLDER ADULTS' MEMORY IMPAIRMENTS

In the laboratory, age-related impairments are most frequently noted on tasks that require older adults to recall specific details of past events or to remember the context in which information was learned. Age-related differences can be minimal on tasks that require only distinguishing events that were experienced from those that are novel, whereas age differences become exaggerated on tasks that require recollection of event details, recounting of contextual elements (Henkel, Johnson, & De Leonardis, 1998), binding of associative detail (Naveh-Benjamin, 2000), or selection of an experienced event among similar lures (Schacter, Koutstaal, & Norman, 1997). Age-related episodic memory impairments have been shown for virtually every stimulus modality and testing procedure. For example, older adults show impairments in source memory tests in which participants are asked to determine which experimentally manipulated details were associated with an item during encoding (e.g., spatial location, color, voice) and in paired associative tests when participants must encode and retrieve stimulus pairs (e.g., face–name, word–word). One exception seems to be episodic memory for emotional or social information, as discussed later in this chapter and in Chapter 6. Nonetheless, given the fairly ubiquitous nature of these impairments, it is likely that they may be explained by age-related changes in brain regions that support episodic memory in a domain-general manner. Numerous structural and functional imaging studies have investigated the underlying neural factors that contribute to older adults' episodic memory impairments. Most studies have focused on the medial temporal lobe (MTL) and the prefrontal cortex (PFC). In this section, we weigh evidence for the contributions of dysfunction in these regions to age-related memory impairments.

Weak Contribution of Core Episodic Network Dysfunction to Older Adults' Episodic Memory Impairments

Evidence from numerous functional magnetic imaging (fMRI) studies has revealed that episodic memory success is dependent on several regions, including the MTL (hippocampus and parahippocampus) and the highly interconnected posterior parietal cortex (Davachi, Mitchell, & Wagner, 2003; Diana, Yonelinas, & Ranganath, 2007; Mitchell & Johnson, 2009; Uncapher & Wagner, 2009; Vilberg & Rugg, 2008). Furthermore, patient studies suggest that these *core episodic network* regions are necessary for episodic memory function with MTL or parietal damage producing amnesia (reviewed in Benoit & Schacter, 2015; Berryhill, Phuong, Picasso, Cabeza, & Olson, 2007; Milner, 2005). Several theories have been proposed to explain the functional role of this network in episodic memory. A common view is that the MTL facilitates the binding of multiple features into unique episodic representations during encoding and in the comparison of those representations with retrieval cues during retrieval (Eichenbaum, Yonelinas, & Ranganath, 2007; Sestieri, Shulman, & Corbetta, 2017; Simons & Spiers, 2003). Regions within the posterior parietal cortex serve a less direct role in memory such as accumulating mnemonic evidence for memory decisions (i.e., male or female voice? intact or rearranged pair?; Wagner, Shannon, Kahn, & Buckner, 2005). Consequently, a reasonable prediction is that dysfunction in this network is a major contributor to episodic memory impairments in healthy older adults. Indeed, functional imaging studies have shown age-related differences, primarily under-recruitment of these regions concomitant with older adults' memory impairments (Cansino, Trejo-Morales, et al., 2015; Dennis, Kim, & Cabeza, 2008).

A few points of evidence argue against the role of MTL dysfunction in age-related episodic memory impairments. First, MTL atrophy is not pronounced until the eighth or ninth decade in healthy older adults but the majority of episodic memory studies have assessed older adults between the ages of 60 and 80 (Salami, Eriksson, & Nyberg, 2012). Furthermore, numerous studies have shown age-related sparing of successful encoding and retrieval-related activity in the MTL and parietal cortex (Duarte, Henson, & Graham, 2008; Dulas & Duarte, 2012; S. L. Miller et al., 2008; Morcom, Li, & Rugg, 2007), particularly when memory performance is experimentally or statistically equivalent equated between age groups (Angel et al., 2013; de Chastelaine, Mattson, Wang, Donley, & Rugg, 2015; Duarte, Ranganath, Trujillo, & Knight, 2006; Duverne, Motamedinia, & Rugg, 2009b; Rugg & Morcom, 2005; Wang, Johnson, de Chastelaine, Donley, & Rugg, 2016). The idea behind equating performance is that group differences in episodic memory activity may be related to dilution by guessing or poor task comprehension rather than aging per se (Rugg & Morcom, 2005). Some studies have implemented study repetitions (Leshikar & Duarte, 2014; Morcom et al., 2007) or reduced memory load (Dulas & Duarte, 2013, 2014) to boost memory performance for older adults, while others have investigated the relationship between neural activity and age after parceling out individual differences in memory performance (de Chastelaine, Mattson, Wang, Donley, & Rugg, 2016). Collectively, these results suggest that dysfunction in the core episodic network is unlikely to be a major contributor to healthy older adults' episodic memory impairments.

Strong Contribution of Prefrontal Dysfunction to Older Adults' Episodic Memory Impairments

Like the core episodic network, the PFC has been implicated in episodic memory success across a number of material domains and task procedures (Blumenfeld, Parks, Yonelinas, & Ranganath, 2011; Gottlieb, Uncapher, & Rugg, 2010; Mitchell & Johnson, 2009). The PFC supports the cognitive control processes that allow information to be processed and behavior to vary in ways that are consistent with one's current task goals (E. K. Miller & Cohen, 2001). Cognitive control functions are diverse and include evaluation of relationships between stimuli or concepts and monitoring retrieved information (Badre, 2008). Damage to the MTL, and potentially also the posterior parietal cortex, results in profound amnesia, whereas damage to the PFC produces subtler episodic memory deficits (Janowsky, Shimamura, & Squire, 1989; Kopelman, Stanhope, & Kingsley, 1997).

Several factors point to PFC dysfunction as a principal source of episodic memory impairments in aging. First, both healthy older adults (Duarte et al., 2006, 2008) and patients with focal lateral or medial PFC lesions (Ciaramelli & Ghetti, 2007; Duarte, Ranganath, & Knight, 2005) can show intact subjective recollection despite impaired objective recollection of experimentally manipulated details. Second, structural imaging studies show disproportionate declines in PFC gray (Raz & Kennedy, 2009) and white matter volume (Nyberg et al., 2010) compared with non-PFC regions across the lifespan. Furthermore, older adults with larger gray matter volumes in lateral PFC regions show better episodic memory performance (Becker et al., 2015). Third, fMRI studies show age-related reductions in PFC activity during encoding (Dennis, Hayes, et al., 2008; Dulas & Duarte, 2011), and retrieval (Dulas & Duarte, 2012; McDonough & Gallo, 2013; Rajah, Languay, & Valiquette, 2010) despite age-equivalent MTL recruitment. Some neural models predict age-related PFC over-recruitment when cognitive demands are low and underrecruitment when demands are high and performance reduced (Morcom et al., 2007; Reuter-Lorenz & Cappell, 2008). The truth is that both PFC under- and over-recruitment are often observed in the aging literature, and the question of how to interpret these patterns is still under debate (Cabeza et al., 2018). Last, even when memory performance is equated between age groups, PFC activity differences may persist during encoding (de Chastelaine et al., 2015; Dulas & Duarte, 2014) and retrieval (Duarte et al., 2008; Dulas & Duarte, 2014; Wang et al., 2016). Collectively, these findings are consistent with the "frontal aging hypothesis," which posits that PFC dysfunction underlies many cognitive impairments including but not limited to episodic memory in aging (West, 1996). Other influential cognitive aging theories such as the *inhibitory deficit hypothesis* suggest that older adults' cognitive impairments arise from an inability to reduce interference from task-irrelevant information (Hasher & Zacks, 1988). Importantly, this theory is not inconsistent with the frontal aging hypothesis. Indeed, it is probable that PFC dysfunction underlies poor inhibitory control and that episodic memory tests that place high demands on inhibition will be particularly difficult for older adults (Jacoby, Bishara, Hessels, & Toth, 2005).

Factors Moderating the Relationship Between the PFC and Episodic Memory in Aging Studies

Our discussion thus far has assumed that young and older adults recruit the same cognitive operations to support their memory performance. Thus, any group differences in neural activity could not be explained by individual differences in the strategies used to encode or retrieve events. However, it is well known that older adults are less likely than young adults to self-initiate effective encoding strategies when they are simply told to memorize events but not given instructional support (Craik & Byrd, 1982; Hertzog, McGuire, Horhota, & Jopp, 2010; Hultsch, Hertzog, & Dixon, 1990; Logan, Sanders, Snyder, Morris, & Buckner, 2002; Naveh-Benjamin, Brav, & Levy, 2007; Perfect & Dasgupta, 1997). Young adults spontaneously use deep encoding strategies such as semantic elaboration and visual imagery, whereas older adults more often use no strategies or shallow ones such as rote repetition, leading to worse memory performance. Importantly, patterns of neural activity underlying these encoding strategies differ in multiple brain regions, including the PFC (Kirchhoff, Anderson, Barch, & Jacoby, 2012; Kirchhoff & Buckner, 2006; Leshikar, Duarte, & Hertzog, 2012). Differential strategy use can also affect neural activity patterns during episodic memory retrieval

(Dulas & Duarte, 2014). Thus, studies that do not constrain the strategies that participants use during encoding or retrieval may conflate age-related differences in strategy utilization with age-related differences in memory-related activity. Indeed, some evidence suggests that when task instructions facilitate elaborative encoding strategies, age-related memory impairments and PFC underrecruitment are reduced (Gutchess et al., 2015; Leshikar & Duarte, 2014; Logan et al., 2002).

Existing findings support the idea that PFC dysfunction is a major contributor to the increasing number of episodic memory failures experienced across the lifespan. However, the PFC is large and functionally heterogeneous. Lesion and human neuroimaging studies suggest dissociations between cognitive control processes within the PFC between hemispheres and along rostral-caudal and dorsal-ventral gradients (Badre, 2008; Petrides, 2005; Ramnani & Owen, 2004; Simons & Spiers, 2003). For example, in most models of PFC function, posterior areas support control over concrete item or action representations (e.g., "Is this a female face?") while rostral areas support control involving abstract representations or rules (e.g., "Are these two faces alike in the same way as these other two faces?"). Although multiple PFC regions have been implicated in episodic memory through neuroimaging and lesion studies, little work has been done to separate the effects of age on distinct PFC subregions and the control functions they support. Future cognitive aging studies that do so may reveal a more precise role of PFC dysfunction in age-related episodic memory impairments than is currently recognized.

INTERACTIONS BETWEEN EMOTION AND MEMORY

Despite losses in episodic memory for neutral events, older adults' ability to remember emotional events appears to be relatively well preserved. This relative preservation was first revealed when examining memories for highly surprising and personally significant public events, events proposed to trigger "flashbulb memories" (Brown & Kulik, 1977). On the whole, these studies demonstrated that older adults retain the ability to form vivid memories that meet the criteria for "flashbulb memory" (reviewed in Kensinger, Allard, & Krendl, 2014) and suggested that memory deficits can sometimes be mitigated when events are highly emotional (e.g., Kvavilashvili, Mirani, Schlagman, Erskine, & Kornbrot, 2010). Because these highly emotional events differ from more mundane experiences on many factors, extensive laboratory research has been conducted to better delineate the effects of age on emotional memory and to understand their neural underpinnings. In this section, we focus on evidence supporting three conclusions about age-related changes in emotional memory and discuss the proposed mechanisms: First, older adults' memories prioritize internal states (e.g., thoughts and feelings) more than younger adults' memories. Second, older adults often are more likely to remember the good times than the bad times, in contrast to younger adults who often show a "negativity bias" in memory. Third, when asked to remember a negative life experience, older adults are more likely than younger adults to find a silver lining or to focus on positive aspects, and they often remember negative events less vividly.

Older Adults Prioritize Thoughts and Feelings

When we think back to a prior event, we can remember may types of details: We can recall what happened during an event, we can think about the context in which the event unfolded—where, when, and with whom the event took place—and we can also think about our own internal state, or the internal state of others, during the event. With age, there appears to be a shift toward reflection on these internal aspects of an event. Older adults tend to remember the thoughts or feelings elicited by previous experiences better than they remember perceptual or semantic features of an event. For instance, when asked to self-report the features that comprise a memory, older adults give higher ratings for thoughts and feelings than do younger adults (e.g., Hashtroudi, Johnson, & Chrosniak, 1990), and they are more likely than younger adults to state that they "remember" an item from a study list because they recollect their emotional reaction (Comblain, D'Argembeau, Van der Linden, & Aldenhoff, 2004). Similarly, older adults remember proportionally more emotional information from prose passages than do young adults: They are more likely to recall portions of the narrative related to a character's affect ("looked very searchingly at Mrs. Oliver . . ."; Carstensen & Turk-Charles, 1994).

Age differences at both encoding and retrieval may underlie these behavioral effects. As noted in the previous section, older adults do not spontaneously engage highly effective encoding strategies. During event encoding, older adults often expend more resources on evaluative processing than young adults. Although this is not the most effective encoding strategy, it may boost their ability to encode the thoughts and feelings elicited by that event. A meta-analysis comparing young and older adults' neural recruitment during successful episodic memory encoding revealed that, relative to younger adults, older adults under-recruit perceptual regions and over-recruit regions of the *default mode network* typically linked to evaluative processing, including portions of the medial prefrontal cortex. Importantly, while recruitment of these "default" regions is typically associated with failed encoding in younger adults, older adults recruit these regions in the service of successful encoding (see the meta-analysis by Maillet & Rajah, 2014).

At retrieval, older adults may benefit from the fact that emotional and evaluative information may require less effort to retrieve than other types of episodic information (Clark-Foos & Marsh, 2008; Zajonc, 1980). As noted in the previous section, the *frontal aging hypothesis* proposes that older adults will be particularly disadvantaged on tasks that place heavy burdens on the PFC. Episodic retrieval typically is such a task, with the PFC implicated in the search and monitoring phases, but there is reason to think that PFC demands may be reduced during the retrieval of emotional information. For instance, divided attention has a lesser impact on retrieval of emotional information than neutral information (Clark-Foos & Marsh, 2008), and event-related potential studies have revealed that retrieval of emotional information increases an early-onsetting frontal old–new affect associated with relatively automatic retrieval of familiarity (for review, see van Strien, Cappaert, & Witter, 2009). Because older adults tend to show the most difficulties on tasks with high retrieval demands (Light, 1991), they may recall more affective and evaluative information simply because it is easier for them to retrieve (for a related discussion, see Burke & Light, 1981).

On many tasks, older adults' prioritization of evaluative processing may be to the detriment of their overall memory ability. Often, older adults who show greater over-recruitment of neural regions associated with evaluative processing are those who show poorer memory performance (Duverne, Motamedinia, & Rugg, 2009a; Düzel, Schütze, Yonelinas, & Heinze, 2011). Moreover, older adults who rely on relatively automatic retrieval processes may be those who have a lesser ability to engage controlled retrieval strategies to recall other affective details, consistent with evidence that older adults' focus on affective tone may come at a cost for memory for other types of details (e.g., Comblain, D'Argembeau, & Van der Linden, 2005; Kensinger, Brierley, Medford, Growdon, & Corkin, 2002). Yet other times, this prioritization likely benefits older adults' memories: For example, older adults are as good as younger adults at remembering whether food is safe to eat (May, Rahhal, Berry, & Leighton, 2005) or whether someone is a good or bad person (Rahhal, May, & Hasher, 2002). This focus on thoughts and feelings also may help to explain why older adults readily form "flashbulb memories" despite their general deficits in creating detailed, episodic memories (reviewed in Kensinger et al., 2014). Thus, older adults' evaluative focusing may be a double-edged sword, enabling them to remember some types of events, or event details, at the cost of others.

Older Adults Remember the Good More Than the Bad

Although the previous section has emphasized that older adults' memories prioritize thoughts and feelings, it is not the case that all types of emotional events are prioritized equally. The *positivity effect* is a widely discussed consequence of aging: While younger adults often show a *negativity bias* in memory, consistent with proposals that "bad is stronger than good" (Baumeister, Bratslavsky, Finkenauer, & Vohs, 2001), older adults do not show the same degree of bias toward the negative, and in fact they often remember positive information more readily than negative (see Chapter 6, this volume).

One of the more surprising revelations about the positivity effect is that it occurs most readily in older adults who have the most cognitive control resources to devote (Knight et al., 2007; Mather & Knight, 2005). Thus, it is the higher functioning older adults who show a memory pattern that diverges from younger adults, while lower functioning older adults are more likely to show the negativity bias typical in younger cohorts. This pattern has led to the proposal that the effect reflects an adaptive change in the way that information is remembered, enabling high-functioning older adults to focus on content that will maximize their well-being and support their emotion-regulation goals (Nashiro & Mather, 2011; Reed & Carstensen, 2012).

This regulatory account has been supported by evidence that not only do older adults sometimes recruit prefrontal regions more on memory tasks than younger adults (as reviewed in the preceding subsection), prefrontal regions are engaged and connected differently depending on the valence of information being remembered. Most notably, aging is associated with greater increases in prefrontal recruitment during negative relative to neutral (Murty et al., 2009) and positive event retrieval (Ford, Morris, & Kensinger, 2014). These effects of age are present over relatively short retention delays, but they may become exaggerated over longer delays (Kalpouzos, Fischer, Rieckmann, Macdonald, & Bäckman, 2012). At least some of the time, these prefrontal processes appear to dampen activity in medial temporal-lobe regions, including both the amygdala (St. Jacques, Dolcos, & Cabeza, 2009) and hippocampus (Ford et al., 2014), broadly consistent with a regulatory account.

Three studies incorporating assessments of individual differences also revealed evidence consistent with a regulatory account. In one study (Erk, Kleczar, & Walter, 2007), older adults who endorsed using reappraisal strategies more frequently showed reduced amygdala activity to negative stimuli. In another study (Waldinger, Kensinger, & Schulz, 2011), only older adults who rated themselves to have high life satisfaction showed stronger connectivity between the amygdala and other nodes of an emotional memory network when successfully encoding positive compared to negative images. Individual differences in neural connectivity also can relate to the prevalence of the positivity effect. Sakaki, Nga, and Mather (2013) demonstrated that the older adults most likely to show enhanced connectivity between the PFC and amygdala at rest (i.e., when no task is instructed) also are those who are most likely to remember positive information disproportionately.

However, there are some lines of work that suggest a regulatory account may not be the sole mechanism of the positivity effect. Most notably, age-by-valence interactions have been revealed early in the time course of retrieval (Newsome, Dulas, & Duarte, 2012), before regulatory processes would be likely to be implemented, as measured with electroencephalography (EEG). Although these early changes could reflect age differences in the processing of an emotional retrieval cue, rather than in mnemonic content elicited by it, they emphasize the need for further research to elucidate whether there are circumstances when older adults' prefrontal engagement is less likely to be tied to regulatory actions.

Older Adults Reflect on Past Negative Events Differently

The previous subsection emphasized that negative events often are less likely to come to mind for an older adult than for a younger adult. Even when they do come to mind, however, age can affect the way that individuals reflect on those past bad experiences. Two primary changes have been noted in this domain. First, older adults are better able to find the good to remember. For instance, when asked to describe autobiographical events from their past, older adults use more positive words to describe a past negative event than do younger adults. Relatedly, when young and older adults were asked to report how often they thought about positive and negative aspects of a highly negative event (the bombings at the 2013 Boston Marathon), older age increased the likelihood of thinking about the positive aspects (e.g., heroism, town pride, capture of suspect) but had no effect on the likelihood of thinking about the negative aspects. Second, older adults can remember negative events less vividly than younger adults, and this reduced memory vividness can be connected to their recruitment of prefrontal regions (Ford & Kensinger, 2018). Specifically, older adults often show an inverse relation between prefrontal activity and medial temporal-lobe activity during the retrieval of negative information, and the recruitment of the prefrontal regions that show this inverse relation with hippocampal activity is both disproportionate during the retrieval of negative information and linked to lower ratings of subjective vividness for those negative memories (Ford & Kensinger, 2018). It is well known that older adults choose to avoid situations that they know will evoke negative affect: *In the moment*, age increases disengagement from offending situations (Charles & Carstensen, 2008). These results may be intertwined with this phenomenon, suggesting that age also increases the likelihood that individuals disengage from remembering events in ways that will evoke negative affect.

CONCLUDING REMARKS

Although we have learned a great deal about age-related changes in episodic memory from neuroscience research to date, there are several relatively unexplored questions that will be important to address in the coming years. For example, human neuroscience methods and analyses are developing exponentially, but many of these approaches have only recently being applied to age-related memory research. In this section, we discuss some of these approaches and offer suggestions for how they might be used to advance the field of age-related memory research.

Implications

The research reviewed in this chapter may elucidate an apparent contradiction: Laboratory assessments paint a somewhat bleak picture of older adults' memory capabilities, yet the older adult participants in these studies lead independent lives and contribute meaningfully to society, often taking on roles (e.g., caretaking) that have high memory demands. What may account for this contradiction?

First, many laboratory assessments exaggerate age-related differences due to a combination of factors. The sterile and potentially intimidating laboratory environment and long lists of briefly presented, unimodal (usually visual), unrelated stimuli may curtail the evaluative and motivationally relevant processes that older adults would excel at using in everyday life (see Chapter 5, this volume, for more on motivated learning). These factors also may exaggerate the attentional and interference-resolution demands of learning and retrieving beyond those typical in everyday life. As technological advances improve the ability to enrich learning contexts and to tailor learning tasks to the experience and goals of each participant, laboratory assessments should better approximate the learning environments of older adults' day-to-day experience. This may provide new insights into the patterns of age-related preservation and decline.

Second, a fundamental insight to be gained from a cognitive neuroscience perspective is that older adults often remember information by recruiting different strategies than those engaged by younger adults, consistent with the centrality of compensation to the conceptualization of cognitive aging (Baltes & Lindenberger, 1997). The efficacy of these compensatory processes can be shaped by the experiences achieved over a lifetime and by the degree of cognitive or brain reserve available to an older adult (Park & Reuter-Lorenz, 2009). As discussed earlier, more longitudinal aging research is necessary to determine whether differential neural recruitment in the PFC or other areas in aging reflects functional compensation. Nonetheless, these age differences should not always be cast as deficits. As we have described, older adults' shift toward evaluative processing can help them to remember the thoughts and feelings associated with past events. Similarly, older adults' shift toward pattern completion or toward gist-based memory can lead them to be more likely than younger adults to extract the high-level importance of an event, including its implications (McGinnis, Goss, Tessmer, & Zelinski, 2008). These shifts may also enable older adults to note connections across experiences, often are considered part of the "wisdom" acquired with age (Baltes & Staudinger, 2000).

Moreover, it is increasingly recognized that the brain retains plasticity into older age, and that older adults can continue to benefit from life experiences (Lövdén, Bäckman, Lindenberger, Schaefer, & Schmiedek, 2010). Newer lines of research suggest a potential for lifestyle interventions—many focused on improving fitness levels, nutrition, and social engagement (for review, see Williams & Kemper, 2010) to benefit older adults' cognitive performance. Similarly, there is speculation that personalized cognitive training interventions may benefit older adults (for commentary, see Mishra & Gazzaley, 2014). Although many open questions remain regarding the efficacy of these interventions (for a review, see Salthouse, 2015), two broad points can be made. First, there are more interconnections between our mental and physical health than many older adults realize, enabling interventions known to convey benefits in one domain (e.g., increased fitness improving physical health) to potentially deliver benefits in the other. Second, a beneficial cycle may be created whereby those older adults who seek new learning opportunities to allow them to stay cognitively active, physically fit, and socially engaged may be those who will find it easier to continue to learn from these experiences.

Future Directions for Age-Related Memory Research

Most neuroimaging and EEG studies have used univariate analyses, which are excellent for determining whether a particular brain region or EEG signal contributes to memory or is affected by age but do not allow for assessments of brain networks. Multivariate analyses, by contrast, can be used to characterize how aging affects functional coherence within and between networks. For example, consistent with older adults' cognitive control impairments, univariate analyses show age-related decreases in lateral PFC recruitment during attempts to perform cognitively demanding emotion regulation strategies, namely, reappraisal (Opitz, Rauch, Terry, & Urry, 2012; Winecoff, Labar, Madden, Cabeza, & Huettel, 2011). Multivariate analyses, however, show that both young and older adults recruit a coherent network of PFC regions while engaging in reappraisal of negative events (Allard & Kensinger, 2014). This example highlights the potential divergence in conclusions reached by univariate and multivariate analyses. Thus, while univariate analyses might suggest reduced availability of PFC regions to support episodic memory functioning in older adults, multivariate analyses show that functional communication between these regions can support memory performance across age. Recently, analyses grounded in graph theory have been used to show that aging is associated with reduced segregation of functional brain networks that support distinct high-order cognitive functions, which in turn is related to impaired long-term memory performance (Chan, Park, Savalia, Petersen, & Wig, 2014). Age-related reductions in within-network connectivity together with increases in between-network connectivity (i.e., segregation) have largely been assessed for resting state data and in association with memory performance measured offline (Antonenko & Flöel, 2014). It will be important for future studies to determine whether age-related desegregation of functional brain networks affects the recruitment of these networks during performance of episodic memory tasks.

Machine-learning-based analyses such as multivariate pattern analysis (MVPA) have become popular in recent years for their ability to detect patterns of activity, within and across brain areas, that are indicative of different cognitive states (reviewed in Norman, Polyn, Detre, & Haxby, 2006). MVPA has been used in young adults to reveal the specificity, measured as the degree of matching between encoding and retrieval brain activity patterns, with which episodic memories are retrieved (Liang & Preston, 2017; Staresina, Henson, Kriegeskorte, & Alink, 2012; Xiao et al., 2017). Specifically, MVPA results show that successful retrieval of previous events is associated with neural reactivation of category (e.g., scene, face, word) or context (e.g., orienting tasks) representations that were observed during encoding (Kuhl, Bainbridge, & Chun, 2012). Even more interestingly, MVPA evidence shows that successful retrieval of word–scene pairs (i.e., "apple"– nature scene) is accompanied by reactivation of encoding activity associated with that specific pair above and beyond reactivation of the category level representations common to all retrieved pairs (Staresina et al., 2012). To date, one study has used MVPA to show category level reinstatement for recollected items is unaffected by age (Wang et al., 2016). As discussed within this chapter, aging is associated with declines in recollection for specific details of previously encoded events. This conclusion has been drawn largely from studies in which memory for details such as spatial location or stimulus color or category is tested, but these are relatively coarse measures. We know little about whether age-related recollection impairments stem from dysfunction in neural reinstatement of specific encoding-related activity or constructive processes that support specific memory retrieval. Brain pattern analyses may prove promising for addressing this issue, but to date, few studies have applied such analyses to aging data.

The majority of aging studies have been cross-sectional and have not examined memory performance and related neural activity in middle-aged adults. Consequently, we know relatively little about what underlies episodic memory changes in middle age or when many of the aforementioned age-related changes in emotional memory begin to emerge. Evidence from lifespan cross-sectional studies suggests that changes in PFC recruitment during encoding (Cansino, Estrada-Manilla, et al., 2015) and retrieval (Ankudowich, Pasvanis, & Rajah, 2016; Cansino, Hernández-Ramos, & Trejo-Morales, 2012; Cansino, Trejo-Morales, et al., 2015; Kwon et al., 2016) contribute to episodic memory decline even in mid-life (~40–60 years of age). It is not clear from this work whether the mechanisms underlying memory decline in middle age are the same as those in old age. Arguably the best approach to investigate neural changes underlying episodic memory decline across the lifespan would be longitudinal assessments of individuals over an extended period of time. Although such studies are costly and face unique issues including subject attrition and practice effects (Salthouse, 2014), a few longitudinal studies have revealed some important findings regarding aging and memory. For example, longitudinal evidence suggests that findings of age-related PFC over-recruitment in cross-sectional studies may be overestimated and that PFC under-recruitment during encoding or retrieval is a more typical response (Nyberg et al., 2010). Furthermore, PFC over-recruitment may be more likely related to declining memory function than to a compensatory mechanism that supports memory performance in older adults (Pudas, Josefsson, Rieckmann, & Nyberg, 2018). With regard to affect, longitudinal behavioral evidence substantiates the decline in negativity bias across the lifespan that has been observed in numerous cross-sectional studies (Charles, Reynolds, & Gatz, 2001). Longitudinal work is needed, however, to determine what underlying neural changes contribute to this positivity shift. We would argue that longitudinal research is needed to more accurately characterize the neural basis of age-related episodic memory decline and the factors that contribute to these changes (i.e., lifestyle, genetics). This is not to suggest that cross-sectional aging studies have no value. Indeed, cross-sectional research is arguably the best method for dissociating cognitive mechanisms that contribute to memory performance, including recollection, familiarity, and various cognitive control operations, and identifying the brain areas and networks that support these mechanisms. A combination of cross-sectional and longitudinal research may be the strongest approach to tackling questions about lifespan changes in memory function.

REFERENCES

Allard, E. S., & Kensinger, E. A. (2014). Age-related differences in functional connectivity during cognitive emotion regulation. *The Journals of Gerontology: Series B. Psychological Sciences and Social Sciences, 69*, 852–860. http://dx.doi.org/10.1093/geronb/gbu108

Angel, L., Bastin, C., Genon, S., Balteau, E., Phillips, C., Luxen, A., . . . Collette, F. (2013). Differential effects of aging on the neural correlates of recollection and familiarity. *Cortex, 49*, 1585–1597. http://dx.doi.org/10.1016/j.cortex.2012.10.002

Ankudowich, E., Pasvanis, S., & Rajah, M. N. (2016). Changes in the modulation of brain activity during context encoding vs. context retrieval across the adult lifespan. *NeuroImage, 139*, 103–113. http://dx.doi.org/10.1016/j.neuroimage.2016.06.022

Antonenko, D., & Flöel, A. (2014). Healthy aging by staying selectively connected: A mini-review. *Gerontology, 60*, 3–9. http://dx.doi.org/10.1159/000354376

Badre, D. (2008). Cognitive control, hierarchy, and the rostro-caudal organization of the frontal lobes. *Trends in Cognitive Sciences, 12*, 193–200. http://dx.doi.org/10.1016/j.tics.2008.02.004

Baltes, P. B., & Lindenberger, U. (1997). Emergence of a powerful connection between sensory and cognitive functions across the adult life span: A new window to the study of cognitive aging? *Psychology and Aging, 12*, 12–21. http://dx.doi.org/10.1037/0882-7974.12.1.12

Baltes, P. B., & Staudinger, U. M. (2000). Wisdom. A metaheuristic (pragmatic) to orchestrate mind and virtue toward excellence. *American Psychologist, 55*, 122–136. http://dx.doi.org/10.1037/0003-066X.55.1.122

Baumeister, R. F., Bratslavsky, E., Finkenauer, C., & Vohs, K. D. (2001). Bad is stronger than good. *Review of General Psychology, 5*, 323–370. http://dx.doi.org/10.1037/1089-2680.5.4.323

Becker, N., Laukka, E. J., Kalpouzos, G., Naveh-Benjamin, M., Bäckman, L., & Brehmer, Y. (2015). Structural brain correlates of associative memory in older adults. *NeuroImage, 118*, 146–153. http://dx.doi.org/10.1016/j.neuroimage.2015.06.002

Benoit, R. G., & Schacter, D. L. (2015). Specifying the core network supporting episodic simulation and episodic memory by activation likelihood estimation. *Neuropsychologia, 75*, 450–457. http://dx.doi.org/10.1016/j.neuropsychologia.2015.06.034

Berryhill, M. E., Phuong, L., Picasso, L., Cabeza, R., & Olson, I. R. (2007). Parietal lobe and episodic memory: Bilateral damage causes impaired free recall of autobiographical memory. *The Journal of Neuroscience, 27*, 14415–14423. http://dx.doi.org/10.1523/JNEUROSCI.4163-07.2007

Blumenfeld, R. S., Parks, C. M., Yonelinas, A. P., & Ranganath, C. (2011). Putting the pieces together: The role of dorsolateral prefrontal cortex in relational memory encoding. *Journal of Cognitive Neuroscience, 23*, 257–265. http://dx.doi.org/10.1162/jocn.2010.21459

Brown, R., & Kulik, J. (1977). Flashbulb memories. *Cognition, 5,* 73–99. http://dx.doi.org/10.1016/0010-0277(77)90018-X

Burke, D. M., & Light, L. L. (1981). Memory and aging: The role of retrieval processes. *Psychological Bulletin, 90,* 513–514. http://dx.doi.org/10.1037/0033-2909.90.3.513

Cabeza, R., Albert, M., Belleville, S., Craik, F. I. M., Duarte, A., Grady, C. L., . . . Rajah, M. N. (2018). Maintenance, reserve and compensation: The cognitive neuroscience of healthy ageing [erratum at http://dx.doi.org/10.1038/s41583-018-0086-0]. *Nature Reviews Neuroscience, 19,* 701–710. http://dx.doi.org/10.1038/s41583-018-0068-2

Cansino, S., Estrada-Manilla, C., Trejo-Morales, P., Pasaye-Alcaraz, E. H., Aguilar-Castañeda, E., Salgado-Lujambio, P., & Sosa-Ortiz, A. L. (2015). fMRI subsequent source memory effects in young, middle-aged and old adults. *Behavioural Brain Research, 280,* 24–35. http://dx.doi.org/10.1016/j.bbr.2014.11.042

Cansino, S., Hernández-Ramos, E., & Trejo-Morales, P. (2012). Neural correlates of source memory retrieval in young, middle-aged and elderly adults. *Biological Psychology, 90,* 33–49. http://dx.doi.org/10.1016/j.biopsycho.2012.02.004

Cansino, S., Trejo-Morales, P., Estrada-Manilla, C., Pasaye-Alcaraz, E. H., Aguilar-Castañeda, E., Salgado-Lujambio, P., & Sosa-Ortiz, A. L. (2015). Brain activity during source memory retrieval in young, middle-aged and old adults. *Brain Research, 1618,* 168–180. http://dx.doi.org/10.1016/j.brainres.2015.05.032

Carstensen, L. L., & Turk-Charles, S. (1994). The salience of emotion across the adult life span. *Psychology and Aging, 9,* 259–264. http://dx.doi.org/10.1037/0882-7974.9.2.259

Chan, M. Y., Park, D. C., Savalia, N. K., Petersen, S. E., & Wig, G. S. (2014). Decreased segregation of brain systems across the healthy adult lifespan. *Proceedings of the National Academy of Sciences of the United States of America, 111,* E4997–E5006. http://dx.doi.org/10.1073/pnas.1415122111

Charles, S. T., & Carstensen, L. L. (2008). Unpleasant situations elicit different emotional responses in younger and older adults. *Psychology and Aging, 23,* 495–504. http://dx.doi.org/10.1037/a0013284

Charles, S. T., Reynolds, C. A., & Gatz, M. (2001). Age-related differences and change in positive and negative affect over 23 years. *Journal of Personality and Social Psychology, 80,* 136–151. http://dx.doi.org/10.1037/0022-3514.80.1.136

Ciaramelli, E., & Ghetti, S. (2007). What are confabulators' memories made of? A study of subjective and objective measures of recollection in confabulation. *Neuropsychologia, 45,* 1489–1500. http://dx.doi.org/10.1016/j.neuropsychologia.2006.11.007

Clark-Foos, A., & Marsh, R. L. (2008). Recognition memory for valenced and arousing materials under conditions of divided attention. *Memory, 16,* 530–537. http://dx.doi.org/10.1080/09658210802007493

Comblain, C., D'Argembeau, A., & Van der Linden, M. (2005). Phenomenal characteristics of autobiographical memories for emotional and neutral events in older and younger adults. *Experimental Aging Research, 31*, 173–189. http://dx.doi.org/10.1080/03610730590915010

Comblain, C., D'Argembeau, A., Van der Linden, M., & Aldenhoff, L. (2004). The effect of ageing on the recollection of emotional and neutral pictures. *Memory, 12*, 673–684. http://dx.doi.org/10.1080/09658210344000477

Craik, F. I. M., & Byrd, M. (1982). Aging and cognitive deficits: The role of attentional resources. In F. Craik & S. Trehub (Eds.), *Aging and cognitive processes* (pp. 191–211). New York, NY: Springer.

Davachi, L., Mitchell, J. P., & Wagner, A. D. (2003). Multiple routes to memory: Distinct medial temporal lobe processes build item and source memories. *Proceedings of the National Academy of Sciences of the United States of America, 100*, 2157–2162. http://dx.doi.org/10.1073/pnas.0337195100

de Chastelaine, M., Mattson, J. T., Wang, T. H., Donley, B. E., & Rugg, M. D. (2015). Sensitivity of negative subsequent memory and task-negative effects to age and associative memory performance. *Brain Research, 1612*, 16–29. http://dx.doi.org/10.1016/j.brainres.2014.09.045

de Chastelaine, M., Mattson, J. T., Wang, T. H., Donley, B. E., & Rugg, M. D. (2016). The neural correlates of recollection and retrieval monitoring: Relationships with age and recollection performance [erratum at https://www.sciencedirect.com/science/article/pii/S1053811917301763?via%3Dihub]. *NeuroImage, 138*, 164–175. http://dx.doi.org/10.1016/j.neuroimage.2016.04.071

Dennis, N. A., Hayes, S. M., Prince, S. E., Madden, D. J., Huettel, S. A., & Cabeza, R. (2008). Effects of aging on the neural correlates of successful item and source memory encoding. *Journal of Experimental Psychology: Learning, Memory, and Cognition, 34*, 791–808. http://dx.doi.org/10.1037/0278-7393.34.4.791

Dennis, N. A., Kim, H., & Cabeza, R. (2008). Age-related differences in brain activity during true and false memory retrieval. *Journal of Cognitive Neuroscience, 20*, 1390–1402. http://dx.doi.org/10.1162/jocn.2008.20096

Diana, R. A., Yonelinas, A. P., & Ranganath, C. (2007). Imaging recollection and familiarity in the medial temporal lobe: A three-component model. *Trends in Cognitive Sciences, 11*, 379–386. http://dx.doi.org/10.1016/j.tics.2007.08.001

Duarte, A., Henson, R. N., & Graham, K. S. (2008). The effects of aging on the neural correlates of subjective and objective recollection. *Cerebral Cortex, 18*, 2169–2180. http://dx.doi.org/10.1093/cercor/bhm243

Duarte, A., Ranganath, C., & Knight, R. T. (2005). Effects of unilateral prefrontal lesions on familiarity, recollection, and source memory. *The Journal of Neuroscience, 25*, 8333–8337. http://dx.doi.org/10.1523/JNEUROSCI.1392-05.2005

Duarte, A., Ranganath, C., Trujillo, C., & Knight, R. T. (2006). Intact recollection memory in high-performing older adults: ERP and behavioral evidence. *Journal of Cognitive Neuroscience, 18*, 33–47. http://dx.doi.org/10.1162/089892906775249988

Dulas, M. R., & Duarte, A. (2011). The effects of aging on material-independent and material-dependent neural correlates of contextual binding. *NeuroImage, 57*, 1192–1204. http://dx.doi.org/10.1016/j.neuroimage.2011.05.036

Dulas, M. R., & Duarte, A. (2012). The effects of aging on material-independent and material-dependent neural correlates of source memory retrieval. *Cerebral Cortex, 22*, 37–50. http://dx.doi.org/10.1093/cercor/bhr056

Dulas, M. R., & Duarte, A. (2013). The influence of directed attention at encoding on source memory retrieval in the young and old: An ERP study. *Brain Research, 1500*, 55–71. http://dx.doi.org/10.1016/j.brainres.2013.01.018

Dulas, M. R., & Duarte, A. (2014). Aging affects the interaction between attentional control and source memory: An fMRI study. *Journal of Cognitive Neuroscience, 26*, 2653–2669. http://dx.doi.org/10.1162/jocn_a_00663

Duverne, S., Motamedinia, S., & Rugg, M. D. (2009a). Effects of age on the neural correlates of retrieval cue processing are modulated by task demands. *Journal of Cognitive Neuroscience, 21*, 1–17. http://dx.doi.org/10.1162/jocn.2009.21001

Duverne, S., Motamedinia, S., & Rugg, M. D. (2009b). The relationship between aging, performance, and the neural correlates of successful memory encoding. *Cerebral Cortex, 19*, 733–744. http://dx.doi.org/10.1093/cercor/bhn122

Düzel, E., Schütze, H., Yonelinas, A. P., & Heinze, H. J. (2011). Functional phenotyping of successful aging in long-term memory: Preserved performance in the absence of neural compensation. *Hippocampus, 21*, 803–814.

Eichenbaum, H., Yonelinas, A. P., & Ranganath, C. (2007). The medial temporal lobe and recognition memory. *Annual Review of Neuroscience, 30*, 123–152. http://dx.doi.org/10.1146/annurev.neuro.30.051606.094328

Erk, S., Kleczar, A., & Walter, H. (2007). Valence-specific regulation effects in a working memory task with emotional context. *NeuroImage, 37*, 623–632. http://dx.doi.org/10.1016/j.neuroimage.2007.05.006

Ford, J. H., & Kensinger, E. A. (2018). Older adults use a prefrontal regulatory mechanism to reduce negative memory vividness of a highly emotional real-world event. *Neuroreport, 29*, 1129–1134. http://dx.doi.org/10.1097/WNR.0000000000001084

Ford, J. H., Morris, J. A., & Kensinger, E. A. (2014). Neural recruitment and connectivity during emotional memory retrieval across the adult life span. *Neurobiology of Aging, 35*, 2770–2784. http://dx.doi.org/10.1016/j.neurobiolaging.2014.05.029

Gottlieb, L. J., Uncapher, M. R., & Rugg, M. D. (2010). Dissociation of the neural correlates of visual and auditory contextual encoding. *Neuropsychologia, 48*, 137–144. http://dx.doi.org/10.1016/j.neuropsychologia.2009.08.019

Gutchess, A. H., Sokal, R., Coleman, J. A., Gotthilf, G., Grewal, L., & Rosa, N. (2015). Age differences in self-referencing: Evidence for common and distinct encoding strategies. *Brain Research, 1612*, 118–127. http://dx.doi.org/10.1016/j.brainres.2014.08.033

Hasher, L., & Zacks, R. (1988). Working memory, comprehension, and aging: A review and a new view. In G. Bower (Ed.), *The psychology of learning and motivation* (pp. 193–225). San Diego, CA: Academic Press. http://dx.doi.org/10.1016/S0079-7421(08)60041-9

Hashtroudi, S., Johnson, M. K., & Chrosniak, L. D. (1990). Aging and qualitative characteristics of memories for perceived and imagined complex events. *Psychology and Aging, 5,* 119–126. http://dx.doi.org/10.1037/0882-7974.5.1.119

Henkel, L. A., Johnson, M. K., & De Leonardis, D. M. (1998). Aging and source monitoring: Cognitive processes and neuropsychological correlates. *Journal of Experimental Psychology: General, 127,* 251–268. http://dx.doi.org/10.1037/0096-3445.127.3.251

Hertzog, C., McGuire, C. L., Horhota, M., & Jopp, D. (2010). Does believing in "use it or lose it" relate to self-rated memory control, strategy use, and recall? *The International Journal of Aging & Human Development, 70,* 61–87. http://dx.doi.org/10.2190/AG.70.1.c

Hultsch, D. F., Hertzog, C., & Dixon, R. A. (1990). Ability correlates of memory performance in adulthood and aging. *Psychology and Aging, 5,* 356–368. http://dx.doi.org/10.1037/0882-7974.5.3.356

Jacoby, L. L., Bishara, A. J., Hessels, S., & Toth, J. P. (2005). Aging, subjective experience, and cognitive control: Dramatic false remembering by older adults. *Journal of Experimental Psychology: General, 134,* 131–148. http://dx.doi.org/10.1037/0096-3445.134.2.131

Janowsky, J. S., Shimamura, A. P., & Squire, L. R. (1989). Source memory impairment in patients with frontal lobe lesions. *Neuropsychologia, 27,* 1043–1056. http://dx.doi.org/10.1016/0028-3932(89)90184-X

Kalpouzos, G., Fischer, H., Rieckmann, A., Macdonald, S. W., & Bäckman, L. (2012). Impact of negative emotion on the neural correlates of long-term recognition in younger and older adults. *Frontiers in Integrative Neuroscience, 6,* 74. http://dx.doi.org/10.3389/fnint.2012.00074

Kensinger, E. A., Allard, E., & Krendl, A. C. (2014). The effects of age on memory for socioemotional material: An affective neuroscience perspective. In P. Verhaeghen & C. Hertzog (Eds.), *The Oxford handbook of emotion, social cognition, and problem solving in adulthood* (pp. 26–46). Oxford, England: Oxford University Press.

Kensinger, E. A., Brierley, B., Medford, N., Growdon, J. H., & Corkin, S. (2002). Effects of normal aging and Alzheimer's disease on emotional memory. *Emotion, 2,* 118–134. http://dx.doi.org/10.1037/1528-3542.2.2.118

Kirchhoff, B. A., Anderson, B. A., Barch, D. M., & Jacoby, L. L. (2012). Cognitive and neural effects of semantic encoding strategy training in older adults. *Cerebral Cortex, 22,* 788–799. http://dx.doi.org/10.1093/cercor/bhr129

Kirchhoff, B. A., & Buckner, R. L. (2006). Functional–anatomic correlates of individual differences in memory. *Neuron, 51,* 263–274. http://dx.doi.org/10.1016/j.neuron.2006.06.006

Knight, M., Seymour, T. L., Gaunt, J. T., Baker, C., Nesmith, K., & Mather, M. (2007). Aging and goal-directed emotional attention: Distraction reverses emotional biases. *Emotion, 7,* 705–714. http://dx.doi.org/10.1037/1528-3542.7.4.705

Kopelman, M. D., Stanhope, N., & Kingsley, D. (1997). Temporal and spatial context memory in patients with focal frontal, temporal lobe, and diencephalic lesions. *Neuropsychologia, 35*, 1533–1545. http://dx.doi.org/10.1016/S0028-3932(97)00076-6

Kuhl, B. A., Bainbridge, W. A., & Chun, M. M. (2012). Neural reactivation reveals mechanisms for updating memory. *The Journal of Neuroscience, 32*, 3453–3461. http://dx.doi.org/10.1523/JNEUROSCI.5846-11.2012

Kvavilashvili, L., Mirani, J., Schlagman, S., Erskine, J. A., & Kornbrot, D. E. (2010). Effects of age on phenomenology and consistency of flashbulb memories of September 11 and a staged control event. *Psychology and Aging, 25*, 391–404. http://dx.doi.org/10.1037/a0017532

Kwon, D., Maillet, D., Pasvanis, S., Ankudowich, E., Grady, C. L., & Rajah, M. N. (2016). Context memory decline in middle aged adults is related to changes in prefrontal cortex function. *Cerebral Cortex, 26*, 2440–2460. http://dx.doi.org/10.1093/cercor/bhv068

Leshikar, E. D., & Duarte, A. (2014). Medial prefrontal cortex supports source memory for self-referenced materials in young and older adults. *Cognitive, Affective & Behavioral Neuroscience, 14*, 236–252. http://dx.doi.org/10.3758/s13415-013-0198-y

Leshikar, E. D., Duarte, A., & Hertzog, C. (2012). Task-selective memory effects for successfully implemented encoding strategies. *PLoS One, 7*, e38160. http://dx.doi.org/10.1371/journal.pone.0038160

Liang, J. C., & Preston, A. R. (2017). Medial temporal lobe reinstatement of content-specific details predicts source memory. *Cortex, 91*, 67–78. http://dx.doi.org/10.1016/j.cortex.2016.09.011

Light, L. L. (1991). Memory and aging: Four hypotheses in search of data. *Annual Review of Psychology, 42*, 333–376. http://dx.doi.org/10.1146/annurev.ps.42.020191.002001

Logan, J. M., Sanders, A. L., Snyder, A. Z., Morris, J. C., & Buckner, R. L. (2002). Under-recruitment and nonselective recruitment: Dissociable neural mechanisms associated with aging. *Neuron, 33*, 827–840. http://dx.doi.org/10.1016/S0896-6273(02)00612-8

Lövdén, M., Bäckman, L., Lindenberger, U., Schaefer, S., & Schmiedek, F. (2010). A theoretical framework for the study of adult cognitive plasticity. *Psychological Bulletin, 136*, 659–676. http://dx.doi.org/10.1037/a0020080

Maillet, D., & Rajah, M. N. (2014). Age-related differences in brain activity in the subsequent memory paradigm: A meta-analysis. *Neuroscience and Biobehavioral Reviews, 45*, 246–257. http://dx.doi.org/10.1016/j.neubiorev.2014.06.006

Mather, M., & Knight, M. (2005). Goal-directed memory: The role of cognitive control in older adults' emotional memory. *Psychology and Aging, 20*, 554–570. http://dx.doi.org/10.1037/0882-7974.20.4.554

May, C. P., Rahhal, T., Berry, E. M., & Leighton, E. A. (2005). Aging, source memory, and emotion. *Psychology and Aging, 20*, 571–578. http://dx.doi.org/10.1037/0882-7974.20.4.571

McDonough, I. M., & Gallo, D. A. (2013). Impaired retrieval monitoring for past and future autobiographical events in older adults. *Psychology and Aging, 28*, 457–466. http://dx.doi.org/10.1037/a0032732

McGinnis, D., Goss, R., Tessmer, C., & Zelinski, E. M. (2008). Inference generation in young, young-old, and old-old adults: Evidence for semantic architecture stability. *Applied Cognitive Psychology, 22,* 171–192. http://dx.doi.org/10.1002/acp.1367

Miller, E. K., & Cohen, J. D. (2001). An integrative theory of prefrontal cortex function. *Annual Review of Neuroscience, 24,* 167–202. http://dx.doi.org/10.1146/annurev.neuro.24.1.167

Miller, S. L., Celone, K., DePeau, K., Diamond, E., Dickerson, B. C., Rentz, D., . . . Sperling, R. A. (2008). Age-related memory impairment associated with loss of parietal deactivation but preserved hippocampal activation. *Proceedings of the National Academy of Sciences of the United States of America, 105,* 2181–2186. http://dx.doi.org/10.1073/pnas.0706818105

Milner, B. (2005). The medial temporal-lobe amnesic syndrome. *Psychiatric Clinics of North America, 28,* 599–611, 609. Retrieved from https://www.sciencedirect.com/science/article/pii/S0193953X05000560?via%3Dihub

Mishra, J., & Gazzaley, A. (2014). Closed-loop rehabilitation of age-related cognitive disorders. *Seminars in Neurology, 34,* 584–590. http://dx.doi.org/10.1055/s-0034-1396011

Mitchell, K. J., & Johnson, M. K. (2009). Source monitoring 15 years later: What have we learned from fMRI about the neural mechanisms of source memory? *Psychological Bulletin, 135,* 638–677. http://dx.doi.org/10.1037/a0015849

Morcom, A. M., Li, J., & Rugg, M. D. (2007). Age effects on the neural correlates of episodic retrieval: Increased cortical recruitment with matched performance. *Cerebral Cortex, 17,* 2491–2506. http://dx.doi.org/10.1093/cercor/bhl155

Murty, V. P., Sambataro, F., Das, S., Tan, H. Y., Callicott, J. H., Goldberg, T. E., . . . Mattay, V. S. (2009). Age-related alterations in simple declarative memory and the effect of negative stimulus valence. *Journal of Cognitive Neuroscience, 21,* 1920–1933. http://dx.doi.org/10.1162/jocn.2009.21130

Nashiro, K., & Mather, M. (2011). Effects of emotional arousal on memory binding in normal aging and Alzheimer's disease. *The American Journal of Psychology, 124,* 301–312. http://dx.doi.org/10.5406/amerjpsyc.124.3.0301

Naveh-Benjamin, M. (2000). Adult age differences in memory performance: Tests of an associative deficit hypothesis. *Journal of Experimental Psychology: Learning, Memory, and Cognition, 26,* 1170–1187. http://dx.doi.org/10.1037/0278-7393.26.5.1170

Naveh-Benjamin, M., Brav, T. K., & Levy, O. (2007). The associative memory deficit of older adults: The role of strategy utilization. *Psychology and Aging, 22,* 202–208. http://dx.doi.org/10.1037/0882-7974.22.1.202

Newsome, R. N., Dulas, M. R., & Duarte, A. (2012). The effects of aging on emotion-induced modulations of source retrieval ERPs: Evidence for valence biases. *Neuropsychologia, 50,* 3370–3384. http://dx.doi.org/10.1016/j.neuropsychologia.2012.09.024

Norman, K. A., Polyn, S. M., Detre, G. J., & Haxby, J. V. (2006). Beyond mind-reading: Multi-voxel pattern analysis of fMRI data. *Trends in Cognitive Sciences, 10,* 424–430. http://dx.doi.org/10.1016/j.tics.2006.07.005

Nyberg, L., Salami, A., Andersson, M., Eriksson, J., Kalpouzos, G., Kauppi, K., . . . Nilsson, L. G. (2010). Longitudinal evidence for diminished frontal cortex function in aging. *Proceedings of the National Academy of Sciences of the United States of America, 107*, 22682–22686. http://dx.doi.org/10.1073/pnas.1012651108

Opitz, P. C., Rauch, L. C., Terry, D. P., & Urry, H. L. (2012). Prefrontal mediation of age differences in cognitive reappraisal. *Neurobiology of Aging, 33*, 645–655. http://dx.doi.org/10.1016/j.neurobiolaging.2010.06.004

Park, D. C., & Reuter-Lorenz, P. (2009). The adaptive brain: Aging and neurocognitive scaffolding. *Annual Review of Psychology, 60*, 173–196. http://dx.doi.org/10.1146/annurev.psych.59.103006.093656

Perfect, T. J., & Dasgupta, Z. R. (1997). What underlies the deficit in reported recollective experience in old age? *Memory & Cognition, 25*, 849–858. http://dx.doi.org/10.3758/BF03211329

Petrides, M. (2005). Lateral prefrontal cortex: Architectonic and functional organization. *Philosophical Transactions of the Royal Society of London: Series B. Biological Sciences, 360*, 781–795. http://dx.doi.org/10.1098/rstb.2005.1631

Pudas, S., Josefsson, M., Rieckmann, A., & Nyberg, L. (2018). Longitudinal evidence for increased functional response in frontal cortex for older adults with hippocampal atrophy and memory decline. *Cerebral Cortex, 28*, 936–948. http://dx.doi.org/10.1093/cercor/bhw418

Rahhal, T. A., May, C. P., & Hasher, L. (2002). Truth and character: Sources that older adults can remember. *Psychological Science, 13*, 101–105. http://dx.doi.org/10.1111/1467-9280.00419

Rajah, M. N., Languay, R., & Valiquette, L. (2010). Age-related changes in prefrontal cortex activity are associated with behavioural deficits in both temporal and spatial context memory retrieval in older adults. *Cortex, 46*, 535–549. http://dx.doi.org/10.1016/j.cortex.2009.07.006

Ramnani, N., & Owen, A. M. (2004). Anterior prefrontal cortex: Insights into function from anatomy and neuroimaging. *Nature Reviews Neuroscience, 5*, 184–194. http://dx.doi.org/10.1038/nrn1343

Raz, N., & Kennedy, K. M. (2009). A systems approach to the aging brain: Neuroanatomic changes, their modifiers, and cognitive correlates. In W. J. Jagust & M. D'Esposito (Eds.), *Imaging the aging brain* (pp. 43–70). New York, NY: Oxford University Press. http://dx.doi.org/10.1093/acprof:oso/9780195328875.003.0004

Reed, A. E., & Carstensen, L. L. (2012). The theory behind the age-related positivity effect. *Frontiers in Psychology, 3*, 339. http://dx.doi.org/10.3389/fpsyg.2012.00339

Reuter-Lorenz, P. A., & Cappell, K. A. (2008). Neurocognitive aging and the compensation hypothesis. *Current Directions in Psychological Science, 17*, 177–182. http://dx.doi.org/10.1111/j.1467-8721.2008.00570.x

Rugg, M. D., & Morcom, A. M. (2005). The relationship between brain activity, cognitive performance and aging: The case of memory. In R. Cabeza, L. Nyberg, & D. C. Park (Eds.), *Cognitive neuroscience of aging: Linking cognitive and cerebral aging* (pp. 132–154). New York, NY: Oxford University Press.

Sakaki, M., Nga, L., & Mather, M. (2013). Amygdala functional connectivity with medial prefrontal cortex at rest predicts the positivity effect in older adults' memory. *Journal of Cognitive Neuroscience, 25*, 1206–1224. http://dx.doi.org/10.1162/jocn_a_00392

Salami, A., Eriksson, J., & Nyberg, L. (2012). Opposing effects of aging on large-scale brain systems for memory encoding and cognitive control. *The Journal of Neuroscience, 32*, 10749–10757. http://dx.doi.org/10.1523/JNEUROSCI.0278-12.2012

Salthouse, T. A. (2014). Why are there different age relations in cross-sectional and longitudinal comparisons of cognitive functioning? *Current Directions in Psychological Science, 23*, 252–256. http://dx.doi.org/10.1177/0963721414535212

Salthouse, T. A. (2015). Do cognitive interventions alter the rate of age-related cognitive change? *Intelligence, 53*, 86–91. http://dx.doi.org/10.1016/j.intell.2015.09.004

Schacter, D. L., Koutstaal, W., & Norman, K. A. (1997). False memories and aging. *Trends in Cognitive Sciences, 1*, 229–236. http://dx.doi.org/10.1016/S1364-6613(97)01068-1

Sestieri, C., Shulman, G. L., & Corbetta, M. (2017). The contribution of the human posterior parietal cortex to episodic memory. *Nature Reviews Neuroscience, 18*, 183–192. http://dx.doi.org/10.1038/nrn.2017.6

Simons, J. S., & Spiers, H. J. (2003). Prefrontal and medial temporal lobe interactions in long-term memory. *Nature Reviews Neuroscience, 4*, 637–648. http://dx.doi.org/10.1038/nrn1178

St. Jacques, P. L., Dolcos, F., & Cabeza, R. (2009). Effects of aging on functional connectivity of the amygdala for subsequent memory of negative pictures: A network analysis of functional magnetic resonance imaging data. *Psychological Science, 20*, 74–84. http://dx.doi.org/10.1111/j.1467-9280.2008.02258.x

Staresina, B. P., Henson, R. N., Kriegeskorte, N., & Alink, A. (2012). Episodic reinstatement in the medial temporal lobe. *The Journal of Neuroscience, 32*, 18150–18156. http://dx.doi.org/10.1523/JNEUROSCI.4156-12.2012

Uncapher, M. R., & Wagner, A. D. (2009). Posterior parietal cortex and episodic encoding: Insights from fMRI subsequent memory effects and dual-attention theory. *Neurobiology of Learning and Memory, 91*, 139–154. http://dx.doi.org/10.1016/j.nlm.2008.10.011

van Strien, N. M., Cappaert, N. L., & Witter, M. P. (2009). The anatomy of memory: An interactive overview of the parahippocampal-hippocampal network. *Nature Reviews Neuroscience, 10*, 272–282. http://dx.doi.org/10.1038/nrn2614

Vilberg, K. L., & Rugg, M. D. (2008). Memory retrieval and the parietal cortex: A review of evidence from a dual-process perspective. *Neuropsychologia, 46*, 1787–1799. http://dx.doi.org/10.1016/j.neuropsychologia.2008.01.004

Wagner, A. D., Shannon, B. J., Kahn, I., & Buckner, R. L. (2005). Parietal lobe contributions to episodic memory retrieval. *Trends in Cognitive Sciences, 9*, 445–453. http://dx.doi.org/10.1016/j.tics.2005.07.001

Waldinger, R. J., Kensinger, E. A., & Schulz, M. S. (2011). Neural activity, neural connectivity, and the processing of emotionally valenced information in older adults: Links with life satisfaction. *Cognitive, Affective & Behavioral Neuroscience, 11*, 426–436. http://dx.doi.org/10.3758/s13415-011-0039-9

Wang, T. H., Johnson, J. D., de Chastelaine, M., Donley, B. E., & Rugg, M. D. (2016). The effects of age on the neural correlates of recollection success, recollection-related cortical reinstatement, and post-retrieval monitoring. *Cerebral Cortex, 26*, 1698–1714. http://dx.doi.org/10.1093/cercor/bhu333

West, R. L. (1996). An application of prefrontal cortex function theory to cognitive aging. *Psychological Bulletin, 120*, 272–292. http://dx.doi.org/10.1037/0033-2909.120.2.272

Williams, K. N., & Kemper, S. (2010). Interventions to reduce cognitive decline in aging. *Journal of Psychosocial Nursing and Mental Health Services, 48*, 42–51. http://dx.doi.org/10.3928/02793695-20100331-03

Winecoff, A., Labar, K. S., Madden, D. J., Cabeza, R., & Huettel, S. A. (2011). Cognitive and neural contributors to emotion regulation in aging. *Social Cognitive and Affective Neuroscience, 6*, 165–176. http://dx.doi.org/10.1093/scan/nsq030

Xiao, X., Dong, Q., Gao, J., Men, W., Poldrack, R. A., & Xue, G. (2017). Transformed neural pattern reinstatement during episodic memory retrieval. *The Journal of Neuroscience, 37*, 2986–2998. http://dx.doi.org/10.1523/JNEUROSCI.2324-16.2017

Zajonc, R. B. (1980). Feeling and thinking. Preferences need no inferences. *American Psychologist, 35*, 151–175. http://dx.doi.org/10.1037/0003-066X.35.2.151

5

MOTIVATED MEMORY, LEARNING, AND DECISION-MAKING IN OLDER AGE: SHIFTS IN PRIORITIES AND GOALS

MARY B. HARGIS, ALEXANDER L. M. SIEGEL, AND ALAN D. CASTEL

Our goals across the lifespan often include gaining new knowledge, building relationships, and staying healthy. A younger adult's goals may center on his or her acquisition of knowledge to succeed in a career, whereas older adults' goals shift toward emotion regulation, and many may seek to build and maintain relationships with loved ones. However, motivation appears to be more complex than a single theory, such as lifespan theory of control (e.g., Heckhausen & Schulz, 1995) or socioemotional selectivity theory (e.g., Carstensen, Isaacowitz, & Charles, 1999), may suggest because older adults also pursue learning for the sake of acquiring knowledge or to satisfy their curiosity and spend time on hobbies such as bird-watching and traveling, and younger adults may spend time in romantic relationships seeking lifelong partners. Thus, younger and older adults are likely to have many

This work was supported in part by the National Institutes of Health (National Institute on Aging), Award Number R01AG044335. We thank Catherine Middlebrooks for her thoughts about reward salience and her comments on an earlier draft.

http://dx.doi.org/10.1037/0000143-006
The Aging Brain: Functional Adaptation Across Adulthood, G. R. Samanez-Larkin (Editor)

goals in common, but the pursuit of these goals may be different, based at least partially on the resources available to pursue such goals.

For instance, in the context of memory, younger and older adults likely have different performance abilities and functional goals. When we are faced with a large amount of information in our environment—when learning about a new medication in a doctor's office, for instance, or when learning a new language—our goals often influence what we attend to and whether we remember it later. A middle-aged or older adult's goal may be to learn Spanish phrases to help them communicate on an upcoming trip to South America with family or friends, while a younger adult in a Spanish language class could be motivated to learn Spanish verb conjugations to attain a high score on the next exam. Older adults may also learn new languages to keep their brain sharp and as a way to challenge themselves. In another context, an older adult may remember the most important information shared by his or her doctor (perhaps that which would lead to dangerous health outcomes), while a younger adult may have more processing resources at hand to remember large amounts of medical information.

In this chapter, we examine how and why motivation changes across the lifespan in the domains of learning, memory, and decision-making. We discuss how goals might change in light of perceived time horizons, particularly shifting toward social and emotional goals with age. However, we also explore the notion that curiosity and interest can be strong motivations to learn new information, in both formal and informal learning environments. We highlight in particular how younger and older people remember information that is made important to them either by the experimenter through the assignment of higher point values to certain items (e.g., Castel, 2008) or as a more practical feature of the stimuli (e.g., dangerous medical outcomes; Hargis & Castel, 2018), including a discussion of the critical role of attentional control during encoding and an exploration of the potential underlying neurocognitive mechanisms. We then explore decision-making and aging in a variety of contexts that reflect how goals and priorities may (or may not) change across the lifespan and how intrinsic versus extrinsic motivational factors may differentially affect cognitive processes during the aging process.

SHIFTING GOALS ACROSS THE LIFESPAN

Socioemotional selectivity theory (SST) focuses on the shift from knowledge acquisition goals in younger adulthood (typically college students under age 30) to emotion regulation goals in older adulthood (typically people over age 65). We perceive our future lifespan as more limited as we age, but also when younger adults experience endings such as graduation

(Ersner-Hershfield, Mikels, Sullivan, & Carstensen, 2008) or are suffering from a serious illness (Carstensen & Fredrickson, 1998). This recognition of the limited nature of the future causes individuals to focus more on emotion-related goals, such as maintaining relationships, and to expend more of their resources (cognitive and social) in pursuit of them. Emotion regulation, a processing component that is largely spared from age-related cognitive decline (Charles & Carstensen, 2007), is thought to be promoted by this shift toward emotional goals. Motivation is intricately tied to memory, especially in aging; if more of older adults' goals are related to emotion, their memory for emotional items may be preserved, in contrast to other declines in memory. For example, older adults more accurately remembered a product's slogan if it included an emotional component (e.g., "Capture those special moments" for a camera advertisement), compared with a nonemotional component (e.g., "Capture the unexplored world"; Fung & Carstensen, 2003). This difference was eliminated, however, if participants were first asked to imagine that a life-extending medication would allow them to live 20 years longer than they expected to live, indicating that perceived time horizons are in fact a major component in this type of processing. SST suggests that self-regulation influences memory and attention, such that cognitive resources in those domains are directed toward emotional information as goals shift in older adulthood.

Carstensen and Mikels (2005) argued that a key factor in processing information as we age is the *positivity effect*, which is closely linked to, and possibly caused by, the shift in goals accounted for by SST (see also Kan, Garrison, Drummey, Emmert, & Rogers, 2018). The positivity effect, or the tendency to focus on positive rather than negative information, is often present in older adults' recall of emotional information (Mather & Carstensen, 2005). Younger adults do not usually show this favoring of positive information; in fact, evidence suggests that they actually display a negativity bias in recall. In line with predictions made by SST, emotional information seems to be processed differently by younger and older adults; because older adults' time horizons are perceived as more limited and the goal of emotional well-being becomes more salient, information may be processed in such a way that positive information is maximized and negative information is minimized (Mather & Knight, 2005). Further, when younger adults are primed to think about their time horizons as limited, they recall positive information at a higher rate than if they think about expansive time horizons (Barber, Opitz, Martins, Sakaki, & Mather, 2016), suggesting a strong connection between perception of future time and the positivity effect. However, when older adults are unable to devote sufficient cognitive resources toward pursuing a goal (e.g., when completing an unrelated task simultaneously during study), the positivity effect is not present in recall. In fact, those who studied under dual-task conditions were actually more likely to recall negative information than positive (Mather & Knight, 2005).

Although the empirical evidence to support a shift in goals from knowledge acquisition to emotion regulation is strong (Carstensen, 1992; Carstensen, Isaacowitz, & Charles, 1999; Fung & Carstensen, 2004; for a more in-depth review of the brain-based mechanisms underlying SST, see Chapter 6, this volume), it is also worth examining the situations in which older adults continue to seek knowledge. Old age does not necessarily lead to a halt in pursuing goals that promote the acquisition of new information in daily lives. For example, older adults, when retired, may travel frequently. If an older adult is planning a trip to a new city to see family, this could be thought of as an emotion-based goal on its surface because the emotional connections with family members will likely be strengthened. However, the additional information that one may learn in preparing for this journey—from the best transportation options to the airport to information about the art history museum they wish to tour—can be considered as acquiring new knowledge that would be in the service of a broader, emotional goal. That is, older adults' lives are often not confined to only the pursuit of emotion regulation. Instead, goals that are less emotional are often pursued, such as learning trivia, becoming an expert birdwatcher, or completing crossword puzzles. Motivation, therefore, is a multifaceted domain in aging, and understanding what motivates older adults in their daily lives can be more complex than a single theory may suggest. We further note that motivation is a significant component in the construction of memory tasks (e.g., Jenkins, 1979), and this can be especially important when considering age-related differences and similarities in how younger and older adults might approach certain memory tasks.

Further, the motivation to engage in a behavior depends on the level of self-determination associated with completing said action. Motivations that are completely self-determined are deemed *intrinsic*, whereas motivations that stem from some external factor(s) are considered *extrinsic*. Actions that are intrinsically motivated arise due to an internal desire and are done so for one's own pleasure, often in the absence of any material reward (e.g., watching a favorite movie). Extrinsically motivated behaviors, on the other hand, arise when there is potential to earn some external reward (e.g., working overtime to earn extra money) or to avoid consequences associated with not completing said behavior (e.g., exercising to mitigate negative health outcomes). Many actions we take are associated with both intrinsic and extrinsic motivational factors that may differentially contribute to younger and older adults' behaviors. Take, for example, younger and older adults' participation in psychological experiments. In the authors' experience, younger adults tend to be extrinsically motivated to come into the lab to participate in experiments, generally to earn course credit (the earning of which is not usually dependent on task performance) or a small monetary reward. In contrast, older adults tend to be intrinsically motivated to participate for the most part: Although they also earn monetary rewards, the small sums that they do earn are often not the main factor in their motivation. Anecdotally, older adults often report being more interested in the "experience" of participating, "exercising" their memory, and being able to contribute to the advancement of science. It is important to note, however, that this is not the case in all circumstances; younger adults can be intrinsically motivated and older adults extrinsically motivated to participate, dependent on various factors, including personal interests, personality characteristics, and socioeconomic factors.

In the context of a classroom learning environment, intrinsically motivated students are more likely to engage in learning to challenge themselves, satisfy their curiosity, and become experts in the given domain (Pintrich, Smith, Garcia, & McKeachie, 1991). Extrinsically motivated students are interested in learning as a means to an end—that is, to earn some external reward (e.g., for external approval, for an increased grade point average). Prior research has examined the relationship between these two types of motivation and academic performance among younger undergraduates. Vansteenkiste and colleagues (2004) found that students assigned to an intrinsic motivation condition were more persistent and ultimately received higher grades than students in an extrinsic motivation condition. Bye, Pushkar, and Conway (2007) extended this research to aging by including in their sample "traditional" undergraduate students (those aged 21 years or younger), as well as "nontraditional" undergraduate students (those aged 28 years or older). Participants ranging in age from 18 to 60 years completed measurements of intrinsic and extrinsic motivation to learn, interest in particular topics, and emotional well-being. Nontraditional (older) students reported more intrinsic motivation to learn (e.g., learning to challenge themselves, satisfy their curiosity, or master a certain topic) than traditional (younger) students, and intrinsic motivation was related to positive affect in both age groups. An earlier study by Donohue and Wong (1997) using a sample ranging in age from 19 to 57 years old also suggested that nontraditional students demonstrate higher achievement motivation than traditional students. Further, Wolfgang and Dowling (1981) suggested that older students (i.e., older than 18–22 years) are strongly motivated by cognitive interest in the subjects they study and weakly motivated by social relationships (e.g., "to make new friends") or external expectations (e.g., "to carry out the recommendation of some authority," p. 642), providing further evidence in support of the possibility that, in some cases, older learners seek knowledge for the sake of attaining it (e.g., McGillivray, Murayama, & Castel, 2015). Prior work has proposed the linkage of emotion, motivation, and cognition among young students (e.g., Meyer & Turner, 2006), and the effects of these components are also important to understand in older learners.

In a complementary line of research, Kim and Merriam (2004) recruited participants from a Learning in Retirement institute to determine the factors underlying their decisions to seek knowledge. According to this survey, interest in learning information was the strongest motivator in attending this institute, followed in strength by social contact, which is in line with previous work regarding the increasing importance of socially and emotionally relevant goals with age (e.g., Carstensen & Mikels, 2005). Somewhat surprisingly, among the lowest endorsed were items that explicitly included emotional-social goals, such as "to keep up with my children/others in my family," while items tapping into information-seeking goals such as "to acquire general knowledge" and "to seek knowledge for its own sake" were among the highest endorsed. Therefore, although pursuing emotional and social goals is undoubtedly important to older adults, their own interest in acquiring knowledge seems to also be a strong motivator, at least in the domain of learning in structured educational courses. In fact, 30% of American older adults participated in some sort of educational program in 1999 (Kim & Merriam, 2004), including those within universities and senior centers, and this percentage is likely to have grown since then with the advent of online educational resources and more senior-friendly university-based programs.

Some of the goals we set, however, are not possible for us to attain. Wrosch, Scheier, Miller, Schulz, and Carver (2003) examined the self-reported ability of younger and older adults to disengage from goals that were proven unattainable and instead engage with other, more attainable goals. For example, if one loses his or her job, the goal of affording a luxurious vacation this year may be put on hold or disengaged from entirely, but other goals such as finding a new source of income or saving more money may become more relevant. Being able to disengage from an impossible goal is a valuable skill, as is the ability to reengage with the next goal that is attainable. Wrosch et al. found that older adults, compared with younger adults, reported more ease in disengaging from unattainable goals and shifting instead to more realistic goals. This can be considered adaptive because older adults recognized that continuing to pursue an unattainable goal would waste resources. The interplay between interest in a goal and its pursuit is worth considering: Perhaps older adults are less able to disengage from emotion regulation or other valuable goals than those in which they do not have a reported interest, which would demonstrate that interest in a set of actions is not always beneficial and can sometimes be detrimental to effective pursuit of said actions.

One's goals can also affect his or her allocation of attention to certain information. Older adults tend to exhibit general impairments in selective and divided attention, as well as switching attention between multiple sources of information, thought to be due to a slowing of information processing (Salthouse, 1995) and a decline in processing resources that occur with advancing age (Craik & Byrd, 1982; for reviews of the effects of aging on attention, see McDowd & Shaw, 1999, as well as Kennedy & Mather, Chapter 2, this volume).

MOTIVATION TO ATTEND TO AND REMEMBER INFORMATION

Although older adults show general deficits in attentional resources, there is evidence that they can effectively allocate attention toward information they deem important. As previously discussed, SST describes older adults' shift to the pursuance of emotion regulation goals from knowledge acquisition goals earlier in life (Carstensen et al., 1999). This overarching goal of emotion regulation is then likely to influence older adults' attention. In one study, younger and older adults were shown two faces on a computer screen, one of which had a neutral expression and the other an emotional expression (positive or negative in various trials; Mather & Carstensen, 2003). After being shown the pair of faces, a dot appeared on one side, and participants were asked to indicate on which side (left or right) the dot was located as quickly as possible. Younger adults' response time did not differ across valence conditions, whereas older adults responded significantly faster for positive faces relative to neutral faces and significantly slower for negative faces relative to neutral faces, which was interpreted as an attentional bias toward the positive information. Similarly, when presented with various models of cars, older adults were more likely to pay attention to the positive features and less likely to pay attention to the negative features, compared with younger adults, indicating that this attentional positivity bias may also be present in more naturalistic settings (Mather, Knight, & McCaffrey, 2005).

When we are faced with more information in our environment than we can hope to remember, we might engage in a strategy to remember that which is most important to us or that which will be most likely to help us achieve our goal(s). Outside of the lab, this may occur when we make decisions about which items we need to bring on a trip: Our toothbrush seems important, but may be less so compared to our passport (McGillivray & Castel, 2017). *Value-directed remembering* (VDR) involves the allocation of more cognitive resources toward remembering important information (e.g., to bring my passport) and less of those resources toward remembering less important information (e.g., to bring my toothbrush; Castel, 2008).

Inside the lab, Castel and colleagues (Castel, Balota, & McCabe, 2009; Castel, Benjamin, Craik, & Watkins, 2002; Castel, Farb, & Craik, 2007) have developed a paradigm that engages such strategies, most commonly using words paired with point values. In the original VDR task (adapted from Watkins & Bloom, 1999), participants are presented with a list of words (often 10–12 words) paired with point values. If participants were to see 12 words, as in Castel et al. (2002), those point values would be from 1 to 12. Participants are told that their goal is to maximize their score, which would be calculated by summing the point values associated with the words they later recall. Study-test phases are repeated for multiple trials, with the hypothesis that strategy use or selectivity (or both) may change with task experience. Feedback is often given in the form of the amount of points associated with the recalled words. Older adults remember less information than younger adults overall, but they tend to recall the items with the highest values equally as well as younger adults when given task experience. Both age groups also tend to be more selective across the task, perhaps as they form appropriate strategies to remember the highest value items. This finding has also been extended to the visuospatial memory domain, suggesting that older adults' ability to selectively attend to and remember high-value information may generalize to areas other than verbal memory (Siegel & Castel, 2018).

If one were to consider only age-related cognitive deficits, particularly in working memory and processing speed (e.g., Salthouse, 1995), the finding that older adults remember less information overall would not be novel. However, when given this goal-oriented framework, older adults can be just as selective (and sometimes more so) than younger adults in remembering the highest value information (Castel, 2008; Castel et al., 2002). Even when the items presented are emotionally salient (e.g., the words *tragedy* or *joyful*), older adults retain cognitive control over their memory and are able to remember what is valuable (Eich & Castel, 2016).

Further evidence for older adults' ability to effectively allocate attention toward information that is important for one's goals stems from research investigating attentional control in a VDR task. Castel and colleagues (2009) investigated whether younger adults, healthy older adults, and older adults with a diagnosis of Alzheimer's disease (AD) could selectively allocate attention toward (and thus later remember) high-value information. AD is typically associated with severe memory impairments, but there is also evidence that these impairments are at least in part due to a reduction in attentional control (Balota & Faust, 2001). Not only did participants with AD recall less information overall, they were also significantly less selective toward high-value information than the healthy older adult controls. This decrease in selectivity in individuals with AD was attributed to impairments in the ability to strategically allocate attention at the initial point of encoding. Importantly, participants with AD were still somewhat selective, remembering a greater proportion of high- than low-value information; however, they were significantly less selective than healthy older adults indicating an issue with effectively allocating attention to execute a value-based strategy but not with recognizing the need for one. Additionally, younger individuals with impairments in attention were unable to perform efficiently on this VDR task (Castel, Lee, Humphreys, & Moore, 2011). As such, healthy older adults' ability to demonstrate optimal selectivity in this context suggests that they are able to effectively allocate attentional resources to information that they are motivated to remember.

Although examining the recall of words paired with point values has been extremely useful in examining value-directed strategies, other VDR work has used perhaps more ecologically valid stimuli. Remembering information about medications, for example, can be important but difficult, especially for older adults (for an example using medication stimuli, see Hargis & Castel, 2018). Older adults tend to struggle in remembering specific events or details (Zacks & Hasher, 2006) and associated items (Naveh-Benjamin, 2000), both of which could harm memory accuracy after leaving a doctor's office with information about a new diagnosis or medication. Friedman, McGillivray, Murayama, and Castel (2015) suggested that "subjective" selectivity—that is, the act of attending to information that is important based on the individual's goals or the setting of the task—could affect memory differently from "objective" selectivity imposed by the experimenter (e.g., by random assignment of point values to items). Relatedly, McGillivray and Castel (2017) allowed participants to assign point values to the items they were to take on a trip, such as a passport and a toothbrush, and found that items that were assigned high point values were in fact recalled more accurately than those assigned low point values.

In addition, recent work by Hargis and Castel (2017) examined how younger and older adults remember valuable social information. Participants studied a series of face–name–occupation items of differing social value to the participant, based on their likelihood of interacting with that person again (see Figure 5.1 for example stimuli) before being tested on that information with four cycles of study and recall, and were ultimately given a final cued recall test. When both age groups were given 3 seconds to study each item, there were no significant differences between younger and older adults' recall accuracy of the most valuable information, and both groups recalled this information relatively accurately (see Figure 5.2). Age differences in accuracy were present in recall of the lowest value information: Younger adults largely outperformed older adults when asked to recall the information about people whom they would not meet again. The likelihood of remembering information about people we meet may in part be due to our motivation to remember those who we consider important; older adults are not subject to established age-related deficits in associative memory when recalling this important information (Naveh-Benjamin, 2000; see also Fung, Lu, &

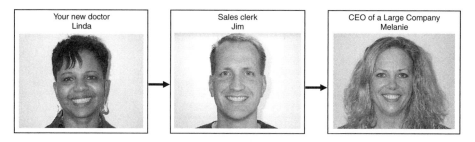

Figure 5.1. Example stimuli from Hargis and Castel (2017) using face stimuli from Minear and Park (2004). There were 20 items that varied with respect to the likelihood of the participant interacting with the given person again (e.g., one's new doctor was considered personally important due to the likelihood of future interaction). Younger and older adults studied each item for 3 seconds before four free-recall tests for name and occupation information and a final and cued-recall test. From "A Lifespan Database of Adult Facial Stimuli," by M. Minear and D. C. Park, 2004, *Behavior Research Methods, Instruments, & Computers, 36*, pp. 630–633. Copyright 2004 by Springer Nature. Adapted with permission.

Isaacowitz, 2018), but deficits do emerge for low-value information, similarly to other VDR tasks (e.g., Castel et al., 2002).

However, memory for a short-term task goal (e.g., recalling this information on the next free recall test) may differ from memory for a task to be done in the future (e.g., mailing in postcards to the experimenter on a specified date; Einstein & McDaniel, 1990). When tested inside the lab, older adults' prospective memory (PM), or memory for things to be done in the future, is often less accurate than younger adults'. When given outside-the-laboratory tasks such as mailing in a postcard, older adults often perform more accurately than younger adults, creating what is known as the "age PM paradox" (Phillips, Henry, & Martin, 2008). This paradox may be better understood when considering how motivation changes with age. More recent work using daily diaries has shown that older adults' PM is more accurate than younger adults' in social and health situations (e.g., "pick up grandchild after kindergarten" or "do one hour of walking"; Schnitzspahn et al., 2016, p. 448), which may reflect older adults' increased motivation to pursue social and health-related goals. An older adult's motivation to perform well on a PM task outside the lab may be more powerful (or perhaps different) from a younger adult's, leading to differences in PM performance. That is, perhaps the reason why younger adults tend not to have superior PM once they leave the lab is because they are not sufficiently motivated to do so. Aberle, Rendell, Rose, McDaniel, and Kliegel (2010) used the possibility of

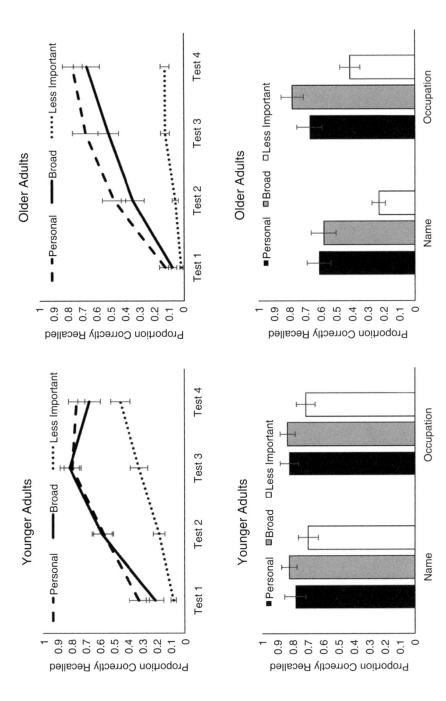

Figure 5.2. The proportion of personally important, broadly important, and less important information correctly recalled by younger adults (left) and older adults (right) in the four free recall tests (top) and final cued recall test (bottom). These results suggest that, given 3 seconds to study each item, participants in both age groups are able to remember the important information with a relatively high level of accuracy, whereas younger adults do perform better than older adults in recalling less important information. Error bars reflect standard error of the mean. Adapted from "Younger and Older Adults' Associative Memory for Social Information: The Role of Information Importance," by M. B. Hargis and A. D. Castel, 2017, *Psychology and Aging, 32,* p. 327. Copyright 2017 by the American Psychological Association.

winning a small lottery to enhance extrinsic motivation to complete a PM task. There were no age differences in accuracy on this task, but the motivational manipulation led to more accurate performance among younger adults compared with no mention of this lottery, and it did not affect older adults' PM performance. This suggests that older adults' completion of such tasks does not depend on an extrinsic monetary incentive to do so, but younger adults' accuracy benefits from such an incentive.

Curiosity and Other Motivations

An individual's subjective interest in acquiring certain types of information over others is an important motivational factor and should not be overlooked. In fact, age-related memory differences can be overcome—or at least reduced—when older adult participants are interested in the information (see Zacks & Hasher, 2006), possibly related to the reduced load on attentional resources that is needed to study interesting material (McDaniel, Waddill, Finstad, & Bourg, 2000). McGillivray and colleagues (2015) examined how subjective interest and metacognitive judgments related to immediate recall of the to-be-learned information, as well as recall at a 1-week delay. Younger and older adults were presented with trivia questions and asked to indicate which ones they felt confident in answering correctly. Following are three of the trivia questions asked to younger and older adults[1]:

- What is the only planet in our solar system that rotates clockwise?
- What note do most American car horns beep in?
- What world capital city has the fewest cinemas in relation to its population?

Participants were not told in advance of any memory test, only that they were to guess the answers and rate their curiosity and their confidence in knowing the answer. Once the answer was presented, participants rated how interesting they found the information that they learned, as well as how likely they thought they would remember the answer at a later time. At the end of the day's testing session, participants completed a surprise cued recall test on half the questions, in which they were presented with the trivia question and asked to remember the answer, and those who responded incorrectly on a particular question were told the correct answer. After a 1-week delay, participants were tested on the other half of the questions. There were no age-related differences in recall at the immediate test or at the 1-week delay, which was somewhat surprising given prior work showing differential effects of delay on younger and older adults' memory (e.g., Zacks, Radvansky, &

---

[1]Answers: Venus; F; and Cairo, Egypt.

Hasher, 1996). Overall, performance after a 1-week delay was significantly less accurate than the immediate test, as expected. Interestingly, older adults' recall was more strongly predicted by the ratings they gave after learning the answers to the trivia questions, whereas younger adults' recall was less strongly predicted by this factor. This underscores the importance of interest in older adults' long-term learning of information. Interest may affect attention because resources are diverted away from items in which the participant is not interested and toward more interesting items, which has notable implications for learning in other domains (e.g., learning Spanish for an upcoming trip to South America versus learning Spanish because you read that learning a new language is good for your cognitive health, although these might evoke different levels of interest from different people, based on their goals and prior knowledge).

Loewenstein (1994) argued that a positive relationship between curiosity and knowledge is a major component in establishing expertise in a particular domain because people become "progressively more curious" (p. 94) about the subject matter they are learning. Interest, as explored by Hidi (1990), is not to be underestimated as a motivation for learning new things. In fact, Hidi argued that interest-based activities involve motivation, attention, increased knowledge, and value. Although Hidi noted that applying individual interest in the educational domain by tailoring curricula to students' interests is difficult, interest may be a more applicable tool for an older adult learner who is empowered to seek out information. That is, older adults may benefit by seeking out interesting material because the attentional control problems that they may face in other areas of learning (i.e., information that they are asked to memorize for a laboratory task, which may not inherently interesting to them) may be greatly decreased, thus improving later recall of the information. Relatedly, higher need for cognition, or the extent to which one values and pursues cognitively demanding activities (Cacioppo, Petty, Feinstein, & Jarvis, 1996), is associated with higher levels of cognitive performance in older age (Salthouse, 2014).

Verbal knowledge may be maintained and used effectively in older age; on tests of vocabulary, younger and older adults often perform equally well (Verhaeghen, 2003). This knowledge is often put to use in proofreading e-mails, letters, or other documents, but one's interest in the material being proofread may vary. Hargis et al. (2017) examined younger and older adults' performance on a proofreading task and found that younger and older adults were similarly motivated to perform the task (as measured by self-report Likert-scale ratings) but that older adults found the passages more interesting overall than did younger adults. Neither proofreading accuracy nor comprehension of the text differed between younger and older adults (cf. Connelly, Hasher, & Zacks, 1991; Stine-Morrow, Shake, Miles, & Noh,

2006), suggesting that interest in the materials may play an important role in performing well on this task.

Noting that memory is "extraordinarily complicated" (p. 430), Jenkins (1979) created a model of how discrete aspects of memory experiments can influence performance, with a particular goal of conceptualizing how these variables interacted with one another in the construction and implementation of memory experiments (see also Roediger, 2008). The original Problem Pyramid (see Figure 5.3) contained the following variables: subjects (including one's abilities and knowledge), orienting tasks (including what the experimenter included as instructions and apparatus), materials (including the organization and sequence of stimuli), and criterial tasks (including the

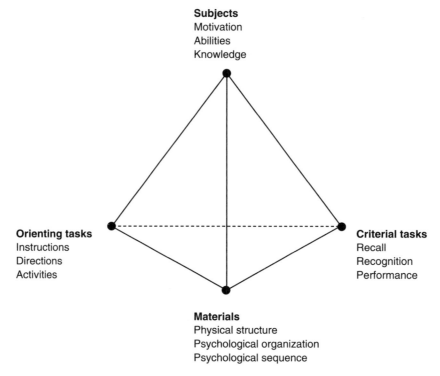

Subjects
Motivation
Abilities
Knowledge

Orienting tasks
Instructions
Directions
Activities

Criterial tasks
Recall
Recognition
Performance

Materials
Physical structure
Psychological organization
Psychological sequence

Figure 5.3. Jenkins's (1979) tetrahedral model of memory experiments, adapted to include "Motivation" within the variable "Subjects." Jenkins suggested that the variables at the vertices interact with each other in significant ways and that experimenters should consider them when designing tasks. We suggest that the explicit inclusion of "Motivation" within the variable "Subjects" reflects its importance in the domain of memory and cognitive aging. From "Four Points to Remember: A Tetrahedral Model of Memory Experiments," by J. J. Jenkins, 1979, in L. S. Cermak and F. I. M. Craik (Eds.), *Levels of processing in human memory* (p. 432), 1979, Hillsdale, NJ: Erlbaum. Copyright 2006 by Taylor & Francis. Adapted with permission.

construction of free- and cued-recall tests). Jenkins suggested that these variables interact with each other in meaningful ways and each should be carefully considered when designing memory tasks. This model has not yet been explicitly extended to the study of cognitive aging and how older adults may be motivated in memory experiments. Motivation can vary quasi-experimentally (as younger and older adults may approach tasks with different goals at hand, including knowledge pursuit and emotion regulation), or the experimenter can vary motivation with between- or within-subjects task construction. Emphasizing motivation in the overall "subjects" variable allows for the consideration of motivation as an important interacting factor with performance and for the examination of how motivation interacts with the other variables in the model. We also note that a participant's background, career, and culture may also influence task performance and motivation. Future research exploring the effects of motivational factors on memory may consider this model in guiding research questions and experimental design.

Reward Salience

One factor that motivates younger and older adults alike is the potential of earning a reward. In many cases, the anticipation of obtaining a reward can enhance explicit memory. Prior research has demonstrated that information associated with a reward may be better consolidated in memory through the activation of dopaminergic reward systems in the midbrain and striatum (for a review, see Shohamy & Adcock, 2010). In a typical task investigating the effects of reward salience on memory, younger adults were shown various scenes preceded by a low-value (e.g., $0.01) or high-value (e.g., $5.00) reward cue indicating the amount that they could later earn by correctly remembering that scene (Adcock, Thangavel, Whitfield-Gabrieli, Knutson, & Gabrieli, 2006). Participants studied the scenes while neural activity was measured using functional magnetic resonance imaging (fMRI). Results indicated that after a 24-hour delay, participants had better memory for the high-value scenes. Further, during encoding, greater activation in the ventral tegmental area (VTA) in the midbrain, the nucleus accumbens (NAcc) in the ventral striatum, and the hippocampus was associated with those high-value scenes that were later remembered, but not forgotten high-value scenes. These findings suggest that the presence of a high reward may increase activation in the midbrain and striatum, which may in turn enhance memory for associated information by increasing hippocampal dopamine release before the encoding of that information.

Advancing age is linked to a decline in dopaminergic modulation (Bäckman, Nyberg, Lindenberger, Li, & Farde, 2006; Kaasinen et al., 2000), and many of the cognitive impairments associated with age have been associated with a degradation of dopaminergic systems (Volkow et al., 1998). As such, it is important to determine whether the effects of reward as a motivational factor on memory are consistent throughout old age. Spaniol, Schain, and Bowen (2014) examined reward-enhanced memory in the context of aging. Using a similar paradigm to Adcock et al. (2006) in younger and older adults, Spaniol and colleagues found that older adults showed a similar pattern to their younger adult counterparts, remembering more high- than low-value scenes after a 24-hour delay, demonstrating an age-independent effect of reward anticipation on intentional episodic memory formation. Importantly, although no neuroimaging data were obtained in this particular study, the authors considered this evidence for reward-enhanced, hippocampus-dependent memory consolidation persisting into older adulthood.

Further, the activation of dopaminergic reward systems has been proposed as a possible explanation for VDR effects, at least in younger adults. Although the previously discussed research used monetary reward as a motivational factor, other research has demonstrated similar effects using a point-based reward system. Cohen, Rissman, Suthana, Castel, and Knowlton (2014) examined the neural correlates of VDR, using pairs of words and point values that were tested via free recall. Younger adults engaged in a VDR task while undergoing fMRI. Similar to results obtained when using monetary rewards, Cohen and colleagues found greater activation in dopaminergic reward regions (i.e., the VTA and NAcc) on high-value trials, even at immediate testing. These results indicate that episodic memory can benefit from reward anticipation even when there is no opportunity for memory consolidation, as previous work found enhanced memory for high-value information only after a 24-hour delay (Adcock et al., 2006; Spaniol et al., 2014). In addition, there was greater activation in the left ventrolateral prefrontal cortex (VLPFC; an area associated with deep semantic processing) when encoding high-value words and a significant correlation of activity in this area with a measure of memory selectivity, suggesting that explicit use of deep semantic processing strategies may also contribute to the selective encoding of high-value information in the context of this task. The same group of researchers extended this research to aging by including an older adult sample and found that similar semantic processing regions were associated with memory selectivity in older adults but that the pattern of activation in such areas differed from younger adults (Cohen, Rissman, Suthana, Castel, & Knowlton, 2016). Specifically, they found that older adults were less likely to engage areas associated with semantic processing (e.g., the left VLPFC) during the presentation of low-value information, whereas younger adults were more likely to engage these areas during the presentation of high-value information (see Figure 5.4). Interestingly, activation in dopaminergic reward regions was not modulated by the value of information in older adults. These findings

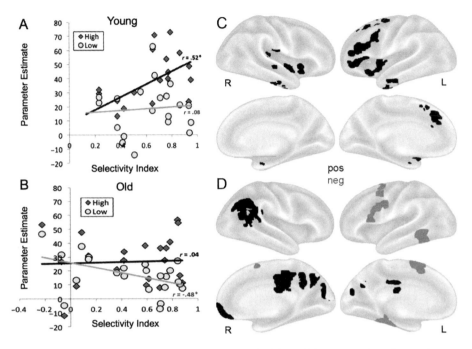

Figure 5.4. Results obtained from younger and older adults on a value-directed remembering task while undergoing functional magnetic resonance imaging depict correlations between a measure of memory selectivity and brain areas associated with semantic processing (i.e., the left ventrolateral prefrontal cortex). On the left, (A) higher memory selectivity in younger adults is associated with higher activation in such areas for high-value but not low-value information, and (B) higher memory selectivity in older adults is associated with lower activation in semantic processing areas for low-value but not high-value information. Activation in dopaminergic reward regions (i.e., the nucleus accumbens and ventral tegmental area) was not significantly modulated by value in older adults. On the right, regions associated with correlations between brain activity during encoding and the selectivity index for (C) high-value information in younger adults and (D) for low-value information in older adults. From "Effects of Aging on Value-Directed Modulation of Semantic Network Activity During Verbal Learning," by M. S. Cohen, J. Rissman, N. A. Suthana, A. D. Castel, and B. J. Knowlton, 2016, *NeuroImage, 125*, pp. 1055, 1058. Copyright 2016 by Elsevier. Adapted with permission.

highlight the importance of semantic processing areas but call into question the role of dopaminergic reward systems, at least for older adults, in VDR tasks. As such, future research should examine the extent to which activation in dopaminergic reward systems and engagement of frontotemporal regions during explicit strategy use contribute to older adults' selectivity on these reward-based tasks. Given that older adults often show equivalent (or in some cases, enhanced) selectivity on VDR tasks (Castel et al., 2002, 2007, 2009), future research should investigate the extent to which activation in dopaminergic reward systems and engagement of frontotemporal regions during explicit strategy use contribute to older adults' selectivity on these reward-based tasks.

MOTIVATION AND MAKING DECISIONS

To achieve our goals, we must make a series of decisions (e.g., deciding to enroll in a class at a local community college to learn a new language with the ultimate goal of communicating, staying cognitively active, or both); the reasons why and the ways in which these decisions are made may change across the lifespan. Although some research has shown that younger and older adults perform equivalently on many decision-making tasks (Kovalchik, Camerer, Grether, Plott, & Allman, 2005), there is also reason to expect that older adults may value time and money differently than younger adults.

Age-related changes in goals influence how we think about the future: Older adults are less likely to commit the sunk cost fallacy (i.e., older participants are not likely to persist with a failed investment; Strough, Mehta, McFall, & Schuller, 2008), which is thought to be related to their limited time horizons and perhaps their tendency to focus on positive, rather than negative, information. Strough et al. (2008) suggested that, due at least in part to this positivity effect, older adults are more likely than younger adults to weigh losses and gains somewhat similarly, thus leading to their lower likelihood of demonstrating the sunk cost fallacy. That is, an older adult is more likely to make the normatively correct decision—for example, spending the same amount of time watching a movie that you do not enjoy whether you paid for it or not.

More recent work suggests that the perception of limited time horizons contributes to this type of decision-making. Strough, Schlosnagle, Karns, Lemaster, and Pichayayothin (2014) limited younger adults' perception of their future time by asking them to imagine having a critical illness that does not allow them much longer to live. This group's decisions about sunk cost scenarios were compared with a group that received an expansive time horizon manipulation and a control group. The participants whose time horizons were limited were significantly less likely to demonstrate the sunk cost fallacy than the expansive and control groups (the lack of difference between the expansive and control groups was explained by noting that younger adults often already have expansive time horizons, and thus the manipulation may not have changed much about their decision-making). Similarly, another study examined older adults' decision-making process when purchasing a new car and found that older adults considered fewer brands, dealers, and models than younger adults and that older adults were more likely to repurchase a brand of car that they had previously owned (Lambert-Pandraud, Laurent, & Lapersonne, 2005). Interpreted via an SST lens (Carstensen et al., 1999), older adults were motivated to repurchase from a particular brand in an effort to maintain and give priority to a close relationship formed with that brand, compared with a new, unfamiliar brand. These findings suggest that the positivity effect and the perceived expansiveness of the future may affect how goals are pursued in a variety of domains.

Prosocial behavior, particularly the giving of time or money, is thought to increase with age and is correlated with well-being across the lifespan (McAdams, de St. Aubin, & Logan, 1993; see also Okun & Schultz, 2003). For older adults, deciding to act prosocially is connected with having a sense of meaning in life (Midlarsky & Hannah, 1989) and is also positively related to social connectedness (Choi & Chou, 2010). Younger adults are often thought to choose to donate time or money because of the personal benefits attained (one can boost one's self-esteem and résumé by volunteering; Choi & Chou, 2010). Bjälkebring, Västfjäll, Dickert, and Slovic (2016) suggested that the motivation to give to charity is motivated at least in part by a positivity bias when considering both past and future donations, such that older adults experience more positivity when giving, and younger adults experience both negative and positive feelings while making decisions about donating. Emotional variables are important in charitable giving but may not entirely explain older adults' decisions, and future research can investigate how, for example, gist-based processing and VDR in older age can affect these decisions (Hargis & Oppenheimer, 2016).

Other research also demonstrates that older adults' decisions about their own health care may be affected by this shift from knowledge acquisition to emotion regulation. Various studies have found that older adults are less likely to request additional information about potential cancer treatment options and make more immediate, less informed decisions both in experimental laboratory scenarios with healthy participants and in actual cancer patient samples (Cassileth, Zupkis, Sutton-Smith, & March, 1980; Meyer, Russo, & Talbot, 1995). These results have been explained, in part, by older adults' tendency to avoid potentially negative knowledge acquisition to maintain emotional well-being (Löckenhoff & Carstensen, 2004). Unsurprisingly, this lack of desire to gain health-related knowledge has been shown to lead to negative health consequences (Morrell, Park, & Poon, 1989; Willis, Dolan, & Bertrand, 1999).

With regard to health-related decision-making, there is also considerable evidence that older adults are more likely to avoid making a decision and instead defer the choice to their physicians or relatives both in laboratory settings (Curley, Eraker, & Yates, 1984; Finucane et al., 2002) and in real-life situations (Beisecker, 1988; Cassileth et al., 1980; Petrisek, Laliberte, Allen,

& Mor, 1997). Given that the decision-making process can elicit negative emotions, especially when the decision has personally relevant consequences (Houston, Sherrill-Mittleman, & Weeks, 2001), it is not surprising that older adults may seek to avoid such processes to maintain successful emotion regulation. It is important to note, however, that this may also represent an adaptive feature of older adults' decision-making, in that they are more likely to delegate a potentially life-dependent decision to someone (e.g., a physician, surgeon, or other health care professional) who has a deeper understanding about the situation and is ultimately more likely to make a beneficial decision.

When older adults do make health-related decisions, however, the manner in which they evaluate their options appears to affect how successful their decisions are. Mikels and colleagues (2010) asked younger and older adults to evaluate and select an option from a list of various fictitious health care options. Each option was presented with a set of attributes, some of which were positive (e.g., "It takes little time to get reimbursed") and some of which were negative (e.g., "No 24-hour phone hotline is available"). In addition to a control group, participants were either instructed to base their decisions on their emotional reactions to the listed options or to base their decisions on the options' specific details. Older adults selected the "better" option (i.e., a higher ratio of positive to negative attributes associated with a particular health care plan, physician, medical treatment, or homecare aid) more frequently in the emotion-focused condition and control conditions, compared with the detail-focused condition. Younger adults, on the other hand, had the best performance in the detail-focused condition.

Other research has demonstrated that focusing on emotional information when making health care decisions may only be beneficial for older adults who themselves are in good health but not for those in poorer health. In a study by English and Carstensen (2015), older adults provided self-report measures of physical health and then reviewed information related to hypothetical health-related decisions (choosing one's physician and health plan) and non–health-related decisions (choosing one's car and neighbor). Each option had characteristics that varied in quality from very good (e.g., very good preventative care associated with a particular health plan) to very poor (e.g., very poor riding comfort associated with a particular car). The results indicated that when making health-related decisions, older adults in good health showed a positivity bias by reviewing more of the positive characteristics, whereas older adults in poor health did not show this bias. Interestingly, this difference in older adults' health did not affect reviewing of characteristics associated with non–health-related decisions, with both groups showing a positivity bias. Taken together, these results suggest that older adults' health-related decision-making may benefit from an emotion-related focus but that personal characteristics such as physical health may also determine what information older adults consider when making health-related decisions.

CONCLUSION

It is clear that as we become older, our motivations and goals tend to change. Underlying much of the research on motivation is the notion that we tend to pursue more socioemotional goals as we age, and with this comes an increase in focusing on positive information (a shift present in memory recall, decision-making, and several other domains). Whereas younger adults may focus more on acquiring knowledge, older adults often seek to build and maintain relationships with loved ones. This pattern is related to a positivity bias in older adults' attention allocation and recall, such that negative information is not often prioritized and positive information is; older adults tend to pursue goals in line with this preference. Not all of older adults' motivations are primarily social and emotional in nature, however; many pursue knowledge for the sake of attaining it or to satisfy their curiosity. Younger and older learners tend be differentially motivated by intrinsic and extrinsic factors, with older learners perhaps more motivated by internal factors (e.g., learning with the goal of challenging themselves) than their younger adult counterparts who may be more motivated by external factors (e.g., learning with the goal of increasing their grade point average). Studies among older undergraduate students and older adults enrolled in lifelong learning programs suggest that learning in a classroom context is appealing to many older people, and perhaps this trend will increase with the increasing accessibility of learning at home via virtual courses given online.

In some goal contexts, it seems that older adults are able to allocate their attention toward information that will help them succeed, even in light of age-related deficits in processing resources. When the information at hand is valuable (e.g., words associated with high point values or social information that we are likely to use again), older adults perform as well as younger adults on recall tests, especially once given task experience. Memory differences are indeed present, such that younger adults often recall more information overall than older adults do, but memory selectivity seems to be possible for older people in several types of tasks.

Certainly, younger and older adults are motivated by a variety of factors to engage in a set of particular behaviors, remember certain information, or make a particular decision. Further research should continue to explore the various intrinsic and extrinsic motivational factors that affect cognition across the lifespan and in what situations these may or may not differ with increasing age. With a greater understanding of the shifts in priorities and goals that occur in later life, we can both further theoretical understanding of cognitive aging and apply this understanding to real-world situations to investigate older adults' cognition in a variety of contexts.

REFERENCES

Aberle, I., Rendell, P. G., Rose, N. S., McDaniel, M. A., & Kliegel, M. (2010). The age prospective memory paradox: Young adults may not give their best outside of the lab. *Developmental Psychology, 46*, 1444–1453. http://dx.doi.org/10.1037/a0020718

Adcock, R. A., Thangavel, A., Whitfield-Gabrieli, S., Knutson, B., & Gabrieli, J. D. E. (2006). Reward-motivated learning: Mesolimbic activation precedes memory formation. *Neuron, 50*, 507–517. http://dx.doi.org/10.1016/j.neuron.2006.03.036

Bäckman, L., Nyberg, L., Lindenberger, U., Li, S. C., & Farde, L. (2006). The correlative triad among aging, dopamine, and cognition: Current status and future prospects. *Neuroscience and Biobehavioral Reviews, 30*, 791–807. http://dx.doi.org/10.1016/j.neubiorev.2006.06.005

Balota, D. A., & Faust, M. E. (2001). Attention in dementia of the Alzheimer's type. In F. Bolla & S. F. Cappa (Eds.), *Handbook of neuropsychology: Vol. 6. Aging and dementia* (2nd ed., pp. 51–80). New York, NY: Elsevier Science.

Barber, S. J., Opitz, P. C., Martins, B., Sakaki, M., & Mather, M. (2016). Thinking about a limited future enhances the positivity of younger and older adults' recall: Support for socioemotional selectivity theory. *Memory & Cognition, 44*, 869–882. http://dx.doi.org/10.3758/s13421-016-0612-0

Beisecker, A. E. (1988). Aging and the desire for information and input in medical decisions: Patient consumerism in medical encounters. *The Gerontologist, 28*, 330–335. http://dx.doi.org/10.1093/geront/28.3.330

Bjälkebring, P., Västfjäll, D., Dickert, S., & Slovic, P. (2016, June 15). Greater emotional gain from giving in older adults: Age-related positivity bias in charitable giving. *Frontiers in Psychology, 7*. Retrieved from https://www.frontiersin.org/articles/10.3389/fpsyg.2016.00846/full

Bye, D., Pushkar, D., & Conway, M. (2007). Motivation, interest, and positive affect in traditional and nontraditional undergraduate students. *Adult Education Quarterly, 57*, 141–158. http://dx.doi.org/10.1177/0741713606294235

Cacioppo, J. T., Petty, R. E., Feinstein, J. A., & Jarvis, W. B. G. (1996). Dispositional differences in cognitive motivation: The life and times of individuals varying in need for cognition. *Psychological Bulletin, 119*, 197–253. http://dx.doi.org/10.1037/0033-2909.119.2.197

Carstensen, L. L. (1992). Social and emotional patterns in adulthood: Support for socioemotional selectivity theory. *Psychology and Aging, 7*, 331–338. http://dx.doi.org/10.1037/0882-7974.7.3.331

Carstensen, L. L., & Fredrickson, B. L. (1998). Influence of HIV status and age on cognitive representations of others. *Health Psychology, 17,* 494–503. http://dx.doi.org/10.1037/0278-6133.17.6.494

Carstensen, L. L., Isaacowitz, D. M., & Charles, S. T. (1999). Taking time seriously. A theory of socioemotional selectivity. *American Psychologist, 54,* 165–181. http://dx.doi.org/10.1037/0003-066X.54.3.165

Carstensen, L. L., & Mikels, J. A. (2005). At the intersection of emotion and cognition aging and the positivity effect. *Current Directions in Psychological Science, 14,* 117–121. http://dx.doi.org/10.1111/j.0963-7214.2005.00348.x

Cassileth, B. R., Zupkis, R. V., Sutton-Smith, K., & March, V. (1980). Information and participation preferences among cancer patients. *Annals of Internal Medicine, 92,* 832–836. http://dx.doi.org/10.7326/0003-4819-92-6-832

Castel, A. D. (2008). The adaptive and strategic use of memory by older adults: Evaluative processing and value-directed remembering. In A. S. Benjamin & B. H. Ross (Eds.), *The psychology of learning and motivation* (Vol. 48, pp. 225–270). London, England: Academic Press.

Castel, A. D., Balota, D. A., & McCabe, D. P. (2009). Memory efficiency and the strategic control of attention at encoding: Impairments of value-directed remembering in Alzheimer's disease. *Neuropsychology, 23,* 297–306. http://dx.doi.org/10.1037/a0014888

Castel, A. D., Benjamin, A. S., Craik, F. I., & Watkins, M. J. (2002). The effects of aging on selectivity and control in short-term recall. *Memory & Cognition, 30,* 1078–1085. http://dx.doi.org/10.3758/BF03194325

Castel, A. D., Farb, N. A., & Craik, F. I. (2007). Memory for general and specific value information in younger and older adults: Measuring the limits of strategic control. *Memory & Cognition, 35,* 689–700. http://dx.doi.org/10.3758/BF03193307

Castel, A. D., Lee, S. S., Humphreys, K. L., & Moore, A. N. (2011). Memory capacity, selective control, and value-directed remembering in children with and without attention-deficit/hyperactivity disorder (ADHD). *Neuropsychology, 25,* 15–24. http://dx.doi.org/10.1037/a0020298

Charles, S. T., & Carstensen, L. L. (2007). Emotion regulation and aging. In J. Gross (Ed.), *Handbook of emotion regulation* (pp. 307–327). New York, NY: Guilford Press.

Choi, N. G., & Chou, R. J. A. (2010). Time and money volunteering among older adults: The relationship between past and current volunteering and correlates of change and stability. *Ageing & Society, 30,* 559–581. http://dx.doi.org/10.1017/S0144686X0999064X

Cohen, M. S., Rissman, J., Suthana, N. A., Castel, A. D., & Knowlton, B. J. (2014). Value-based modulation of memory encoding involves strategic engagement of fronto-temporal semantic processing regions. *Cognitive, Affective & Behavioral Neuroscience, 14,* 578–592. http://dx.doi.org/10.3758/s13415-014-0275-x

Cohen, M. S., Rissman, J., Suthana, N. A., Castel, A. D., & Knowlton, B. J. (2016). Effects of aging on value-directed modulation of semantic network activity during verbal learning. *NeuroImage, 125,* 1046–1062. http://dx.doi.org/10.1016/j.neuroimage.2015.07.079

Connelly, S. L., Hasher, L., & Zacks, R. T. (1991). Age and reading: The impact of distraction. *Psychology and Aging, 6,* 533–541. http://dx.doi.org/10.1037/0882-7974.6.4.533

Craik, F. I. M., & Byrd, M. (1982). Aging and cognitive deficits: The role of attentional resources. In F. I. M. Craik & S. Trehub (Eds.), *Aging and cognitive processes* (pp. 191–211). New York, NY: Plenum.

Curley, S. P., Eraker, S. A., & Yates, J. F. (1984). An investigation of patients' reactions to therapeutic uncertainty. *Medical Decision Making, 4,* 501–511. http://dx.doi.org/10.1177/0272989X8400400412

Donohue, T. L., & Wong, E. H. (1997). Achievement motivation and college satisfaction in traditional and nontraditional students. *Education, 118,* 237–243.

Eich, T. S., & Castel, A. D. (2016). The cognitive control of emotional versus value-based information in younger and older adults. *Psychology and Aging, 31,* 503–512. http://dx.doi.org/10.1037/pag0000106

Einstein, G. O., & McDaniel, M. A. (1990). Normal aging and prospective memory. *Journal of Experimental Psychology: Learning, Memory, and Cognition, 16,* 717–726. http://dx.doi.org/10.1037/0278-7393.16.4.717

English, T., & Carstensen, L. L. (2015). Does positivity operate when the stakes are high? Health status and decision making among older adults. *Psychology and Aging, 30,* 348–355. http://dx.doi.org/10.1037/a0039121

Ersner-Hershfield, H., Mikels, J. A., Sullivan, S. J., & Carstensen, L. L. (2008). Poignancy: Mixed emotional experience in the face of meaningful endings. *Journal of Personality and Social Psychology, 94,* 158–167. http://dx.doi.org/10.1037/0022-3514.94.1.158

Finucane, M. L., Slovic, P., Hibbard, J. H., Peters, E., Mertz, C. K., & MacGregor, D. G. (2002). Aging and decision-making competence: An analysis of comprehension and consistency skills in older versus younger adults considering health-plan options. *Journal of Behavioral Decision Making, 15,* 141–164. http://dx.doi.org/10.1002/bdm.407

Friedman, M. C., McGillivray, S., Murayama, K., & Castel, A. D. (2015). Memory for medication side effects in younger and older adults: The role of subjective and objective importance. *Memory & Cognition, 43,* 206–215. http://dx.doi.org/10.3758/s13421-014-0476-0

Fung, H. H., & Carstensen, L. L. (2003). Sending memorable messages to the old: Age differences in preferences and memory for advertisements. *Journal of Personality and Social Psychology, 85,* 163–178. http://dx.doi.org/10.1037/0022-3514.85.1.163

Fung, H. H., & Carstensen, L. L. (2004). Motivational changes in response to blocked goals and foreshortened time: Testing alternatives to socioemotional selectivity theory. *Psychology and Aging, 19,* 68–78. http://dx.doi.org/10.1037/0882-7974.19.1.68

Fung, H. H., Lu, M., & Isaacowitz, D. M. (2018). Aging and attention: Meaningfulness may be more important than valence. *Psychology and Aging.* Advance online publication. http://dx.doi.org/10.1037/pag0000304

Hargis, M. B., & Castel, A. D. (2017). Younger and older adults' associative memory for social information: The role of information importance. *Psychology and Aging, 32,* 325–330. http://dx.doi.org/10.1037/pag0000171

Hargis, M. B., & Castel, A. D. (2018). Younger and older adults' associative memory for medication interactions of varying severity. *Memory, 26,* 1151–1158. http://dx.doi.org/10.1080/09658211.2018.1441423

Hargis, M. B., & Oppenheimer, D. M. (2016, July 14). Commentary: Greater emotional gain from giving in older adults: Age-related positivity bias in charitable giving. *Frontiers in Psychology, 7,* 1075. http://dx.doi.org/10.3389/fpsyg.2016.01075

Hargis, M. B., Yue, C. L., Kerr, T., Ikeda, K., Murayama, K., & Castel, A. D. (2017). Metacognition and proofreading: The roles of aging, motivation, and interest. *Neuropsychology, Development, and Cognition: Section B. Aging, Neuropsychology and Cognition, 24,* 216–226. http://dx.doi.org/10.1080/13825585.2016.1182114

Heckhausen, J., & Schulz, R. (1995). A life-span theory of control. *Psychological Review, 102,* 284–304.

Hidi, S. (1990). Interest and its contribution as a mental resource for learning. *Review of Educational Research, 60,* 549–571. http://dx.doi.org/10.3102/00346543060004549

Houston, D. A., Sherrill-Mittleman, D., & Weeks, M. (2001). The enhancement of feature salience in dichotomous choice dilemmas. In E. U. Weber & J. Baron (Eds.), *Conflict and tradeoffs in decision making* (pp. 65–85). New York, NY: Cambridge University Press.

Jenkins, J. J. (1979). Four points to remember: A tetrahedral model of memory experiments. In L. S. Cermak & F. I. M. Craik (Eds.), *Levels of processing in human memory* (pp. 429–446). Hillsdale, NJ: Erlbaum.

Kaasinen, V., Vilkman, H., Hietala, J., Någren, K., Helenius, H., Olsson, H., . . . Rinne, J. (2000). Age-related dopamine D2/D3 receptor loss in extrastriatal regions of the human brain. *Neurobiology of Aging, 21,* 683–688. http://dx.doi.org/10.1016/S0197-4580(00)00149-4

Kan, I. P., Garrison, S. L., Drummey, A. B., Emmert, B. E., Jr., & Rogers, L. L. (2018). The roles of chronological age and time perspective in memory positivity. *Neuropsychology, Development, and Cognition: Section B. Aging, Neuropsychology and Cognition, 25,* 598–612. http://dx.doi.org/10.1080/13825585.2017.1356262

Kim, A., & Merriam, S. B. (2004). Motivations for learning among older adults in a learning in retirement institute. *Educational Gerontology, 30,* 441–455. http://dx.doi.org/10.1080/03601270490445069

Kovalchik, S., Camerer, C. F., Grether, D. M., Plott, C. R., & Allman, J. M. (2005). Aging and decision making: A comparison between neurologically healthy elderly and young individuals. *Journal of Economic Behavior & Organization, 58,* 79–94. http://dx.doi.org/10.1016/j.jebo.2003.12.001

Lambert-Pandraud, R., Laurent, G., & Lapersonne, E. (2005). Repeat purchasing of new automobiles by older consumers: Empirical evidence and interpretations. *Journal of Marketing, 69,* 97–113. http://dx.doi.org/10.1509/jmkg.69.2.97.60757

Löckenhoff, C. E., & Carstensen, L. L. (2004). Socioemotional selectivity theory, aging, and health: The increasingly delicate balance between regulating emotions and making tough choices. *Journal of Personality, 72,* 1395–1424. http://dx.doi.org/10.1111/j.1467-6494.2004.00301.x

Loewenstein, G. (1994). The psychology of curiosity: A review and reinterpretation. *Psychological Bulletin, 116,* 7–98. http://dx.doi.org/10.1037/0033-2909.116.1.75

Mather, M., & Carstensen, L. L. (2003). Aging and attentional biases for emotional faces. *Psychological Science, 14,* 409–415. http://dx.doi.org/10.1111/1467-9280.01455

Mather, M., & Carstensen, L. L. (2005). Aging and motivated cognition: The positivity effect in attention and memory. *Trends in Cognitive Sciences, 9,* 496–502. http://dx.doi.org/10.1016/j.tics.2005.08.005

Mather, M., & Knight, M. (2005). Goal-directed memory: The role of cognitive control in older adults' emotional memory. *Psychology and Aging, 20,* 554–570. http://dx.doi.org/10.1037/0882-7974.20.4.554

Mather, M., Knight, M., & McCaffrey, M. (2005). The allure of the alignable: Younger and older adults' false memories of choice features. *Journal of Experimental Psychology: General, 134,* 38–51. http://dx.doi.org/10.1037/0096-3445.134.1.38

McAdams, D. P., de St. Aubin, E., & Logan, R. L. (1993). Generativity among young, midlife, and older adults. *Psychology and Aging, 8,* 221–230. http://dx.doi.org/10.1037/0882-7974.8.2.221

McDaniel, M. A., Waddill, P. J., Finstad, K., & Bourg, T. (2000). The effects of text-based interest on attention and recall. *Journal of Educational Psychology, 92,* 492–502. http://dx.doi.org/10.1037/0022-0663.92.3.492

McDowd, J. M., & Shaw, R. J. (1999). Attention and aging: A functional perspective. In F. I. M. Craik & T. A. Salthouse (Eds.), *The handbook of aging and cognition* (2nd ed., pp. 221–292). Mahwah, NJ: Erlbaum.

McGillivray, S., & Castel, A. D. (2017). Older and younger adults' strategic control of metacognitive monitoring: The role of consequences, task experience and prior knowledge. *Experimental Aging Research, 43,* 233–256. http://dx.doi.org/10.1080/0361073X.2017.1298956

McGillivray, S., Murayama, K., & Castel, A. D. (2015). Thirst for knowledge: The effects of curiosity and interest on memory in younger and older adults. *Psychology and Aging, 30,* 835–841. http://dx.doi.org/10.1037/a0039801

Meyer, B. J. F., Russo, C., & Talbot, A. (1995). Discourse comprehension and problem solving: Decisions about the treatment of breast cancer by women across the life span. *Psychology and Aging, 10,* 84–103. http://dx.doi.org/10.1037/0882-7974.10.1.84

Meyer, D. K., & Turner, J. C. (2006). Re-conceptualizing emotion and motivation to learn in classroom contexts. *Educational Psychology Review, 18,* 377–390. http://dx.doi.org/10.1007/s10648-006-9032-1

Midlarsky, E., & Hannah, M. E. (1989). The generous elderly: Naturalistic studies of donations across the life span. *Psychology and Aging, 4,* 346–351. http://dx.doi.org/10.1037/0882-7974.4.3.346

Mikels, J. A., Löckenhoff, C. E., Maglio, S. J., Goldstein, M. K., Garber, A., & Carstensen, L. L. (2010). Following your heart or your head: Focusing on emotions versus information differentially influences the decisions of younger and older adults. *Journal of Experimental Psychology: Applied, 16,* 87–95. http://dx.doi.org/10.1037/a0018500

Minear, M., & Park, D. C. (2004). A lifespan database of adult facial stimuli. *Behavior Research Methods, Instruments, & Computers, 36,* 630–633. http://dx.doi.org/10.3758/BF03206543

Morrell, R. W., Park, D. C., & Poon, L. W. (1989). Quality of instructions on prescription drug labels: Effects on memory and comprehension in young and old adults. *The Gerontologist, 29,* 345–354. http://dx.doi.org/10.1093/geront/29.3.345

Naveh-Benjamin, M. (2000). Adult age differences in memory performance: Tests of an associative deficit hypothesis. *Journal of Experimental Psychology: Learning, Memory, and Cognition, 26,* 1170–1187. http://dx.doi.org/10.1037/0278-7393.26.5.1170

Okun, M. A., & Schultz, A. (2003). Age and motives for volunteering: Testing hypotheses derived from socioemotional selectivity theory. *Psychology and Aging, 18,* 231–239. http://dx.doi.org/10.1037/0882-7974.18.2.231

Petrisek, A. C., Laliberte, L. L., Allen, S. M., & Mor, V. (1997). The treatment decision-making process: Age differences in a sample of women recently diagnosed with nonrecurrent, early-stage breast cancer. *The Gerontologist, 37,* 598–608. http://dx.doi.org/10.1093/geront/37.5.598

Phillips, L., Henry, J., & Martin, M. (2008). Adult aging and prospective memory: The importance of ecological validity. In M. Kliegal, M. McDaniel, & O. Einstein (Eds.), *Prospective memory: Cognitive, neuroscience, developmental, and applied perspectives* (pp. 161–186). New York: Erlbaum.

Pintrich, P. R., Smith, D. A., Garcia, T., & McKeachie, W. J. (1991). *A manual for the use of the Motivated Strategies for Learning Questionnaire (MLSQ).* Ann Arbor: University of Michigan, National Center for Research to Improve Postsecondary Teaching and Learning.

Roediger, H. L., III. (2008). Relativity of remembering: Why the laws of memory vanished. *Annual Review of Psychology, 59,* 225–254. http://dx.doi.org/10.1146/annurev.psych.57.102904.190139

Salthouse, T. A. (1995). Processing capacity and its role on the relations between age and memory. In F. E. Weinert & W. Schneider (Eds.), *Memory performance and competencies: Issues in growth and development* (pp. 111–125). Hillsdale, NJ: Erlbaum.

Salthouse, T. A. (2014). Correlates of cognitive change. *Journal of Experimental Psychology: General, 143*, 1026–1048. http://dx.doi.org/10.1037/a0034847

Schnitzspahn, K. M., Scholz, U., Ballhausen, N., Hering, A., Ihle, A., Lagner, P., & Kliegel, M. (2016). Age differences in prospective memory for everyday life intentions: A diary approach. *Memory, 24*, 444–454. http://dx.doi.org/10.1080/09658211.2015.1018276

Shohamy, D., & Adcock, R. A. (2010). Dopamine and adaptive memory. *Trends in Cognitive Sciences, 14*, 464–472. http://dx.doi.org/10.1016/j.tics.2010.08.002

Siegel, A. L. M., & Castel, A. D. (2018). Memory for important item-location associations in younger and older adults. *Psychology and Aging, 33*, 30–45. http://dx.doi.org/10.1037/pag0000209

Spaniol, J., Schain, C., & Bowen, H. J. (2014). Reward-enhanced memory in younger and older adults. *The Journals of Gerontology: Series B. Psychological Sciences and Social Sciences, 69*, 730–740. http://dx.doi.org/10.1093/geronb/gbt044

Stine-Morrow, E. A., Shake, M. C., Miles, J. R., & Noh, S. R. (2006). Adult age differences in the effects of goals on self-regulated sentence processing. *Psychology and Aging, 21*, 790–803. http://dx.doi.org/10.1037/0882-7974.21.4.790

Strough, J., Mehta, C. M., McFall, J. P., & Schuller, K. L. (2008). Are older adults less subject to the sunk-cost fallacy than younger adults? *Psychological Science, 19*, 650–652. http://dx.doi.org/10.1111/j.1467-9280.2008.02138.x

Strough, J., Schlosnagle, L., Karns, T., Lemaster, P., & Pichayayothin, N. (2014). No time to waste: Restricting life-span temporal horizons decreases the sunk-cost fallacy. *Journal of Behavioral Decision Making, 27*, 78–94. http://dx.doi.org/10.1002/bdm.1781

Vansteenkiste, M., Simons, J., Lens, W., Soenens, B., Matos, L., & Lacante, M. (2004). Less is sometimes more: Goal content matters. *Journal of Educational Psychology, 96*, 755–764. http://dx.doi.org/10.1037/0022-0663.96.4.755

Verhaeghen, P. (2003). Aging and vocabulary scores: A meta-analysis. *Psychology and Aging, 18*, 332–339. http://dx.doi.org/10.1037/0882-7974.18.2.332

Volkow, N. D., Gur, R. C., Wang, G. J., Fowler, J. S., Moberg, P. J., Ding, Y. S., . . . Logan, J. (1998). Association between decline in brain dopamine activity with age and cognitive and motor impairment in healthy individuals. *The American Journal of Psychiatry, 155*, 344–349.

Watkins, M. J., & Bloom, L. C. (1999). *Selectivity in memory: An exploration of willful control over the remembering process.* Unpublished manuscript.

Willis, S. L., Dolan, M. M., & Bertrand, R. M. (1999). Problem solving on health-related tasks of daily living. In D. C. Park & R. W. Morrell (Eds.), *Processing of medical information in aging patients: Cognitive and human factors perspectives* (pp. 199–219). Mahwah, NJ: Erlbaum.

Wolfgang, M. E., & Dowling, W. D. (1981). Differences in motivation of adult and younger undergraduates. *The Journal of Higher Education, 52*, 640–648. http://dx.doi.org/10.2307/1981772

Wrosch, C., Scheier, M. F., Miller, G. E., Schulz, R., & Carver, C. S. (2003). Adaptive self-regulation of unattainable goals: Goal disengagement, goal reengagement, and subjective well-being. *Personality and Social Psychology Bulletin, 29,* 1494–1508. http://dx.doi.org/10.1177/0146167203256921

Zacks, R., & Hasher, L. (2006). Aging and long-term memory: Deficits are not inevitable. In E. Bialystok & F. I. Craik (Eds.), *Lifespan cognition: Mechanisms of change* (pp. 162–177). New York, NY: Oxford University Press. http://dx.doi.org/10.1093/acprof:oso/9780195169539.003.0011

Zacks, R. T., Radvansky, G., & Hasher, L. (1996). Studies of directed forgetting in older adults. *Journal of Experimental Psychology: Learning, Memory, and Cognition, 22,* 143–156. http://dx.doi.org/10.1037/0278-7393.22.1.143

6

SOCIAL FUNCTION AND MOTIVATION IN THE AGING BRAIN

ANGELA GUTCHESS AND GREGORY R. SAMANEZ-LARKIN

In this chapter, we review some themes from the emerging literature on the social neuroscience of aging. Much of the research thus far focuses on abilities at the intersection of social function and emotion, such as empathy or thinking about the self or other people. Intriguingly, findings from social and motivational tasks largely depart from the lessons about brain aging derived from cognitive tasks. There are hints that strategy or goal shifts may underlie some of the age differences, which illustrates the importance of considering task context and motivation across the lifespan.

Still underappreciated are the connections between social and motivational processes. In this chapter, we review how aging affects social abilities. We then review major themes from the literature on the effects of aging on motivation and consider how social and motivational processes can inform each other. Investigating the intersection of these domains has the potential to advance understanding of the psychology and neuroscience of aging, and such work is in its infancy.

http://dx.doi.org/10.1037/0000143-007

The Aging Brain: Functional Adaptation Across Adulthood, G. R. Samanez-Larkin (Editor)

SOCIAL NEUROSCIENCE OF AGING

Older adults are motivated for social interaction. We examine this through a review of three socioemotional topics that have been the subject of several studies of aging.

Thinking About Self and Others

People-watching at a café on a street in a foreign city might invoke different ways of thinking about other people. One way people might think about others involves impression formation, which is "sizing up" others in terms of the types of traits and behaviors we might expect from them. For example, if a woman bumps another as she rushes past and fails to apologize, you might infer that she is rude. Younger and older adults tend to form converging opinions of others (e.g., Hess & Tate, 1991; Krendl, Rule, & Ambady, 2014; Zebrowitz, Franklin, Hillman, & Boc, 2013). When receiving information that is diagnostic about one's traits, neural activation patterns also converge, with both younger (Mitchell, 2008) and older (Cassidy, Shih, & Gutchess, 2012) adults activating the mentalizing network, including dorsal and ventral medial prefrontal cortex. However, the ways in which this region is engaged across age groups differ in line with socioemotional selective theory. Older adults exhibit more of a positivity bias, with the medial prefrontal cortex (mPFC) more responsive when impressions of others are positive rather than negative, whereas young adults exhibit a negativity bias such that the mPFC is more engaged for negative than positive information (Cassidy, Leshikar, Shih, Aizenman, & Gutchess, 2013). This pattern for the social process of impression formation mirrors findings from the emotion literature (Leclerc & Kensinger, 2008).

Age differences in thinking about others seem to influence how one thinks about the self. Overall, younger and older adults activate similar neural regions, particularly the mPFC, when judging whether words describe oneself (e.g., am I vain?) compared with judgments about another person (e.g., is Albert Einstein cautious?; Gutchess, Kensinger, & Schacter, 2007). This convergence with age extends to encoding self-referenced words into memory (Gutchess et al., 2015). However, making judgments about other people seems to affect the similarity of neural activity with age. When participants encoded words judged in reference to someone other than the self, this dramatically altered the patterns of neural activity for younger and older adults, such that the regions that contribute to the encoding of self-referential information into memory (i.e., more active for words judged about the self, that were successfully remembered on a later memory test) for older adults were associated with encoding words judged about *another person* for younger adults (Gutchess, Kensinger, & Schacter, 2010).

To resolve the inconsistencies across the two encoding studies, making judgments only about the self was directly compared with making judgments across different trials about the self as well as another person in a behavioral study. Whether judgments should be made relative to others (e.g., "am I smart?" vs. "relative to others, am I smart?") was also manipulated, and participants gave judgments on a scale, rather than simply endorsing "yes" or "no." Whereas young adults' memory was relatively unaffected across these manipulations, older adults' memory differed depending on the presence of others, the relative nature of the judgment, and the strength of the endorsement (Gutchess et al., 2015). Younger adults' memories seemed impervious to the context, whereas older adults may be more affected by others such that they encoded information into memory in a more *relative* fashion. These results may also account for the neural differences, suggesting that younger and older adults qualitatively differ in how they think about the self, potentially influenced by the social context.

Mentalizing and Empathizing

Another way of thinking about others while people-watching involves *mentalizing*, or attempting to infer the mental state of another person. For example, while people-watching from the café, you may spot a man looking distraught, staring at his cell phone. You might infer that he received unwelcome news; you might even empathize, feeling some of the same emotion of disappointment or frustration that he is experiencing. *Theory of mind*, the ability to understand and experience events from another person's perspective, encompasses both cognitive (mentalizing; e.g., do I understand what information the character in this story has access to, compared with others?) and affective (empathy; e.g., can I feel the emotions that this character is experiencing?) components. Research indicates that theory of mind overall is impaired with age (e.g., Henry, Phillips, Ruffman, & Bailey, 2013; Maylor, Moulson, Muncer, & Taylor, 2002; Moran, 2013; Sullivan & Ruffman, 2004), although there is some evidence that the deficits may be larger for the cognitive than affective aspects. For example, once overall cognitive ability differences are accounted for, performance on an empathy measure is not impaired with age (Phillips, MacLean, & Allen, 2002). This indicates that cognitive demands such as integrating different cues (e.g., different facial movements, tone of voice) can affect the ability to experience another person's emotion. Performance on some economic tasks shows that older adults may experience more empathy than younger adults. For example, in one study younger and older adults assigned money to an opponent in an economic game. When empathy was induced for the opponent, who revealed a recent skin cancer diagnosis, older adults assigned more money to the opponent than did younger adults (Beadle, Sheehan, Dahlben,

& Gutchess, 2015). The amount of money transferred served as a measure of prosocial behavior, suggesting that older adults experienced more empathy than young in this task. Several behavioral economic studies have documented more equitable divisions of money between self and other or increased giving in older age (Bailey, Ruffman, & Rendell, 2013; Ebner, Bailey, Horta, Joiner, & Chang, 2017; Lim & Yu, 2015; Roalf, Mitchell, Harbaugh, & Janowsky, 2012). Preservation of empathy with age indicates that older adults are motivated to experience the mental state of another person.

There has been little investigation of the effects of aging on the neural response to affective components of empathy, but one functional magnetic resonance (fMRI) study suggests some impairment with age. Younger, middle-aged, and older adults viewed pictures of body parts in pain (e.g., a syringe stuck in a hand), intended to induce empathy compared with a "no pain" control picture (e.g., a hand holding a syringe). Younger and middle-aged adults activated the anterior insula more than did older adults to the painful stimuli, and middle-aged adults also activated the posterior insula (Chen, Chen, Decety, & Cheng, 2014). The response of these regions was thought to reflect a more robust empathic response in the younger and middle-aged adults than in older adults, although further investigation with a variety of tasks, including active ones requiring a judgment, is needed.

Age differences in the neural regions underlying mentalizing have emerged across multiple tasks. One study compared younger and older adults on three social cognitive tasks compared with nonsocial control tasks (Moran, Jolly, & Mitchell, 2012). Across all three tasks, older adults exhibited decreased activity in dorsomedial prefrontal cortex, accompanied by increases in errors or decreases in using relevant information to inform social judgments, compared with younger adults. Whether these results generally capture effects of aging on mentalizing or may reflect the more cognitive nature of the tasks or emphasis on negative information (as for the moral judgment task, as discussed in Cassidy et al., 2013) will require additional work in these areas. Another study used a less cognitive task in which individuals select the word that describes another person's mental state by reading the expression displayed in the eye region (Castelli et al., 2010). Although much of the mentalizing network was activated by both younger and older adults, some differences in discrete regions emerged that were suggested to reflect strategy differences (e.g., older adults may rely more on language, based on heightened activation of regions associated with verbal processing).

Response to Stigmatized Individuals

From your seat at the posh café, you may also see homeless people in the street, panhandling for change. Seeing stigmatized individuals, such as individuals with amputations or who are homeless, may invoke feelings of discomfort, disgust, or fear. Like younger adults, research suggests that older adults are motivated to regulate their response to seeing stigmatized individuals. Regulating this response requires cognitive control to overcome one's initial negative reaction. Behaviorally, older adults' executive function capacity predicted their ability to regulate their response to stigmatized individuals (Krendl, 2018). A similar effect emerged for younger adults. When tested under divided-attention conditions, young adults were less able to regulate their negative reactions. These results indicate the importance of executive function in regulating one's response to stigmatized individuals and the negative results when this ability is disrupted with aging, at least for older adults with limited executive function ability. The brain regions activated while undergoing fMRI were consistent with the pattern of behavioral results. Both younger and older adults activated brain regions implicated in automatic (e.g., amygdala) and controlled (e.g., inferior frontal gyrus) processes in response to viewing stigmatized individuals (Krendl, Heatherton, & Kensinger, 2009). Prefrontal regions implicated in executive function were activated the most by older adults with higher levels of executive function ability, suggesting the importance of using regulatory processes for controlling older adults' response to stigmatized individuals. Some of the research on responses to stigmatized individuals connects to the literature on empathy. Stigmatized individuals were depicted as either responsible or not responsible for their situation, in an attempt to manipulate pity and empathy. Older adults with higher levels of global cognitive function showed greater insula activation when viewing stigmatized individuals not responsible for their status (Krendl & Kensinger, 2016). Under these conditions, older adults with lower levels of cognitive function engaged anterior cingulate cortex. Although both brain regions are associated with empathy, these results indicate individual differences in how aging affects pity responses. Krendl and Kensinger speculated that insula activity may reflect empathy, as in seeing a situation through another person's eyes, whereas anterior cingulate activation could reflect one's own personal distress, although additional work is needed to substantiate these claims. Taken together, the literature on responses to stigmatized individuals also serves as an indication of older adults' interest in others and attempt to preserve positive social interactions across the lifespan.

EMERGING THEMES IN SOCIAL NEUROSCIENCE

On the basis of this brief sampling of some of the findings related to the social neuroscience of aging, we discuss observations of patterns that seem to be heightened in the social domain, compared with research on cognitive changes with age. For cognitive tasks, individuals may be constrained in the operations they apply to tasks, taxed by the cognitive load, time limits, and other task demands. It is possible that tasks can be approached more flexibly and with a variety of strategies in the social domain, potentially allowing for age differences of a different nature to materialize (see Gutchess, 2019).

Many Neural Differences With Age May Reflect Changes to Strategy, Rather Than Ability

Age differences in the recruitment of neural regions that emerge for social tasks largely do not reflect the canon of literature based on more cognitive tasks (Gutchess, 2014). In many studies, there are not clear patterns of underactivation of the same networks used by younger adults or additional, perhaps compensatory, activation of prefrontal regions (for reviews of these ideas, see Buckner, 2004; Cabeza, 2002; Cabeza & Dennis, 2013). Rather, many of the age differences seem to reflect the adoption of different strategies for younger and older adults. From the literature reviewed in the preceding text, the age differences in regions recruited during theory of mind (Castelli et al., 2010) or when encoding information in reference to the self or another person (Gutchess et al., 2010, 2015) may reflect the use of different strategies (e.g., verbal processing vs. mentalizing) or different ways of thinking about the targets (e.g., thinking about the self in a more relative, other-focused way).

Ultimately the recruitment of different networks and processes across age groups may reflect some role of capacity or cognitive demand. Perhaps older adults recruit different strategies than younger adults out of necessity, lacking the resources to employ successfully the strategies used during young adulthood. For example, the greater engagement of cognitive control regions in older adults with high levels of executive function in response to viewing stigmatized individuals may reflect an age-related failure (Krendl et al., 2009). Other systems may be able to regulate the negative reaction in young adults but are not adequate to do so for older adults. Addressing the interplay of flexible social and constrained cognitive abilities will require investigation into social processes in much more depth, testing abilities under a variety of instructions and task constraints. At present, the dearth of research applying a social neuroscience approach to the study of aging makes it impossible to resolve the role of cognitive capacity.

Context Contributes to When Age-Related Impairments Emerge

The malleability of strategies and orientations that can be adopted when making social judgments may make the social domain particularly prone to context effects. According to this perspective, age differences may reflect what type of information is more motivating, or prioritized for additional process-ing, in one age group compared with the other. One example of this is reversals in how conditions activate a region with age, such as the engagement of mPFC for positive versus negative information, presented earlier in the chapter. The region is more engaged by negative information for young adults but positive information for older adults, and this occurs for emotional objects (Leclerc & Kensinger, 2010) as well as impressions of other people (Cassidy et al., 2013).

Motivational factors may also affect task performance and engagement of neural networks such that age differences can be reduced when strategies or task orientations are aligned with older adults' goals. Compared with younger adults, older adults show disrupted activity in midline cortical regions, including the mPFC, when thinking about personal goals (K. J. Mitchell et al., 2009). These age differences are magnified specifically when thinking about promotion-focused goals (i.e., those related to hopes and aspirations) compared with when thinking about prevention-focused goals, related to duties and obligations. This pattern of age differences that are decreased or increased depending on the approach to thinking about goals may reflect motivational differences with age. Age differences may be reduced when task orientation is aligned with older adults' perspective.

One intriguing observation from the literature involves the effects of aging on cortical midline activation, including mPFC. As we have discussed at points throughout the chapter, the region can be robustly activated with age when thinking about the self, others, or emotionally valenced informa-tion. Yet a large literature demonstrates impairments in engagement of this same network when individuals are at rest, or not performing a task (e.g., Grady et al., 2010; Persson, Lustig, Nelson, & Reuter-Lorenz, 2007). Under these conditions, the network is often referred to as the default mode net-work, indicating the heightened activity during baseline periods (between trials) compared with during cognitively demanding, externally focused tasks. Is it possible that performing social or personally motivating tasks mitigates these age differences? Or does the apparent preservation of these regions with aging during social and self-relevant tasks reflect methods used thus far (e.g., smaller, higher functioning samples or less demanding tasks)?

CONNECTION TO COGNITION AND EMOTION

Given the long-standing focus on the study of cognitive processes with aging, it is not surprising that the intersection between socioemotional and cognitive domains has been explored to some extent. There are purported to be bidirectional connections between social and cognitive domains that reflect shared and distinct processes and neural networks. As discussed in

Kensinger and Gutchess (2017), models from the cognitive domain that consider the availability of resources (e.g., level of fluid cognition predicts emotion regulation ability; Opitz, Lee, Gross, & Urry, 2014) or compensatory activation (e.g., the shift with age to engage anterior brain regions rather than posterior brain regions occurs not only for cognitive processes but also affective ones; Ford, Morris, & Kensinger, 2014) have some utility in accounting for how aging affects socioemotional abilities with age. However, there is also a need to recognize the ways in which socioemotional domains influence cognition (e.g., orienting to the personal relevance could eliminate age differences in memory for character information; Cassidy & Gutchess, 2012), as well as the ways in which the domains are separate (e.g., environmental support, reducing cognitive demands by relying on the environment, may be more robust for socioemotional abilities).

What about distinguishing social from emotional abilities, which were treated in tandem in the previous section under the umbrella of *socioemotional*? One theory that has shaped a substantial amount of research in this field emerged at the intersection of social and emotional processes. Socioemotional selectivity theory (SST) initially emphasized older adults' preference to spend time with family and friends in contrast to young adults' preference for information seeking (Carstensen, Isaacowitz, & Charles, 1999). These choices were thought to reflect older adults' heightened awareness of the limited time available in one's life, as preferences for emotionally meaningful social partners emerge for younger as well as older adults as perceived endings approach (Fung, Carstensen, & Lutz, 1999). The theory was later extended to encompass age differences in attention to positive information for older adults compared with negative information for young adults, including attentional biases (Mather & Carstensen, 2003) and the valence of recalled autobiographical memories (Kennedy, Mather, & Carstensen, 2004). These differences in orientation to positive versus negative information were suggested to reflect older adults' motivation to regulate emotions and limit emotionally negative experiences (Mather & Carstensen, 2005). According to SST, social preferences can have a direct impact on emotional processes.

A neural approach reveals largely distinct networks supporting memory for social and emotionally valenced information (Macrae, Moran, Heatherton, Banfield, & Kelley, 2004). However, the same regions, such as the amygdala, can emerge in both domains (as discussed in Kensinger & Gutchess, 2015). It seems important to consider its role in tasks and its connectivity with other regions in distinguishing the domains, as the amygdala may operate more automatically and in conjunction with lower level regions (e.g., visual cortex) for emotional processes but in a more resource-intensive manner, and with higher level regions (e.g., prefrontal cortex) for social processes (Sakaki, Niki, & Mather, 2012).

Kensinger and Gutchess (2017) proposed some future directions for examining how social and affective processes influence each other, as well as intersect with cognition. But importantly, they more broadly raise questions as to how these domains intersect with motivation. In the next section, we discuss the effects of aging on motivation and related neural systems. Then we will consider why the combined study of social and motivational processes is an important future direction.

CONNECTION TO MOTIVATION AND REWARD

The neuroscience of aging literature has only somewhat recently begun to focus on adult age differences in motivational brain systems. The vast majority of studies on motivation and aging use monetary incentives or points-based performance feedback in cognitive tasks (Samanez-Larkin & Knutson, 2015). For example, a number of studies have examined how the structure and function of frontostriatal circuits are differentially involved in reward processing, reinforcement learning, and decision-making in older age (Samanez-Larkin & Knutson, 2015). Some of these studies document age-related impairments whereby older adults have more difficulty learning from reward feedback and show less activation in frontostriatal circuits (Eppinger, Hämmerer, & Li, 2011). Others demonstrate that basic reward signals are intact well into old age, especially in reward-based tasks where older adults perform better or no differently from younger adults (Samanez-Larkin & Knutson, 2015). Importantly, although most of these studies use monetary incentives to motivate performance, studies (Jimura et al., 2011; Seaman et al., 2016) have identified domain effects such that adult age differences in decision-making, for example, differ depending on the reward domain (e.g., food, money, social reward, health). Thus, it appears that motivational systems may be differentially engaged across adulthood depending on the type of task or reward being offered. The strong focus on monetary reward in the current neuroimaging literature is a limitation for our understanding of broader motivational function in the aging brain.

Although most existing studies use fMRI and thus cannot directly measure specific neurotransmitters, often age differences in these circuits are assumed to be related to age differences in the dopamine system. The dopamine system is composed of an interconnected network of structures in the midbrain, striatum, and cortex (Haber & Knutson, 2010). In the midbrain, the substantia nigra and ventral tegmental area serve as the core source of dopamine for the striatum and other cortical and subcortical regions. Beyond these initial projections, these regions are organized into ascending anatomical loops through glutamatergic and GABAergic direct connections and relays through the globus pallidus and thalamus (Alexander, DeLong, & Strick, 1986). The connectivity of these circuits, drawn from early studies in nonhuman primates (Haber, 2003) recently replicated in humans using diffusion tensor imaging (Cohen, Schoene-Bake, Elger, & Weber, 2009; Draganski et al., 2008), verifies the strong connectivity between the striatum and cortex. The lateral cortical circuit has been referred to as a cognitive–executive loop whereas the ventral striatal, medial temporal, and ventromedial cortical circuit has been referred to as a motivational loop (Lawrence, Sahakian, & Robbins, 1998; Seger, Peterson, Cincotta, Lopez-Paniagua, & Anderson, 2010).

Many theories of cognitive aging are centered on age-related change in neuromodulation, focusing specifically on dopamine. Although a number of theoretical accounts link dopamine function with age-related cognitive decline (Braver & Barch, 2002; Li, Lindenberger, & Sikström, 2001), there has been little attempt to explore the potential role of the dopamine system and these ventromedial corticostriatal circuits for supporting motivation across adulthood. Dopamine clearly also plays an important role in motivation. Midbrain and striatal dopamine function is associated with several motivational individual difference characteristics such as reward sensitivity, novelty seeking, and impulsivity (Buckholtz, Treadway, Cowan, Woodward, Benning, et al., 2010, Buckholtz, Treadway, Cowan, Woodward, Li, et al., 2010; Zald et al., 2008). Theories suggesting a link between mesolimbic dopamine and positive emotional experience and improvements in cognitive control (Ashby, Isen, & Turken, 1999) have not been thoroughly tested or applied to understanding age differences in motivation.

Although theories of cognitive aging are not only supported by but also are based on neurobiological evidence for age-related change (e.g., Braver & Barch, 2002; Li et al., 2001), the same is currently not the case for motivational theories of aging (e.g., Carstensen, Isaacowitz, & Charles, 1999; Freund, 2006). In addition to the work cited earlier on reward processing, other related neuroscientific research has begun to investigate affective and emotional functioning in the aging brain (Samanez-Larkin & Carstensen, 2011), but there has been little to no neurobiological theory development around motivation. There is currently no established neuropsychological model of the adult development and aging of motivational function. Although not previously articulated by existing theories of aging, dopamine might also play an important role in these motivational age effects. Overall, the relation between age-related declines in dopamine functioning and motivational factors have received little study, and no studies have explored the potential overlap of, or dissociations in, dopamine's influence on neurobiological systems that are associated with motivation across adulthood.

A potential neurobiological theory of motivation and aging is complicated by the strong neural evidence for declines in the dopamine system (Bäckman, Nyberg, Lindenberger, Li, & Farde, 2006; Karrer, Josef, Mata, Morris, & Samanez-Larkin, 2017) and behavioral evidence for mostly preservation in many forms of motivational function (Mather & Carstensen, 2005). However, recent research has identified preservation in some aspects of dopamine function and the ventromedial corticostriatal–midbrain circuit in old age. A meta-analytic study revealed that synthesis capacity (the potential to produce dopamine in presynaptic neurons) does not appear to decline with age (Karrer et al., 2017). Additionally, both structural and functional neuroimaging studies have documented preservation or even enhancement with age within the midbrain and striatum (Samanez-Larkin & Knutson, 2015) and preserved or enhanced connectivity between these regions and medial prefrontal regions, such as the anterior cingulate cortex (Schott et al., 2007). Thus, it is possible that relative preservation within aspects in these systems supports both social and motivational function in older age, although this has not yet been directly assessed.

Interplay Between Social Context and Motivation

Because the medial prefrontal cortex (mPFC) is a region that features prominently in our review of findings from the social literature, contributing to mentalizing, forming impressions of others, and making judgments about the self, we focus on this region in considering connections between social and motivational processes. Thus far, we have largely considered the effects of aging on this region in terms of its role in social cognition. However, the region has multiple functions, including regulation of emotion and computation of value (Delgado et al., 2016). There are several subdivisions of mPFC; the most general subdivision into three segments identifies the posterior region as reflecting motor function, the middle region as reflecting affective and cognitive control functions, and the anterior region as reflecting social cognition, as well as reward and memory processes, although each of these segments can be partitioned more finely into further subdivisions (de la Vega, Chang, Banich, Wager, & Yarkoni, 2016; see also Dixon, Thiruchselvam, Todd, & Christoff, 2017). The dorsomedial prefrontal region identified in some studies likely maps on to the middle region, and the ventromedial prefrontal region strongly implicated in studies of self and other falls into the anterior region.

The ventromedial prefrontal cortex region that in humans is implicated in thinking about self and others is most strongly implicated in rodents in reward, such as cocaine seeking (e.g., Moorman, James, McGlinchey, & Aston-Jones, 2015). Lesions of mPFC lead to deficits in making choices, particularly in terms of recognizing the consequences of choices (Kennerley & Walton, 2011). These findings converge with those from the fMRI literature (see the review by Rushworth, Noonan, Boorman, Walton, & Behrens, 2011), including multivoxel pattern analysis methods (as reviewed by Kahnt, 2018), which show that patterns of activity in the region reflect information about value, including predictive information about gains and losses.

It may be that different subcircuits (Moorman, James, McGlinchey, & Aston-Jones, 2015), cortical subdivisions (de la Vega et al., 2016), or white matter pathways connecting regions (Rushworth et al., 2011) are implicated in different processes. More research has broached the idea of differing functional connectivity, demonstrating that a region can operate as part of multiple networks, working in conjunction with different regions for different processes (Delgado et al., 2016). It is also possible, however, that age differences in ventromedial prefrontal cortical activity reflect differences in what social information motivates younger and older adults. The potential intersection of social and reward domains with age has been investigated little. In the remainder of this section, we review literature bridging social and reward in younger adults that holds promise for the study of aging.

A role for mPFC has been recognized across typical decision-making tasks (e.g., economic decisions involving money or other consumables, e.g., food) as well as social ones, perhaps distinguishing better and worse outcomes of choices (Lee & Harris, 2013). Some research, however, suggests that different regions of mPFC are sensitive to social and nonsocial evaluation. For example, the posterior anterior cingulate cortex responds to stimulus valence, regardless of whether tasks are social or nonsocial (Harris, McClure, van den Bos, Cohen, & Fiske, 2007; van den Bos, McClure, Harris, Fiske, & Cohen, 2007). In contrast, anterior regions of mPFC are selective for people, responding to positive over negative information regardless of whether the judgment is evaluative (Harris et al., 2007) or to social contexts (e.g., whether feedback is from a computer or another person; van den Bos et al., 2007). The mPFC response is consistent with findings that viewing negative outgroup members (e.g., those that elicit disgust) decreases the response of the region (Harris & Fiske, 2006, 2007).

Although this section focuses narrowly on mPFC and adjacent regions, an important direction for future work is to probe the interactions of explicit learning (e.g., hippocampal), implicit learning (e.g., striatal), and social valuation (e.g., mPFC) systems to understand how one makes decisions and learns socially relevant information. Interestingly, there is substantial spatial overlap in the subcortical and medial frontal neural systems proposed to underlie social behavior and reward motivation. For example, the striatum, strongly implicated in reward learning, also responds to expectancy violations for social information, suggesting that social and reward systems overlap in some situations

(Harris & Fiske, 2010). Delineating under what circumstances the systems work together, and how these systems, or their interactions, are affected by aging is an important direction for future work. Indeed, Lee and Harris (2013) noted the lack of consideration of social contexts in the neuroeconomic literature and the lack of consideration of economic contexts in the social neuroscience literature. This is particularly true for the study of older adults.

One interesting direction for future work concerns the effects of aging on the interaction of reward systems with self and other. The ventral mPFC region implicated in reward is also the region that responds to thinking about oneself. Some work has suggested that thinking about oneself is highly rewarding. When young adults self-disclosed their own opinions or thoughts about their own personality traits, regions associated with reward and the striatal system, including the nucleus accumbens and the ventral tegmental area, as well as mPFC, were engaged more than when they judged the disclosures of another person (Tamir & Mitchell, 2012). It is possible that older adults are less motivated by self-relevant information than young adults. Earlier, we discussed evidence that older adults may be more sensitive than younger adults to the social context when making judgments about oneself and others (Gutchess et al., 2015). Combined with evidence that older adults may play economic games with more of a prosocial orientation than younger adults (Bailey, Ruffman, & Rendell, 2013; Beadle et al., 2015), a promising hypothesis may be that the discrepancy in valuing self above other in youth may be reduced with age. This suggests the possibility of differences across the lifespan in the motivational value of self and other, which could be in line with socioemotional selectivity theory's recognition of the heightened value placed on meaningful interactions with social partners with age (Carstensen et al., 1999).

A better understanding of the neurobiology of social function and motivation across adulthood has great potential for not only a more comprehensive understanding of brain aging in general but also for bringing together cognitive, social, and motivational theories of the psychology and neuroscience of aging.

REFERENCES

Alexander, G. E., DeLong, M. R., & Strick, P. L. (1986). Parallel organization of functionally segregated circuits linking basal ganglia and cortex. *Annual Review of Neuroscience, 9*, 357–381. http://dx.doi.org/10.1146/annurev.ne.09.030186.002041

Ashby, F. G., Isen, A. M., & Turken, A. U. (1999). A neuropsychological theory of positive affect and its influence on cognition. *Psychological Review, 106*, 529–550. http://dx.doi.org/10.1037/0033-295X.106.3.529

Bäckman, L., Nyberg, L., Lindenberger, U., Li, S. C., & Farde, L. (2006). The correlative triad among aging, dopamine, and cognition: Current status and future prospects. *Neuroscience & Biobehavioral Reviews, 30*, 791–807. http://dx.doi.org/10.1016/j.neubiorev.2006.06.005

Bailey, P. E., Ruffman, T., & Rendell, P. G. (2013). Age-related differences in social economic decision making: The ultimatum game. *The Journals of Gerontology: Series B. Psychological Sciences and Social Sciences, 68*, 356–363. http://dx.doi.org/10.1093/geronb/gbs073

Beadle, J. N., Sheehan, A. H., Dahlben, B., & Gutchess, A. H. (2015). Aging, empathy, and prosociality. *The Journals of Gerontology: Series B. Psychological Sciences and Social Sciences, 70*, 213–224. http://dx.doi.org/10.1093/geronb/gbt091

Braver, T. S., & Barch, D. M. (2002). A theory of cognitive control, aging cognition, and neuromodulation. *Neuroscience and Biobehavioral Reviews, 26*, 809–817. http://dx.doi.org/10.1016/S0149-7634(02)00067-2

Buckholtz, J. W., Treadway, M. T., Cowan, R. L., Woodward, N. D., Benning, S. D., Li, R., . . . Zald, D. H. (2010). Mesolimbic dopamine reward system hypersensitivity in individuals with psychopathic traits. *Nature Neuroscience, 13*, 419–421. http://dx.doi.org/10.1038/nn.2510

Buckholtz, J. W., Treadway, M. T., Cowan, R. L., Woodward, N. D., Li, R., Ansari, M. S., . . . Zald, D. H. (2010). Dopaminergic network differences in human impulsivity. *Science, 329*, 532. http://dx.doi.org/10.1126/science.1185778

Buckner, R. L. (2004). Memory and executive function in aging and AD: Multiple factors that cause decline and reserve factors that compensate. *Neuron, 44*, 195–208. http://dx.doi.org/10.1016/j.neuron.2004.09.006

Cabeza, R. (2002). Hemispheric asymmetry reduction in older adults: The HAROLD model. *Psychology and Aging, 17*, 85–100. http://dx.doi.org/10.1037/0882-7974.17.1.85

Cabeza, R., & Dennis, N. A. (2013). Frontal lobes and aging: Deterioration and compensation. In D. T. Stuss & R. T. Knight (Eds.), *Principles of frontal lobe function* (2nd ed., pp. 628–652). New York, NY: Oxford University Press.

Carstensen, L. L., Isaacowitz, D. M., & Charles, S. T. (1999). Taking time seriously. A theory of socioemotional selectivity. *American Psychologist, 54*, 165–181. http://dx.doi.org/10.1037/0003-066X.54.3.165

Cassidy, B. S., & Gutchess, A. H. (2012). Social relevance enhances memory for impressions in older adults. *Memory, 20*, 332–345. http://dx.doi.org/10.1080/09658211.2012.660956

Cassidy, B. S., Leshikar, E. D., Shih, J. Y., Aizenman, A., & Gutchess, A. H. (2013). Valence-based age differences in medial prefrontal activity during impression formation. *Social Neuroscience, 8*, 462–473. http://dx.doi.org/10.1080/17470919.2013.832373

Cassidy, B. S., Shih, J. Y., & Gutchess, A. H. (2012). Age-related changes to the neural correlates of social evaluation. *Social Neuroscience, 7*, 552–564. http://dx.doi.org/10.1080/17470919.2012.674057

Castelli, I., Baglio, F., Blasi, V., Alberoni, M., Falini, A., Liverta-Sempio, O., . . . Marchetti, A. (2010). Effects of aging on mindreading ability through the eyes: An fMRI study. *Neuropsychologia, 48,* 2586–2594. http://dx.doi.org/10.1016/ j.neuropsychologia.2010.05.005

Chen, Y. C., Chen, C. C., Decety, J., & Cheng, Y. (2014). Aging is associated with changes in the neural circuits underlying empathy. *Neurobiology of Aging, 35,* 827–836. http://dx.doi.org/10.1016/j.neurobiolaging.2013.10.080

Cohen, M. X., Schoene-Bake, J. C., Elger, C. E., & Weber, B. (2009). Connectivity-based segregation of the human striatum predicts personality characteristics. *Nature Neuroscience, 12,* 32–34. http://dx.doi.org/10.1038/nn.2228

de la Vega, A., Chang, L. J., Banich, M. T., Wager, T. D., & Yarkoni, T. (2016). Large-scale meta-analysis of human medial frontal cortex reveals tripartite functional organization. *The Journal of Neuroscience, 36,* 6553–6562. http://dx.doi.org/ 10.1523/JNEUROSCI.4402-15.2016

Delgado, M. R., Beer, J. S., Fellows, L. K., Huettel, S. A., Platt, M. L., Quirk, G. J., & Schiller, D. (2016). Viewpoints: Dialogues on the functional role of the ventromedial prefrontal cortex. *Nature Neuroscience, 19,* 1545–1552. http:// dx.doi.org/10.1038/nn.4438

Dixon, M. L., Thiruchselvam, R., Todd, R., & Christoff, K. (2017). Emotion and the prefrontal cortex: An integrative review. *Psychological Bulletin, 143,* 1033–1081. http://dx.doi.org/10.1037/bul0000096

Draganski, B., Kherif, F., Klöppel, S., Cook, P. A., Alexander, D. C., Parker, G. J., . . . Frackowiak, R. S. (2008). Evidence for segregated and integrative connectivity patterns in the human basal ganglia. *The Journal of Neuroscience, 28,* 7143–7152. http://dx.doi.org/10.1523/JNEUROSCI.1486-08.2008

Ebner, N. C., Bailey, P. E., Horta, M., Joiner, J. A., & Chang, S. W. C. (2017). Multidisciplinary perspective on prosociality in aging. In J. A. Sommerville & J. Decety (Eds.), *Social cognition: Development across the life span* (pp. 303–325). New York, NY: Routledge.

Eppinger, B., Hämmerer, D., & Li, S. C. (2011). Neuromodulation of reward-based learning and decision making in human aging. *Annals of the New York Academy of Sciences, 1235,* 1–17. http://dx.doi.org/10.1111/j.1749-6632.2011.06230.x

Ford, J. H., Morris, J. A., & Kensinger, E. A. (2014). Neural recruitment and connectivity during emotional memory retrieval across the adult life span. *Neurobiology of Aging, 35,* 2770–2784. http://dx.doi.org/10.1016/j.neurobiolaging. 2014.05.029

Freund, A. M. (2006). Age-differential motivational consequences of optimization versus compensation focus in younger and older adults. *Psychology and Aging, 21,* 240–252. http://dx.doi.org/10.1037/0882-7974.21.2.240

Fung, H. H., Carstensen, L. L., & Lutz, A. M. (1999). Influence of time on social preferences: Implications for life-span development. *Psychology and Aging, 14,* 595–604. http://dx.doi.org/10.1037/0882-7974.14.4.595

Grady, C. L., Protzner, A. B., Kovacevic, N., Strother, S. C., Afshin-Pour, B., Wojtowicz, M., . . . McIntosh, A. R. (2010). A multivariate analysis of age-related differences in default mode and task-positive networks across multiple cognitive domains. *Cerebral Cortex, 20,* 1432–1447. http://dx.doi.org/10.1093/cercor/bhp207

Gutchess, A. (2014). Plasticity of the aging brain: New directions in cognitive neuroscience. *Science, 346,* 579–582. http://dx.doi.org/10.1126/science.1254604

Gutchess, A. H. (2019). *Cognitive and social neuroscience of aging.* New York, NY: Cambridge University Press.

Gutchess, A. H., Kensinger, E. A., & Schacter, D. L. (2007). Aging, self-referencing, and medial prefrontal cortex. *Social Neuroscience, 2,* 117–133. http://dx.doi.org/10.1080/17470910701399029

Gutchess, A. H., Kensinger, E. A., & Schacter, D. L. (2010). Functional neuroimaging of self-referential encoding with age. *Neuropsychologia, 48,* 211–219. http://dx.doi.org/10.1016/j.neuropsychologia.2009.09.006

Gutchess, A. H., Sokal, R., Coleman, J. A., Gotthilf, G., Grewal, L., & Rosa, N. (2015). Age differences in self-referencing: Evidence for common and distinct encoding strategies. *Brain Research, 1612,* 118–127. http://dx.doi.org/10.1016/j.brainres.2014.08.033

Haber, S. N. (2003). The primate basal ganglia: Parallel and integrative networks. *Journal of Chemical Neuroanatomy, 26,* 317–330. http://dx.doi.org/10.1016/j.jchemneu.2003.10.003

Haber, S. N., & Knutson, B. (2010). The reward circuit: Linking primate anatomy and human imaging. *Neuropsychopharmacology, 35,* 4–26. http://dx.doi.org/10.1038/npp.2009.129

Harris, L. T., & Fiske, S. T. (2006). Dehumanizing the lowest of the low: Neuroimaging responses to extreme out-groups. *Psychological Science, 17,* 847–853. http://dx.doi.org/10.1111/j.1467-9280.2006.01793.x

Harris, L. T., & Fiske, S. T. (2007). Social groups that elicit disgust are differentially processed in mPFC. *Social Cognitive and Affective Neuroscience, 2,* 45–51. http://dx.doi.org/10.1093/scan/nsl037

Harris, L. T., & Fiske, S. T. (2010). Neural regions that underlie reinforcement learning are also active for social expectancy violations. *Social Neuroscience, 5,* 76–91. http://dx.doi.org/10.1080/17470910903135825

Harris, L. T., McClure, S. M., van den Bos, W., Cohen, J. D., & Fiske, S. T. (2007). Regions of the MPFC differentially tuned to social and nonsocial affective evaluation. *Cognitive, Affective & Behavioral Neuroscience, 7,* 309–316. http://dx.doi.org/10.3758/CABN.7.4.309

Henry, J. D., Phillips, L. H., Ruffman, T., & Bailey, P. E. (2013). A meta-analytic review of age differences in theory of mind. *Psychology and Aging, 28,* 826–839. http://dx.doi.org/10.1037/a0030677

Hess, T. M., & Tate, C. S. (1991). Adult age differences in explanations and memory for behavioral information. *Psychology and Aging, 6*, 86–92. http://dx.doi.org/10.1037/0882-7974.6.1.86

Jimura, K., Myerson, J., Hilgard, J., Keighley, J., Braver, T. S., & Green, L. (2011). Domain independence and stability in young and older adults' discounting of delayed rewards. *Behavioural Processes, 87*, 253–259. http://dx.doi.org/10.1016/j.beproc.2011.04.006

Kahnt, T. (2018). A decade of decoding reward-related fMRI signals and where we go from here. *NeuroImage, 180*, 324–333.

Karrer, T. M., Josef, A. K., Mata, R., Morris, E. D., & Samanez-Larkin, G. R. (2017). Reduced dopamine receptors and transporters but not synthesis capacity in normal aging adults: A meta-analysis. *Neurobiology of Aging, 57*, 36–46. http://dx.doi.org/10.1016/j.neurobiolaging.2017.05.006

Kennedy, Q., Mather, M., & Carstensen, L. L. (2004). The role of motivation in the age-related positivity effect in autobiographical memory. *Psychological Science, 15*, 208–214. http://dx.doi.org/10.1111/j.0956-7976.2004.01503011.x

Kennerley, S. W., & Walton, M. E. (2011). Decision making and reward in frontal cortex: Complementary evidence from neurophysiological and neuropsychological studies. *Behavioral Neuroscience, 125*, 297–317. http://dx.doi.org/10.1037/a0023575

Kensinger, E. A., & Gutchess, A. H. (2015). Memory for emotional and social information in adulthood and old age. In A. Duarte, M. Barense, & D. R. Addis (Eds.), *The Wiley handbook on the cognitive neuroscience of human memory* (pp. 393–414). Chichester, England: Wiley Blackwell. http://dx.doi.org/10.1002/9781118332634.ch19

Kensinger, E. A., & Gutchess, A. H. (2017). Cognitive aging in a social and affective context: Advances over the past 50 years. *The Journals of Gerontology: Series B. Psychological Sciences and Social Sciences, 72*, 61–70. http://dx.doi.org/10.1093/geronb/gbw056

Krendl, A. C. (2018). Reduced cognitive capacity impairs the malleability of older adults' negative attitudes to stigmatized individuals. *Experimental Aging Research, 44*, 271–283. Advance online publication. http://dx.doi.org/10.1080/0361073X.2018.1475152

Krendl, A. C., Heatherton, T. F., & Kensinger, E. A. (2009). Aging minds and twisting attitudes: An fMRI investigation of age differences in inhibiting prejudice. *Psychology and Aging, 24*, 530–541. http://dx.doi.org/10.1037/a0016065

Krendl, A. C., & Kensinger, E. A. (2016). Does older adults' cognitive function disrupt the malleability of their attitudes toward outgroup members? An fMRI investigation. *PLoS One, 11*, e0152698. http://dx.doi.org/10.1371/journal.pone.0152698

Krendl, A. C., Rule, N. O., & Ambady, N. (2014). Does aging impair first impression accuracy? Differentiating emotion recognition from complex social inferences. *Psychology and Aging, 29,* 482–490. http://dx.doi.org/10.1037/a0037146

Lawrence, A. D., Sahakian, B. J., & Robbins, T. W. (1998). Cognitive functions and corticostriatal circuits: Insights from Huntington's disease. *Trends in Cognitive Sciences, 2,* 379–388. http://dx.doi.org/10.1016/S1364-6613(98)01231-5

Leclerc, C. M., & Kensinger, E. A. (2008). Age-related differences in medial prefrontal activation in response to emotional images. *Cognitive, Affective & Behavioral Neuroscience, 8,* 153–164. http://dx.doi.org/10.3758/CABN.8.2.153

Leclerc, C. M., & Kensinger, E. A. (2010). Age-related valence-based reversal in recruitment of medial prefrontal cortex on a visual search task. *Social Neuroscience, 5,* 560–576. http://dx.doi.org/10.1080/17470910903512296

Lee, V. K., & Harris, L. T. (2013). How social cognition can inform social decision making. *Frontiers in Neuroscience, 7,* 259. http://dx.doi.org/10.3389/fnins.2013.00259

Li, S. C., Lindenberger, U., & Sikström, S. (2001). Aging cognition: From neuromodulation to representation. *Trends in Cognitive Sciences, 5,* 479–486. http://dx.doi.org/10.1016/S1364-6613(00)01769-1

Lim, K. T. K., & Yu, R. (2015). Aging and wisdom: Age-related changes in economic and social decision making. *Frontiers in Aging Neuroscience, 7,* 120. http://dx.doi.org/10.3389/fnagi.2015.00120

Macrae, C. N., Moran, J. M., Heatherton, T. F., Banfield, J. F., & Kelley, W. M. (2004). Medial prefrontal activity predicts memory for self. *Cerebral Cortex, 14,* 647–654. http://dx.doi.org/10.1093/cercor/bhh025

Mather, M., & Carstensen, L. L. (2003). Aging and attentional biases for emotional faces. *Psychological Science, 14,* 409–415. http://dx.doi.org/10.1111/1467-9280.01455

Mather, M., & Carstensen, L. L. (2005). Aging and motivated cognition: The positivity effect in attention and memory. *Trends in Cognitive Sciences, 9,* 496–502. http://dx.doi.org/10.1016/j.tics.2005.08.005

Maylor, E. A., Moulson, J. M., Muncer, A. M., & Taylor, L. A. (2002). Does performance on theory of mind tasks decline in old age? *British Journal of Psychology, 93,* 465–485. http://dx.doi.org/10.1348/000712602761381358

Mitchell, J. P. (2008). Contributions of Functional Neuroimaging to the Study of Social Cognition. *Current Directions in Psychological Science, 17,* 142–146. http://dx.doi.org/10.1111/j.1467-8721.2008.00564.x

Mitchell, K. J., Raye, C. L., Ebner, N. C., Tubridy, S. M., Frankel, H., & Johnson, M. K. (2009). Age-group differences in medial cortex activity associated with thinking about self-relevant agendas. *Psychology and Aging, 24,* 438–449. http://dx.doi.org/10.1037/a0015181

Moorman, D. E., James, M. H., McGlinchey, E. M., & Aston-Jones, G. (2015). Differential roles of medial prefrontal subregions in the regulation of drug seeking. *Brain Research, 1628,* 130–146. http://dx.doi.org/10.1016/j.brainres.2014.12.024

Moran, J. M. (2013). Lifespan development: The effects of typical aging on theory of mind. *Behavioural Brain Research, 237*, 32–40. http://dx.doi.org/10.1016/j.bbr.2012.09.020

Moran, J. M., Jolly, E., & Mitchell, J. P. (2012). Social-cognitive deficits in normal aging. *Journal of Neuroscience, 32*, 5553–5561. http://dx.doi.org/10.1523/jneurosci.5511-11.2012

Opitz, P. C., Lee, I. A., Gross, J. J., & Urry, H. L. (2014). Fluid cognitive ability is a resource for successful emotion regulation in older and younger adults. *Frontiers in Psychology, 5*, 609. http://dx.doi.org/10.3389/fpsyg.2014.00609

Persson, J., Lustig, C., Nelson, J. K., & Reuter-Lorenz, P. A. (2007). Age differences in deactivation: A link to cognitive control? *Journal of Cognitive Neuroscience, 19*, 1021–1032. http://dx.doi.org/10.1162/jocn.2007.19.6.1021

Phillips, L. H., MacLean, R. D., & Allen, R. (2002). Age and the understanding of emotions: Neuropsychological and sociocognitive perspectives. *The Journals of Gerontology: Series B. Psychological Sciences and Social Sciences, 57*, 526–530. http://dx.doi.org/10.1093/geronb/57.6.P526

Roalf, D. R., Mitchell, S. H., Harbaugh, W. T., & Janowsky, J. S. (2012). Risk, reward, and economic decision making in aging. *The Journals of Gerontology: Series B. Psychological Sciences and Social Sciences, 67*, 289–298. http://dx.doi.org/10.1093/geronb/gbr099

Rushworth, M. F., Noonan, M. P., Boorman, E. D., Walton, M. E., & Behrens, T. E. (2011). Frontal cortex and reward-guided learning and decision-making. *Neuron, 70*, 1054–1069. http://dx.doi.org/10.1016/j.neuron.2011.05.014

Sakaki, M., Niki, K., & Mather, M. (2012). Beyond arousal and valence: The importance of the biological versus social relevance of emotional stimuli. *Cognitive, Affective & Behavioral Neuroscience, 12*, 115–139. http://dx.doi.org/10.3758/s13415-011-0062-x

Samanez-Larkin, G. R., & Carstensen, L. L. (2011). Socioemotional functioning and the aging brain. In J. Decety & J. T. Cacioppo (Eds.), *The Oxford handbook of social neuroscience* (pp. 507–521). New York, NY: Oxford University Press.

Samanez-Larkin, G. R., & Knutson, B. (2015). Decision making in the ageing brain: Changes in affective and motivational circuits. *Nature Reviews Neuroscience, 16*, 278–289. http://dx.doi.org/10.1038/nrn3917

Schott, B. H., Niehaus, L., Wittmann, B. C., Schütze, H., Seidenbecher, C. I., Heinze, H. J., & Düzel, E. (2007). Ageing and early-stage Parkinson's disease affect separable neural mechanisms of mesolimbic reward processing. *Brain: A Journal of Neurology, 130*, 2412–2424. http://dx.doi.org/10.1093/brain/awm147

Seaman, K. L., Gorlick, M. A., Vekaria, K. M., Hsu, M., Zald, D. H., & Samanez-Larkin, G. R. (2016). Adult age differences in decision making across domains: Increased discounting of social and health-related rewards. *Psychology and Aging, 31*, 737–746. http://dx.doi.org/10.1037/pag0000131

Seger, C. A., Peterson, E. J., Cincotta, C. M., Lopez-Paniagua, D., & Anderson, C. W. (2010). Dissociating the contributions of independent corticostriatal systems to visual categorization learning through the use of reinforcement learn-ing modeling and Granger causality modeling. *NeuroImage, 50,* 644–656. http://dx.doi.org/10.1016/j.neuroimage.2009.11.083

Sullivan, S., & Ruffman, T. (2004). Social understanding: How does it fare with advancing years? *British Journal of Psychology, 95,* 1–18. http://dx.doi.org/10.1348/000712604322779424

Tamir, D. I., & Mitchell, J. P. (2012). Disclosing information about the self is intrin-sically rewarding. *Proceedings of the National Academy of Sciences of the United States of America, 109,* 8038–8043. http://dx.doi.org/10.1073/pnas.1202129109

van den Bos, W., McClure, S. M., Harris, L. T., Fiske, S. T., & Cohen, J. D. (2007). Dissociating affective evaluation and social cognitive processes in the ventral medial prefrontal cortex. *Cognitive, Affective & Behavioral Neuroscience, 7,* 337–346. http://dx.doi.org/10.3758/CABN.7.4.337

Zald, D. H., Cowan, R. L., Riccardi, P., Baldwin, R. M., Ansari, M. S., Li, R., . . . Kessler, R. M. (2008). Midbrain dopamine receptor availability is inversely associated with novelty-seeking traits in humans. *The Journal of Neuroscience, 28,* 14372–14378. http://dx.doi.org/10.1523/JNEUROSCI.2423-08.2008

Zebrowitz, L. A., Franklin, R. G., Hillman, S., & Boc, H. (2013). Older and younger adults' first impressions from faces: Similar in agreement but different in posi-tivity. *Psychology and Aging, 28,* 202–212. http://dx.doi.org/10.1037/a0030927

7

COMPENSATION AND BRAIN AGING: A REVIEW AND ANALYSIS OF EVIDENCE

LAURA B. ZAHODNE AND PATRICIA A. REUTER-LORENZ

A recurrent theme in research on cognitive aging is the large variability not only in cross-sectional cognitive performance but also in rates of late-life cognitive change. This variability reflects, in part, individual differences in susceptibility to adverse effects of age on brain structure and function. The concept of *brain maintenance* describes individual differences in brain preservation that can contribute to successful cognitive aging (Nyberg, Lövdén, Riklund, Lindenberger, & Bäckman, 2012). Indeed, a recent investigation of "superagers" (i.e., older adults whose memory resembles that of individuals 20–30 years younger) characterized patterns of neuroanatomical preservation within the cerebral cortex and hippocampus, which correlated with better memory performance (Sun et al., 2016). Although this cross-sectional study cannot rule out that superagers start out with a higher level of brain integrity but evidence the same amount of atrophy as other older adults, it may suggest that superagers are able to resist age-related brain atrophy.

http://dx.doi.org/10.1037/0000143-008
The Aging Brain: Functional Adaptation Across Adulthood, G. R. Samanez-Larkin (Editor)

Although not all older adults are able to resist age-related neural deterioration or the accumulation of age-related neuropathology, many display a remarkable ability to cope with it. Substantial overlap in the distributions of both regional cortical thickness and hippocampal volume among superagers and other older adults indicates that some superagers are able to achieve above-average cognitive performance despite having average brain structural integrity (Sun et al., 2016). An early clinicopathological study reported on 10 older women whose brains, on postmortem analysis, contained extensive AD pathology but who had normal cognition in life (Katzman et al., 1988). We now know that up to 67% of older adults classified as "cognitively normal" in longitudinal studies meet full pathological criteria for dementia at autopsy (Crystal et al., 1988; Neuropathology Group, 2001; Price & Morris, 1999). Thus, some older adults seem able to compensate for age-related neural decline, including neuropathology.

Behavioral evidence for compensation comes from a large epidemiological cohort in France followed for 20 years (Amieva et al., 2014). Among highly educated participants who developed Alzheimer's disease (AD) over the course of the study (i.e., incident cases), prediagnosis trajectories showed two discrete periods of decline. The first, occurring 15 to 16 years before dementia diagnosis, was characterized by subtle cognitive declines that did not extend to activities of daily living. The second, occurring 7 years before dementia diagnosis, was characterized by more global cognitive decline accompanied by functional impairment. In contrast, participants with incident AD who had low educational attainment showed only a single, continuous period of decline before diagnosis. The authors concluded that highly educated participants were able to compensate for the initial occurrence of AD pathology (corresponding to the first period of decline) for approximately 8 to 9 years before showing more widespread clinical decline.

Compensation has long been recognized as a cornerstone of successful late-life development, figuring prominently in behavioral research and theory on cognitive aging (Baltes & Baltes, 1990). According to this traditional view of "behavioral" compensation, it typically manifests as self-initiated cognitive and behavioral strategies that forge alternative means for maintaining everyday functioning. Such compensatory practices need not be conscious or deliberate and may consist of changes in behavior such as writing things down, selecting less noisy restaurants, or adopting external aids, such as reading glasses or hearing aids, all of which aim to offset cognitive and physical declines.

In this chapter, we focus on what is best referred to as *neural compensation*, in contrast to behavioral compensation. By neural compensation, we mean alterations in neural functioning that offset the effects of age-related neural decline or pathology to preserve high levels of cognitive and behavioral output. To the extent that the capacity for neural compensation exists in the aging brain, it constitutes a vital avenue for successful cognitive aging and an alternative to brain maintenance where the relative absence of neural decline presumably obviates the need for compensation. Identifying neural compensatory processes and understanding their implementation are therefore critical to the cognitive neuroscience of aging. Over the past 20 years, many advances have been made toward identifying compensatory processes in the aging brain, and the goal of this chapter is to review and synthesize that progress with respect to both normal and pathological aging.

CHALLENGES IN RESEARCH ON NEURAL COMPENSATION IN AGING

With the increased use of neuroscience approaches to study cognitive aging, compensation has gained prominence as an important explanatory construct for understanding age-related differences, or changes, in neural measures that are associated with relatively preserved behavioral performance. This has been especially true in the functional neuroimaging literature (e.g., positron emission tomography [PET]; functional magnetic resonance imaging [fMRI]) where the notion of compensation has often been applied to explain age differences in brain activity during cognitive task performance (for a review of theories explaining age differences in brain activation, see Festini, Zahodne, & Reuter-Lorenz, 2018). More specifically, the frequent finding of greater or more widespread brain activation in older than younger adults during cognitive tasks involving memory, attention, and other forms of executive control has been interpreted as a sign of neural compensation, especially when behavioral performance shows minimal signs of age-related decline.

Although the compensation interpretation has appeal for a variety of reasons that are discussed in this chapter, there are also challenges that first need to be considered in order to apply it appropriately to brain-based results. We review several of them here, including distinguishing compensation from brain maintenance, distinguishing direct functional consequences of brain aging from reactive (compensatory) responses, navigating limits on the capacity for compensation, and integrating research findings across heterogeneous studies. We believe that each of these challenges highlights specific opportunities for advancing knowledge about compensatory processes in the aging brain.

Distinguishing Compensation From Brain Maintenance

The notion of compensation requires that there is something to compensate for—that is, that some neural compromise or insufficiency is affecting

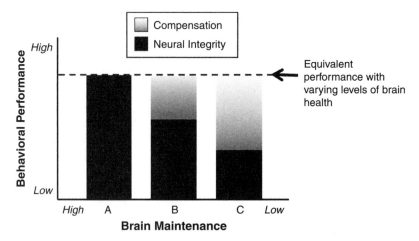

Figure 7.1. Equivalent behavioral performance across different states of brain maintenance. Within an individual across time and age, or across individuals of the same age, the same level of behavioral performance can be accomplished despite different degrees of brain maintenance and neural compromise. This figure depicts Individual A with a high level of brain maintenance, performing well on a generic behavioral task. With decreased brain maintenance, as depicted by declining integrity in hypothetical Individuals B and C, compensation may offset the effects of decline, to produce approximately equivalent performance, within limits (thus the gradient associated with the portion of performance supported by compensation). "Superagers" may be those with exceptional maintenance, or youth-like neural integrity, like Individual A. As task demands increase, the effectiveness of compensation in offsetting neural decline will diminish and behavioral performance will suffer, resulting in measurable performance differences among our three prototypes.

brain function.[1] Interpretations of neural compensation cannot rely solely on behavioral markers because the same level of performance can be attained via different routes. Some older adults achieve high levels of performance due to the absence of neural compromise (e.g., brain maintenance), whereas others achieve comparable levels of performance through different combinations of neural compromise and compensatory processes that offset these neural declines (see Figure 7.1). Therefore, objective characterization of neural compromise (e.g., via structural or functional brain measures) is ultimately an important component of research on compensation. Because cross-sectional studies are limited in their ability to distinguish acquired neural compromise (i.e., within-person declines in brain structural integrity) from long-standing individual differences, longitudinal studies are particularly critical for identifying neural processes that function in a compensatory role. This challenge

---

[1]Capacity limits (i.e., supply–demand mismatch; Lövdén, Bäckman, Lindenberger, Schaefer, & Schmiedek, 2010) in young adults can also promote compensatory recruitment, as we discuss further in the section "Limits on the Capacity for Compensation."

is analogous to the difficulty of measuring psychological resilience in the absence of adversity (Masten, 2007). Specifically, individuals may achieve comparable levels of psychological well-being due to the absence of adversity or through different combinations of adversity and psychological resilience.

One implication of this issue is that compensatory brain activity may not always correlate with better performance in a between-subjects design that includes older adults with varying degrees of brain health. Older adults who show more compensation may have greater need for it (i.e., greater degree of neural compromise), and their performance may therefore be worse than older adults who show less compensation due to the absence of a neural compromise. In low-performing older adults, greater brain activity may allow them to perform better than if they did not generate this additional activity, although not as well as they performed before the onset of neural compromise. Consequently, in this example, more compensation could be associated with poorer performance across subjects. Therefore, in a between-subjects design, it can be challenging to interpret a finding of greater neural activity as compensatory based on its relationship with performance without also considering brain structure or pathology. Within-subjects designs that incorporate longitudinal measurement provide a powerful tool for distinguishing between brain maintenance and compensation.

Distinguishing Direct Functional Consequences From Reactive Responses

A major challenge in studying compensation in aging lies in interpreting whether brain signals, such as those measured using fMRI, arise from primary or secondary consequences of brain aging (Lövdén, Bäckman, Lindenberger, Schaefer, & Schmiedek, 2010). Specifically, primary signs of "normal" age-related neural deterioration must be distinguished from signs of compensation that are secondary or responsive to neural deterioration. For example, is overactivation[2] in a group of older adults, relative to their younger counterparts, a direct indication of age-related dysfunction or a compensatory response to dysfunction?

During "normal" aging, gross brain volume decreases on the order of 0.2% to 0.5% per year (Hedman, van Haren, Schnack, Kahn, & Hulshoff Pol, 2012), with the most significant atrophy occurring in the frontal and temporal lobes (Fjell, McEvoy, Holland, Dale, & Walhovd, 2014). Thus, some patterns of brain activity likely reflect primary changes that correspond directly to typical structural effects of normal aging. Indeed, in the early days

---

[2]In this chapter, the term *overactivation* is used to describe levels of activation that are higher relative to a specific reference group (e.g., young adults).

of task-related functional imaging studies, it was anticipated that older adults would generally show less activation that younger adults (Reuter-Lorenz et al., 2001), based on widely documented age-related reductions in cortical volume (Raz, 2000). Although not the pervasive result (Cabeza, 2002; Reuter-Lorenz & Lustig, 2005), such associations have been reported (Hedden & Gabrieli, 2004; Maillet & Rajah, 2013). For example, cortical hypometabolism in a group of older adults with mild cognitive impairment (MCI) correlated with degree of basal forebrain atrophy, measured using high-resolution MRI, and mediated the association between atrophy and memory performance (Grothe, Heinsen, Amaro, Grinberg, & Teipel, 2016).

An analogous challenge exists in research on compensation in pathological aging. That is, primary signs of pathological deterioration must be distinguished from signs of compensation that are secondary to neuropathology (e.g., plaques and tangles, cerebrovascular disease). Some patterns of brain activity appear to reflect primary changes associated with age-related neurodegenerative disease. For example, medial prefrontal cortex hypometabolism in AD correlated with β-amyloid deposition in that region (Laforce et al., 2014). As described subsequently, these different patterns of response (i.e., primary vs. secondary) can be detected in the same subjects, within the same experiment.

Limits on the Capacity for Compensation

A related challenge for identifying compensatory processes is that there appear to be limits on the capacity for compensation. These limits can be understood as a mismatch between supply (i.e., the functional capacity of the system given brain integrity and available compensatory repertoire) and demand (i.e., task difficulty; Lövdén et al., 2010). The size of one's functional compensatory repertoire may reflect one's level of cognitive reserve, which has been purported to increase with engagement in a variety of cognitive activities (e.g., formal education, cognitively demanding leisure activities) over the life course (Barulli & Stern, 2013). Once a neural compromise passes a certain threshold, compensatory responses may be insufficient to meet current task demands, and their inadequacy could result in plummeting performance.

Apart from low supply, a mismatch may also result from high demand. Specifically, even when supply is high, compensatory responses may prove insufficient in the face of skyrocketing task demands. As a result, there may not be a linear association between brain activity and behavioral performance. As described by the compensation-related utilization of neural circuits hypothesis (CRUNCH; Reuter-Lorenz & Cappell, 2008; Reuter-Lorenz & Mikels, 2006), older adults need to recruit more neural resources and are likely to meet their resource ceiling at lower levels of task demand than

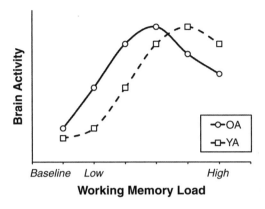

Figure 7.2. Brain activity may index compensation under varying levels of task demand. Neuroimaging indices have documented greater levels of brain activity (referred to as *overactivation*) in older adults compared with younger adults at low levels of task demand, and in association with approximately equivalent performance. As task demands increase, activity increases regardless of age; however, older adults will reach asymptotic levels at lower levels of demand than will younger adults. At this inflection point, task performance suffers because the necessary circuitry can no longer be engaged effectively. These ideas have been articulated in the compensation-related utilization of neural circuits hypothesis (Reuter-Lorenz & Cappell, 2008). In this depiction, the maximal activity is equated across age; however, this assumption is not obligatory in that some populations of older adults may have a lower activity ceiling due to neural pathology, for example. These activity profiles may pertain to task-specific regions but have generally been associated with more domain-general frontoparietal networks. OA = older adults; YA = young adults.

younger adults (see Figure 7.2). According to CRUNCH, older adults may overactivate relative to young adults at a low level of task demand, where age differences in performance may be minimal, and underactivate relative to young adults at higher levels of demand, where performance differences will favor young adults. Accordingly, both neural activation and performance can be lowest for older adults at the highest level of task demand. The implication of this phenomenon is that group differences in brain activation may be especially ambiguous in studies that include only a single level of task demand. The terms *attempted compensation, unsuccessful compensation,* and *successful compensation* have been introduced to facilitate interpreting seemingly paradoxical associations of hyperactivation[3] and performance and to reconcile contradictory interpretations of hyperactivation across studies (Cabeza & Dennis, 2013).

---

[3]In this chapter, the term *hyperactivation* is used to describe generally high levels of activation that are not explicitly compared to an identified reference group.

Heterogeneity in Research on Compensation

Finally, challenges to synthesizing the literature on neural compensation among older adults lie in the heterogeneity of (a) neural compromises (e.g., normal aging, neurodegenerative vs. cerebrovascular pathology) that have been purported to trigger compensation, (b) the specific cognitive or performance task under investigation, and (c) the region(s) or network(s) in which functional response is being inferred. It is possible that the nature of compensation differs depending on the type and location of neural compromise; the specific demands of a cognitive, perceptual, or motor task; and the characteristics of the core neural network typically engaged by each task. Throughout this chapter, we discuss studies that differ with respect to each of these elements and highlight how similarities and differences across studies shed light on various aspects of compensatory processes in aging. We do not review evidence pertaining to motor performance, although age-related compensatory processes have been inferred in that domain as well. For a comprehensive review of motor control and brain aging, the reader is referred to Seidler et al. (2010).

VARIETIES OF EVIDENCE TESTING THE COMPENSATION INTERPRETATION

Brain Activity–Performance Associations

Perhaps the most straightforward evidence favoring a compensatory account of functional imaging data is finding a positive correlation between magnitude of activation and cognitive performance. Studies of task-related activity that provide this type of evidence typically involve at least two analytic steps. First, a contrast is conducted between task and minimal or nontask conditions to identify regions in which activity differs between a group of interest (e.g., healthy older adults) and a comparison group (e.g., healthy young adults). This step demonstrates that the magnitude or spatial extent (or both) of activity is not seen in the comparison group at the same level of task demand. Next, activity within network(s) identified through the first step is correlated with behavioral performance within the group of interest or both groups. This step can be used to interpret whether unique patterns of brain response (e.g., hyperactivation) that characterize the group of interest are detrimental, facilitative, or inconsequential. Importantly, the evidence for compensation in this framework is the positive, within-group correlation between brain response and performance, not whether the group of interest performs better than, worse than, or similarly to the comparison group. It is rare to find examples in which a compromised group performs better than a comparison group because the putative goal of compensation is to restore functioning close to the level achieved before the neural compromise, not to attain a previously unrealized level of functioning.

Studies of Healthy Adults

Numerous fMRI studies of healthy old and young adults have examined task-related brain activity and reported a positive association between degree of overactivation and cognitive performance (Reuter-Lorenz & Cappell, 2008). In a representative study, a flexible go/no-go paradigm was used to explore the conditions in which healthy older adults recruited more neural resources to achieve better task performance (Vallesi, McIntosh, & Stuss, 2011). Older adults in that study overactivated a frontoparietal network during the most difficult task condition involving the acquisition of novel and complex rules. Critically, this frontoparietal overengagement correlated positively with performance among older adults.

Even stronger evidence is provided by studies that integrate not just measures of brain activity and behavioral performance but also direct measures of neural compromise. For example, a positive correlation between frontal hyperactivation and speech discrimination in a noisy environment was linked to overall phoneme dedifferentiation in the auditory cortex of older adults (Du, Buchsbaum, Grady, & Alain, 2016). This study generates within the same experimental paradigm the compensation hypothesis and the dedifferentiation hypothesis, which proposes that aging is associated with a breakdown in specificity of neural representations (Carp, Gmeindl, & Reuter-Lorenz, 2010; S. C. Li, Lindenberger, & Sikström, 2001; Park et al., 2004).

Studies reporting a positive association between degree of frontoparietal hyperactivation and cognitive performance have used a variety of cognitive tasks, including measures of attention and inhibition, episodic memory, lexical–semantic knowledge, and speech perception (Berlingeri et al., 2010; Reuter-Lorenz & Cappell, 2008). The consistency of findings across such disparate cognitive domains suggests that the frontoparietal control network may represent a relatively domain-general processing resource that can be recruited by older adults to enhance performance on a variety of tasks, although the precise frontal and parietal regions used appear to depend on the task at hand (Turner & Spreng, 2012). This domain-general processing resource may involve the deployment of executive abilities. A study using event-related potentials (ERPs) reported that healthy older adults showed more bilateral activity than younger adults during an episodic memory task, and greater bilaterality was associated with better performance among the older adults (Angel, Fay, Bouazzaoui, & Isingrini, 2011). Importantly, this study further demonstrated that age-related differences in the degree of bilaterality within the older adult group were mediated by level of executive functioning (assessed by a battery of neuropsychological tests), supporting the suggestion that age-related compensatory activation is driven by domain-general executive abilities subserved by the frontoparietal network (Bouazzaoui et al., 2014).

In addition to studies of functional activity, correlational evidence for compensation is also emerging in studies of functional connectivity, which measures the associations between levels of brain activity in different (including remote) brain regions over time. Compared with young adults, older adults showed greater changes in functional connectivity when transitioning from a task-free resting state to a working memory task (Gallen, Turner, Adnan, & D'Esposito, 2016). Within the older adult group, an increase in the functional connectivity between subnetworks (i.e., modules) was positively associated with task performance.

Studies of Older Adults With Preclinical or Clinical Dementia

Positive associations between cortical hyperactivation and better cognitive performance have also been reported in studies of older adults with and without AD pathology. Because of the nature of the disease under study, these investigations typically use measures of episodic memory. An early PET study of older adults with and without AD documented a pattern of greater activation in an expanded set of (mostly frontal) cortical regions in the patients compared with healthy older adults, and greater activation was associated with better episodic memory performance (Becker et al., 1996). This result was found in the context of decreased activation within the hippocampus, consistent with their diagnoses. Similarly, hyperactivation of bilateral dorsolateral prefrontal and posterior cortices correlated with better performance on both semantic and episodic memory tasks among individuals with AD (Grady et al., 2003). Subsequent studies have documented similar patterns of results in MCI samples (Lenzi et al., 2011) and in cognitively healthy older adults with PET evidence of high amyloid-β, a marker of preclinical AD (Elman et al., 2014).

Secondary/compensatory brain activity has been documented in the context of primary/pathological brain activity among the same individuals. In one study of memory encoding, hippocampal activity correlated positively with performance in healthy older adults, but not older adults with MCI (Mandzia, McAndrews, Grady, Graham, & Black, 2009). This pattern of results suggests that hippocampal activity was beneficial for healthy older adults, but not for individuals with MCI. However, activity within Brodmann's area 20 correlated positively with performance only in the MCI group, suggesting that alternative temporal lobe circuitry may have provided compensation for dysfunction within the canonical parahippocampal encoding network (Protzner, Mandzia, Black, & McAndrews, 2011).

Individuals may not begin to engage compensatory networks until neural compromise exceeds a certain threshold. For example, one study divided a group of AD patients by memory ability and found that only those with low memory ability recruited an alternate network, compared with both AD patients with high memory ability and healthy older adult controls (Stern et al., 2000). Within this group of low-performing patients, activation of this alternate network was positively correlated with memory ability. Longitudinal evidence that dysfunction within the core memory network drives subsequent increases in alternate network activity comes from a study of 130 older adults followed with serial cognitive testing and MRI scans (Pudas, Josefsson, Rieckmann, & Nyberg, 2018). In that study, only participants with declining memory and smaller hippocampal volumes evidenced an increase in prefrontal activity during a memory task over a 4-year period.

Stroke and Other Neural Compromises

Evidence that hyperactivation correlates with better performance can also be found in the stroke literature. For example, increased activation of dorsal frontoparietal regions correlated with better language comprehension among individuals with aphasia following left-hemisphere stroke (Meltzer, Wagage, Ryder, Solomon, & Braun, 2013). The consistency of findings across studies of healthy aging, MCI, AD, and stroke suggests that the frontoparietal control network may be recruited in response to a variety of neural compromises. Further, a recent study that pushed participants to their individualized working memory capacity limit demonstrated that contralateral prefrontal regions are similarly recruited by both healthy young and healthy older adults in response to increasing subjective difficulty (Höller-Wallscheid, Thier, Pomper, & Lindner, 2017). Together, the results reviewed in the preceding sections on healthy adults, adults with preclinical or clinical dementia, and stroke suggest that relatively domain-general, age-independent frontoparietal networks can be activated to cope with increased cognitive demands due to either task characteristics or neural compromise.

Nonlinear Activity–Performance Associations

As discussed in the previous section on challenges in interpreting compensation in aging, limits on the brain's capacity for compensation could lead to nonlinear brain activity–performance associations. According to CRUNCH, the aging brain must recruit more neural resources to produce cognitive performance equivalent to that of a younger brain even when engaged in a task with relatively low levels of task demand (Reuter-Lorenz &

Cappell, 2008). As task demands increase, an aging brain will hit a resource ceiling such that it is unable to rally sufficient neural resources to maintain a high level of performance. Because older brains will recruit more resources at lower levels of task demand, they will reach their resource limit at lower loads than younger adults. The implication of this phenomenon is that the results of comparisons across individuals with and without neural compromise (e.g., old vs. young) are highly dependent on task demands: At low levels of task demand, compromised individuals show greater activation and perform similarly. At higher levels of task demand, compromised individuals show less activation and perform worse. Indeed, this pattern of results has been reported in multiple studies of healthy young and older adults that have varied working memory load and observed brain function with fMRI (Cappell, Gmeindl, & Reuter-Lorenz, 2010; Mattay et al., 2006) and electroencephalogram (McEvoy, Pellouchoud, Smith, & Gevins, 2001). Positive, linear brain activity–performance associations are most likely to be seen in the context of a reasonable supply–demand mismatch—that is, when task demands exceed the capacity of an established brain network but do not exceed the absolute functional capacity of the system.

Although CRUNCH was largely developed through working memory paradigms that lend themselves to parametric variation of task demand, it has also been used recently as a framework for interpreting disparate research findings in the language domain (Diaz, Rizio, & Zhuang, 2016). Specifically, language comprehension tasks are typically considered to be less demanding than language production tasks, and age-related differences in performance are more frequently observed for production tasks, compared with comprehension tasks. Further, age-related compensation interpretations (e.g., of positive correlations between hyperactivation and performance) are more frequently reported for comprehension tasks, compared with production tasks. Therefore, it is possible that compensation is more successful during less difficult comprehension tasks than during more difficult production tasks, in which the supply–demand mismatch often proves insurmountable for older adults.

Evidence for an inverted U-shaped relationship between activation and level of neural compromise has also been reported along the MCI–AD continuum. During an associative memory task, high-performing individuals with MCI showed overactivation within medial temporal lobe structures compared with healthy older adults, whereas low-performing individuals with MCI and individuals with mild AD showed underactivation within these same regions (Celone et al., 2006). Thus, relative mismatch between supply and demand, which depends on both the extent of neural compromise and the difficulty of the task at hand, appears to be more important in determining the limits of compensation than either supply or demand alone.

Negative Activity–Performance Associations

Not all studies exclusively find positive associations between frontal hyperactivity and behavioral performance in older adults. Indeed, the pattern of associations may depend on the nature of the task or the specific region investigated. In an fMRI study of naming, accuracy correlated positively with hyperactivity in the right inferior frontal gyrus (IFG), but negatively with hyperactivity in the right precentral gyrus in older adults (Wierenga et al., 2008). Thus, up-regulation of right frontal regions during word retrieval may represent unsuccessful attempts at compensation under certain conditions (Meinzer et al., 2012) or a disinhibition of brain regions whose activity disrupts performance.

Correlation With Degree of Neural Compromise in the Context of Matched Performance

In a between-subjects design in which participants all demonstrate approximately similar performance regardless of age or subgroup, a positive correlation between magnitude of activation and extent of a neural compromise (e.g., neuropathology) provides evidence for compensation (see Figure 7.3). This pattern of results suggests that individuals contending with a greater neural compromise are relying on increased activation to maintain cognitive performance at the same level as their noncompromised peers.

Studies of Healthy Adults

In many studies, the extent of neural compromise is inferred solely on the basis of participants' advanced age. In one representative study, older adults showed more activation in frontal, subcortical, and parietal regions than young adults during proactive inhibition in the context of matched behavioral performance (Kleerekooper et al., 2016). One of the most recent and comprehensive meta-analyses of cross-sectional, task-based fMRI studies of healthy young and older adults to date identified 92 studies that met their rigorous inclusion criteria and reported sufficient behavioral data to calculate effect sizes. Of these 92 studies, 11 reported similar behavioral performance across young and older adults. In these studies where performance was age-equivalent, older adults showed increased activation exclusively in the frontoparietal control network, suggesting that recruitment of this network supported the older adults' behavioral performance at the level of their younger peers (H. J. Li et al., 2015). A similar conclusion was reached in an ERP study, which documented greater anterior ERP indices in older adults in the context of age-equivalent performance on a novelty detection task (Alperin, Mott, Rentz, Holcomb, & Daffner, 2014).

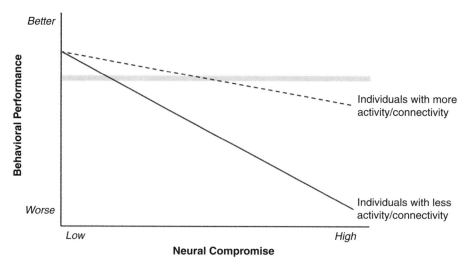

Figure 7.3. Theoretical rendering of two varieties of evidence for compensation. At any given level of behavioral performance (gray line), individuals who show compensatory brain activity/connectivity have more severe neural compromise than individuals who do not show compensatory activity. That is, their performance trajectory will cross the dashed line at a later point on the x-axis. This pattern of results would suggest that neural compensation buffers the negative association between neural compromise and behavioral performance such that individuals who show compensatory activity or connectivity have a weaker negative association (shallower slope) than individuals who lack compensatory activity or connectivity.

Stronger evidence for compensation in studies showing greater activation in older adults compared with younger adults with similar behavioral performance involves linking older adults' overactivation to objective indices of neural compromise. In the language domain, older adults showed greater activation of right hemisphere frontotemporal regions than young adults in the context of age-equivalent performance on a syntactic processing task (Tyler et al., 2010). Critically, greater right hemisphere frontotemporal activity among older adults was associated with lower gray matter density in the canonical left hemisphere frontotemporal network that was activated by the young adults, suggesting that right hemisphere overactivation represented a compensatory response to a structural insufficiency in the core, left hemisphere network.

A pattern of increasing activation to maintain cognitive performance has also been documented in cognitively healthy older adults who are risk of cognitive decline due to their having at least one *APOE-e4* allele. For example, older *APOE-e4* carriers showed more activity over a greater spatial extent of cortical regions than noncarriers during picture encoding despite similar performance (Bondi, Houston, Eyler, & Brown, 2005). A similar pattern of results was found for frontal resting-state activity, suggesting that differences in neural resources available for compensation can also be detected among *APOE-e4* carriers (Lin et al., 2017). Another recent study (Scheller et al., 2017) found equivalent performance between *APOE-e4* carriers and noncarriers on an N-back measure of working memory, but there were regions of prefrontal cortex that were positively associated with performance only among carriers, consistent with a compensatory account.

A 5-year longitudinal study of older *APOE-e4* carriers and noncarriers initially matched on cognitive function demonstrates the dynamic nature of compensation over time. In this study, researchers used fMRI to measure brain activity during a semantic judgment task at baseline and 18 and 57 months later (Rao et al., 2015). *APOE-e4* carriers and noncarriers did not differ on age or any cognitive measures at baseline, but the high-risk group (i.e., *APOE-e4* carriers) showed greater task-related activity than the low risk group (i.e., *APOE-e4* noncarriers). Over time, the high-risk group showed precipitous memory decline, along with declining brain activity during semantic judgments, whereas the low-risk group maintained relatively stable memory performance and showed increasing activation. These patterns suggest that the high-risk group engaged compensatory processes at a younger age than the low-risk group, but with high risk, the capacity to compensate dropped off over the course of the 5-year study. The low-risk group eventually drew on these additional neural resources, but this occurred years later and thus at an older chronological age than in the high-risk group.

Studies of Older Adults With Preclinical or Clinical Dementia

Several studies have developed cognitive tasks in which healthy older adults and older adults with MCI or AD perform similarly. A consistent pattern across these studies is that individuals with MCI or AD show greater frontal activation than healthy control participants, and this frontal activation is positively associated with their performance (Bokde et al., 2010; Clément & Belleville, 2010; Clément, Belleville, & Mellah, 2010; Grady et al., 1993). Thus, even individuals who show clinical impairments can successfully recruit compensatory regions to accomplish certain tasks at the level of their unaffected peers.

One potential consequence of recruiting additional neural resources at relatively low levels of task demands relative to one's peers is a restriction in the range of task demands over which the requisite neural systems can be engaged. This restricted range can also be manifest in the form of reduced modulation of brain activity in response to varying levels of task demand. In a cross-sectional, lifespan sample, Kennedy and her colleagues (2015) demonstrated that activation of cognitive control networks during a semantic judgment task was positively associated with age. However, demand-related modulation of this network was negatively associated with age, consistent with resource limitations, as proposed by the CRUNCH hypothesis. Follow-up work by Kennedy's group has linked reduced modulation to Alzheimer's risk (*APOE-e4* carriers) and to poorer task performance (Foster et al., 2017).

Absence of Association Between Extent of Compromise and Performance

A less commonly reported pattern of results providing evidence for compensation is the finding that a neural compromise does not lead to impaired performance in the presence of greater activity or connectivity. In other words, greater activity or connectivity buffers the negative effect of a neural compromise on performance (see Figure 7.3). In one recent study, levels of amyloid-β in cerebrospinal fluid (CSF) only predicted worse episodic memory among individuals with low frontal resting-state activity (Lin et al., 2017). Among individuals with greater frontal activity, CSF amyloid-β had no impact on memory. A study of preclinical AD (i.e., individuals with both MCI and neuroimaging evidence of amyloid-β pathology) reported a significant interaction between frontal cortex connectivity and precuneus hypometabolism on episodic memory performance (Franzmeier, Duering, Weiner, Dichgans, & Ewers, 2017). Specifically, precuneus hypometabolism was associated with poor episodic memory but not for individuals with high frontal cortex connectivity who appeared to be protected from the deleterious impact of precuneus hypometabolism. These results suggest that greater frontal resting-state activity and connectivity may index an individual's capacity to resist the deleterious effects of amyloid pathology.

Temporary Disruption of Activity

Disruption of Core Network Activity

Recent studies have used repetitive transcranial magnetic stimulation (rTMS) to disrupt activity within a core task network in healthy, young adult samples. These studies have observed subsequent functional changes in brain regions outside the core task network that may be interpreted as compensation. Temporarily disrupting activity within the left posterior superior temporal gyrus (Wernicke's area) during a language comprehension task resulted in increased synchronization of the contralateral homolog, regions surrounding the rTMS site, and the medial frontal gyrus (Mason, Prat, & Just, 2014). Importantly, the extent of this additional activation correlated positively with cognitive performance in the stimulated group. Similarly, temporarily disrupting activity within the left IFG during a speech-processing task led to increased activity in the contralateral homolog (right IFG; Hartwigsen et al., 2013). Importantly, facilitatory drive from the right IFG to the left IFG correlated positively with performance. These studies indicate brain adaptivity and compensation in young adults by demonstrating that certain cognitive tasks can be successfully carried out by alternative networks when core network contributions are diminished.

Disruption of Putative Compensatory Network Activity

Strong evidence that increased bilateral activation represents compensation comes from within-subject experimental designs in which cognitive performance is measured before and after the temporary inhibition of bilateral activation. In a study of healthy young and older adults, only disruption of right dorsolateral prefrontal cortex (DLPFC) activity (via rTMS) resulted in worse visuospatial memory in young adults, whereas disruption of either left or right DLPFC activity had similar negative effects in older adults (Rossi et al., 2004). This experiment shows that contralateral activation among older adults was causally related to successful performance. In another experiment using transcranial direct current stimulation (tDCS), young adults and older adults who performed similarly on episodic memory and executive functioning tasks demonstrated bilateral recruitment of DLPFC and parietal cortex (Brambilla, Manenti, Ferrari, & Cotelli, 2015). In contrast, older adults who performed worse on cognitive tasks demonstrated more asymmetrical recruitment of frontal regions. Importantly, degree of bilateral recruitment correlated positively with performance on tasks of episodic memory and executive functioning in that study.

Similar experimental paradigms have been used to demonstrate the compensatory nature of contralateral frontal activity among older adults compromised by stroke. In a study of individuals with poststroke aphasia, disruption of right IFG by rTMS resulted in worse language performance among patients who demonstrated functional activation of bilateral IFG during language tasks (Winhuisen et al., 2005). Patients who demonstrated only left IFG activation during language tasks were not affected by right IFG disruption. Together, these findings indicate that right IFG can be successfully recruited by patients who are unable to recover left hemisphere function following stroke.

Disruption of Brain Responses That Do Not Benefit Behavior

The studies reviewed in this section have so far been supportive of the view that hyperactivity within certain higher cortical regions, particularly frontal areas, is beneficial to cognitive performance among individuals compromised by aging or stroke. However, hyperactivity in other brain regions may not indicate successful compensation. For example, hippocampal hyperactivity in amnestic MCI was inferred to be disadvantageous in a study documenting improved memory performance in patients following the reduction of excessive hippocampal activity by an antiepileptic drug (Bakker et al., 2012). Rather than unsuccessful attempts at compensation, hippocampal hyperactivity in this context may reflect a loss of hippocampal inhibitory function due to preclinical disease (Andrews-Zwilling et al., 2010). Together, these studies highlight the regional specificity of different types of brain responses in aging and neurodegenerative disease.

Strength of Evidence Testing the Compensation Interpretation

Several efforts have been made to lay out optimal approaches to characterizing compensation in cognitive neuroscience studies of aging. For example, Cabeza and Dennis (2013) emphasized four relevant components of studies on compensation: (a) brain deterioration, (b) brain activity, (c) task demands, and (d) behavioral performance. These authors further suggested patterns of association among two or more of these variables that could be interpreted as evidence for compensation. For example, they proposed that inverted U-shaped relationships between brain activity and brain deterioration or task demands provide evidence for *attempted compensation*, and a positive correlation between activation and performance within a compromised group provides evidence for "successful" compensation. Gregory and colleagues (2017) described expected trajectories of brain deterioration, brain activity, and behavioral performance over time, emphasizing discrete epochs defining relationships among these trajectories. For example, they described an inverted U-shaped trajectory for brain activity, a quadratic decline in behavioral performance, and a linear progression of brain deterioration. In this section, we extend these attempts to highlight key variables and study design characteristics in research on compensation to offer both recommendations and cautions.

In line with previous authors, we emphasize the importance of including measures of brain deterioration, brain activity, task demand, behavioral performance, and time in cognitive neuroscience studies of compensation. Although many studies infer brain deterioration based on chronological age, we advocate for including an objective measure of neural compromise (e.g., brain deterioration) in light of high interindividual variability in brain health among older adults of the same age. In addition, statistically demonstrating a relationship between activation patterns and neural compromise provides greater evidence that a particular brain response is not just beneficial but also reactive to a specific process related to aging or disease (Du et al., 2016). Including more than one level of task demand can reveal the limits of different compensatory processes and the nature of associations among supply, demand, and compensation (Reuter-Lorenz & Cappell, 2008). In addition, considering task demands can facilitate comparisons across studies and potentially reconcile conflicting findings. Finally, although most cognitive neuroscience studies of compensation make inferences about processes of aging and disease based on cross-sectional age, we advocate for within-subjects designs (Raz & Lindenberger, 2011) that allow researchers to (a) distinguish between long-standing individual differences and acquired compensatory responses and (b) track how compensatory responses emerge and evolve in the context of brain aging or disease. A within-subjects, longitudinal design is especially needed in studies comparing risk groups (e.g., APOE-e4 carriers and noncarriers) due to differing selection pressures across groups. Specifically, because a risk factor decreases the likelihood that an individual enters the study population, those who do enter the study population are more likely to possess potentially unmeasured resilience factors than individuals without the risk factor. In this case, age cannot be assumed to mean the same thing among individuals with different levels of risk.

One type of evidence for compensation that we take to be especially strong is longitudinal data that directly correlate changes in brain structure, brain function, and performance over multiple time points in the same individuals. Across a reasonably sized population, we would expect to see subsets of individuals with at least three patterns of change (see Figure 7.4): (a) relative preservation of brain structure, function, and performance, characterizing the prototype of brain and cognitive maintenance (see Figure 7.4a); (b) neural decline, a relative absence of hyperactivity (and perhaps decreasing activity), along with performance decline, corresponding to a pattern of unsuccessful aging (see Figure 7.4b); and (c) declining brain structure, age-specific indices of functional change (i.e., increased activation across time) coupled with relatively preserved performance, providing support for compensation as a means for successful aging (see Figure 7.4c).

A longitudinal study of APOE-e4 carriers and noncarriers described earlier comes closest to providing this type of evidence (Rao et al., 2015). That study defined, a priori, two subsets of initially cognitively healthy older adults based on APOE-e4 carrier status and described these groups' differing trajectories of structure, function, and performance. Carriers showed neural decline, performance decline, and decreasing brain activity (corresponding to the second subgroup described earlier), and noncarriers showed relative neural and performance preservation in the context of increasing brain activity (exhibiting characteristics of both the first and third subgroups described earlier). Increasing activity in the noncarriers was interpreted as compensation based on the assumption that the passage of time increased

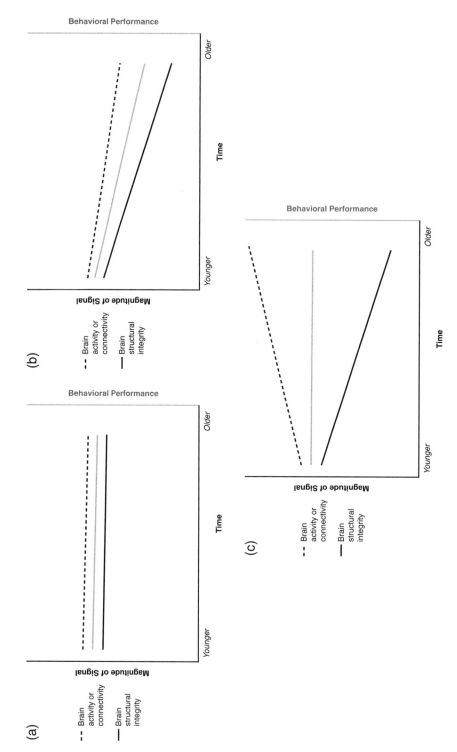

Figure 7.4. Theoretical predictions for three groups of older adults, although an individual older adult may show more than one pattern of change if observed across different stages of older adulthood. Age-related increases in neural compromise (reduced brain structural integrity) can potentially be offset by neural compensation (brain activity or connectivity), contributing to different trajectories of cognition (behavioral performance): (a) older adults who are able to maintain brain structural integrity, brain activity/connectivity, and behavioral performance over time; (b) older adults who show declining brain structural integrity and behavioral performance without showing a concomitant increase in compensatory brain activity/connectivity; (c) older adults whose rate of decline in brain structural integrity is similar to older adults in (b) but who maintain behavioral performance in the context of increased brain activity/connectivity (i.e., compensation). These relationships are affected by varying task demand, which is not depicted here.

the degree of neural compromise in noncarriers, but neural decline was not detected with the study's measures of hippocampal volume or regional cortical thickness. A future longitudinal study without a priori classification of a large sample of initially healthy older adults may reveal the three proposed subgroups more distinctly. An additional component of such a longitudinal study that would provide especially strong evidence for a compensatory interpretation would involve direct associations of changes in structure, function, and performance.

Another study design that we endorse involves causal logic, which is generally more compelling than correlational approaches. In this paradigmatic example, a hyperactive region that is unique to older adults and localized individually is temporarily disrupted by applying localized TMS. This TMS-induced deactivation is accompanied by a significant drop in performance that does not occur after deactivation of a control region or in young adults, who presumably have no need for compensation. This pattern of results has been reported in a TMS study of visuospatial memory in healthy young and older adults (Rossi et al., 2004). At least three additional components within the same study would provide even stronger evidence for a compensatory interpretation: (a) demonstrating (e.g., with functional neuroimaging) that hyperactivity within the region is observed when the older adults, but not the younger adults, completed the task; (b) longitudinal evidence that the TMS findings for older adults were not observed at an early point in time (i.e., recruitment of the region was *acquired*); and (c) demonstrating that TMS findings for older adults are linked to a measurable neural compromise among older adults (i.e., recruitment of the region was *reactive*).

Although varying in design and persuasiveness, the evidence summarized in these sections supports the compensation interpretation as a potentially viable explanatory construct worthy of continued interrogation. Specifically, the reviewed studies provide several types of evidence that favors compensation over alternative interpretations of the brain responses documented in these studies. These alternative interpretations may include the following: They are counterproductive to cognition, they are nonfunctional, they represent preexisting advantages unrelated to acquired neural compromise, or they are statistical artifacts. Ultimately, we recommend additional research to further evaluate the compensation interpretation. To that end, we advocate for study designs that formally test comprehensive models of longitudinal or causal associations among brain structure, brain function, and cognitive performance during multiple task conditions to provide more definitive evidence for neural compensation in aging and clarify underlying mechanisms. In the following paragraphs, we outline additional future directions for research.

In discussing the need to distinguish neural compensation from brain maintenance in the context of challenges in research on neural compensation in aging, we noted that the notion of compensation requires that there is something to compensate for—that is, that some neural compromise is impeding brain function. Thus, one answer to the question "Who compensates?" must acknowledge this prerequisite of a neural compromise. Compensation represents an alternative pathway to preserved cognitive functioning for those individuals who experience a decline in the integrity of their neural network(s).

Among individuals experiencing a neural compromise, there appear to be substantial individual differences in the capacity for compensatory activity. Research examining the concept of cognitive reserve has revealed individual and environmental characteristics that support the capacity to compensate for processes that compromise neural integrity, such as aging and disease (Barulli & Stern, 2013). Experiences found to build cognitive reserve (i.e., buffer against the negative impact of aging and disease processes on cognitive performance) include educational and occupational exposures, as well as engagement in leisure and social activities. Evidence that cognitive reserve proxies such as education predict the brain's potential to generate compensatory activity in response to neural compromise is provided by the study by Lin et al. (2017) in which levels of CSF amyloid-β only predicted worse episodic memory among individuals with low frontal resting-state activity. In this study, the interaction between frontal resting-state activity and the effect of amyloid-β on memory was more pronounced among individuals with higher education.

Several studies have directly linked cognitive reserve proxies to increased cortical activation during cognitive performance among healthy older adults. In a recent study, only older adults with high education demonstrated greater recruitment of the DLPFC during a working memory task, but the authors did not report a direct test of the association between DLPFC recruitment and behavioral performance (Boller, Mellah, Ducharme-Laliberté, & Belleville, 2017). Nevertheless, these results are consistent with previous studies showing greater recruitment of frontoparietal networks in healthy older adults with high levels of education, compared with those with lower levels of education (Scarmeas et al., 2003; Springer, McIntosh, Winocur, & Grady, 2005).

Although much research on compensation has focused on functional brain activity, preserved structural integrity of the brain may be a key predictor of the brain's potential for compensation. In a postmortem study of brains containing pathological levels of plaques and tangles, several structural features differentiated the brains of individuals with and without clinical AD in life (Perez-Nievas et al., 2013). Specifically, brains from individuals with AD pathology but without clinical dementia had preserved neuron numbers, synaptic markers, and axonal geometry, compared with brains from individuals with AD pathology who met clinical criteria for dementia in life. Thus, individuals who were able to resist the clinical impact of AD pathology showed less neural deterioration (i.e., more brain maintenance). Alternatively, those individuals may have had the advantage of better brain structure throughout life (i.e., more brain reserve). Evidence that preserved brain structure provides a foundation for neural compensation also comes from the study by Gallen et al. (2016), described earlier, in which greater task-related functional connectivity among neural subnetworks was positively associated with task performance. In that study, increased functional connectivity was also positively associated with integrity of the superior longitudinal fasciculus, a white matter tract connecting prefrontal cortex and more posterior cortices.

It is possible that the same experiences that contribute to cognitive reserve also promote structural brain integrity. For example, education is positively associated not only with increased functional recruitment but also with greater volume in frontoparietal regions (Boller et al., 2017) and greater white matter integrity (Teipel et al., 2009). This notion is embodied in the revised scaffolding theory of aging and cognition, which posits that life course experiential factors can influence both brain structure/function and compensatory activity (Reuter-Lorenz & Park, 2014). Characterizing individual differences is a relatively understudied area in research on compensation in cognitive aging. Further research delineating individual-level factors that predict the capacity for or extent of compensation (and how) is needed to refine research paradigms and inform the development of individualized interventions and policies to promote successful compensation not only in the context of normal aging but also in the context of age-related disease.

IMPLICATIONS FOR INTERVENTION

Understanding the mechanisms, limits, and facilitators of compensation in cognitive aging may ultimately allow us to harness the brain's natural capacity to combat a variety of normative and pathological changes. Facilitating the recruitment of contralateral brain activity in regions shown to subserve adaptive compensatory responses may expand the functional range of older adults contending with neurodegenerative changes, thereby allowing them to successfully perform more difficult tasks than they would otherwise be capable of performing. High-frequency rTMS over task-positive cortical regions has been shown to improve episodic memory performance among healthy older adults (Sandrini et al., 2014), as well as among older adults with MCI (Drumond Marra et al., 2015). Future studies could explore whether applying high-frequency rTMS over alternative cortical regions that provide compensatory scaffolding results in even greater benefit and whether enhancing the activity of the primary task network reduces the need for compensation. Neurostimulation methods may reveal new strategies to promote healthy adaptation to aging and disease.

Another potential application of knowledge regarding compensatory brain activity is in the area of neurofeedback. Real-time neurofeedback using fMRI or near-infrared spectroscopy (NIRS) has been shown to successfully enhance functioning in healthy adults and individuals with clinical disorders (Stoeckel et al., 2014). In a recent controlled study, NIRS neurofeedback on prefrontal activity during cognitive training resulted in improved executive function performance after only four sessions in healthy adults (Hosseini, Pritchard-Berman, Sosa, Ceja, & Kesler, 2016). Future studies could explore the utility of neurofeedback guided by research on cognitive compensation among older adults with and without age-related disease.

A future research direction that has clear potential to inform interventions lies in linking behavioral and neural compensation. For example, could neural compensation be fostered by strategic behavioral choices to encourage its automaticity? A long-term goal of intervention development guided by research on compensation in cognitive aging will be to design treatment protocols that induce enduring brain and cognitive changes.

In summary, compensatory brain responses may be able to expand the functional range of individuals whose brains are compromised by aging and disease processes. A fruitful direction of future research is examining whether compensatory processes reflect purely functional adaptations (i.e., brain flexibility) or structural changes (i.e., brain plasticity; Lövdén et al., 2010). Conceivably, neural compensation may reflect or even drive more enduring plastic changes in brain structure in response to brain aging. Understanding how to harness any capacities for plasticity that persist into older age is a critical frontier for promoting successful cognitive aging. Compensation may be the most prominent putative indicator of plasticity to date, but perhaps not the only potential avenue for overcoming the adverse effects of age-related decline.

REFERENCES

Alperin, B. R., Mott, K. K., Rentz, D. M., Holcomb, P. J., & Daffner, K. R. (2014). Investigating the age-related "anterior shift" in the scalp distribution of the P3b component using principal component analysis. *Psychophysiology, 51,* 620–633. http://dx.doi.org/10.1111/psyp.12206

Amieva, H., Mokri, H., Le Goff, M., Meillon, C., Jacqmin-Gadda, H., Foubert-Samier, A., . . . Dartigues, J. F. (2014). Compensatory mechanisms in higher-educated subjects with Alzheimer's disease: A study of 20 years of cognitive decline. *Brain, 137*, 1167–1175. http://dx.doi.org/10.1093/brain/awu035

Andrews-Zwilling, Y., Bien-Ly, N., Xu, Q., Li, G., Bernardo, A., Yoon, S. Y., . . . Huang, Y. (2010). Apolipoprotein E4 causes age- and Tau-dependent impairment of GABAergic interneurons, leading to learning and memory deficits in mice. *The Journal of Neuroscience, 30*, 13707–13717. http://dx.doi.org/10.1523/JNEUROSCI.4040-10.2010

Angel, L., Fay, S., Bouazzaoui, B., & Isingrini, M. (2011). Two hemispheres for better memory in old age: Role of executive functioning. *Journal of Cognitive Neuroscience, 23*, 3767–3777. http://dx.doi.org/10.1162/jocn_a_00104

Bakker, A., Krauss, G. L., Albert, M. S., Speck, C. L., Jones, L. R., Stark, C. E., . . . Gallagher, M. (2012). Reduction of hippocampal hyperactivity improves cognition in amnestic mild cognitive impairment. *Neuron, 74*, 467–474. http://dx.doi.org/10.1016/j.neuron.2012.03.023

Baltes, P. B., & Baltes, M. M. (1990). Psychological perspectives on successful aging: The model of selective optimization with compensation. In P. B. Baltes & M. M. Baltes (Eds.), *Successful aging: Perspectives from the behavioral sciences* (pp. 1–34). New York, NY: Cambridge University Press. http://dx.doi.org/10.1017/CBO9780511665684.003

Barulli, D., & Stern, Y. (2013). Efficiency, capacity, compensation, maintenance, plasticity: Emerging concepts in cognitive reserve. *Trends in Cognitive Sciences, 17*, 502–509. http://dx.doi.org/10.1016/j.tics.2013.08.012

Becker, J. T., Mintun, M. A., Aleva, K., Wiseman, M. B., Nichols, T., & DeKosky, S. T. (1996). Compensatory reallocation of brain resources supporting verbal episodic memory in Alzheimer's disease. *Neurology, 46*, 692–700. http://dx.doi.org/10.1212/WNL.46.3.692

Berlingeri, M., Bottini, G., Danelli, L., Ferri, F., Traficante, D., Sacheli, L., . . . Paulesu, E. (2010). With time on our side? Task-dependent compensatory processes in graceful aging. *Experimental Brain Research, 205*, 307–324. http://dx.doi.org/10.1007/s00221-010-2363-7

Bokde, A. L., Karmann, M., Born, C., Teipel, S. J., Omerovic, M., Ewers, M., . . . Hampel, H. (2010). Altered brain activation during a verbal working memory task in subjects with amnestic mild cognitive impairment [erratum at http://dx.doi.org/10.3389/fnagi.2016.00060]. *Journal of Alzheimer's Disease, 21*, 103–118. http://dx.doi.org/10.3233/JAD-2010-091054

Boller, B., Mellah, S., Ducharme-Laliberté, G., & Belleville, S. (2017). Relationships between years of education, regional grey matter volumes, and working memory-related brain activity in healthy older adults. *Brain Imaging and Behavior, 11*, 304–317.

Bondi, M. W., Houston, W. S., Eyler, L. T., & Brown, G. G. (2005). fMRI evidence of compensatory mechanisms in older adults at genetic risk for Alzheimer disease. *Neurology, 64,* 501–508. http://dx.doi.org/10.1212/01.WNL.0000150885.00929.7E

Bouazzaoui, B., Angel, L., Fay, S., Taconnat, L., Charlotte, F., & Isingrini, M. (2014). Does the greater involvement of executive control in memory with age act as a compensatory mechanism? *Canadian Journal of Experimental Psychology, 68,* 59–66. http://dx.doi.org/10.1037/cep0000005

Brambilla, M., Manenti, R., Ferrari, C., & Cotelli, M. (2015). Better together: Left and right hemisphere engagement to reduce age-related memory loss. *Behavioural Brain Research, 293,* 125–133. http://dx.doi.org/10.1016/j.bbr.2015.07.037

Cabeza, R. (2002). Hemispheric asymmetry reduction in older adults: The HAROLD model. *Psychology and Aging, 17,* 85–100. http://dx.doi.org/10.1037/0882-7974.17.1.85

Cabeza, R., & Dennis, N. A. (2013). Frontal lobes and aging: Deterioration and compensation. In D. T. Stuss & R. T. Knight (Eds.), *Principles of frontal lobe function* (2nd ed., pp. 628–652). New York, NY: Oxford University Press.

Cappell, K. A., Gmeindl, L., & Reuter-Lorenz, P. A. (2010). Age differences in prefontal recruitment during verbal working memory maintenance depend on memory load. *Cortex, 46,* 462–473. http://dx.doi.org/10.1016/j.cortex.2009.11.009

Carp, J., Gmeindl, L., & Reuter-Lorenz, P. A. (2010). Age differences in the neural representation of working memory revealed by multi-voxel pattern analysis. *Frontiers in Human Neuroscience, 4,* 217. http://dx.doi.org/10.3389/fnhum.2010.00217

Celone, K. A., Calhoun, V. D., Dickerson, B. C., Atri, A., Chua, E. F., Miller, S. L., . . . Sperling, R. A. (2006). Alterations in memory networks in mild cognitive impairment and Alzheimer's disease: An independent component analysis. *The Journal of Neuroscience, 26,* 10222–10231. http://dx.doi.org/10.1523/JNEUROSCI.2250-06.2006

Clément, F., & Belleville, S. (2010). Compensation and disease severity on the memory-related activations in mild cognitive impairment. *Biological Psychiatry, 68,* 894–902. http://dx.doi.org/10.1016/j.biopsych.2010.02.004

Clément, F., Belleville, S., & Mellah, S. (2010). Functional neuroanatomy of the encoding and retrieval processes of verbal episodic memory in MCI. *Cortex, 46,* 1005–1015. http://dx.doi.org/10.1016/j.cortex.2009.07.003

Crystal, H., Dickson, D., Fuld, P., Masur, D., Scott, R., Mehler, M., . . . Wolfson, L. (1988). Clinico-pathologic studies in dementia: Nondemented subjects with pathologically confirmed Alzheimer's disease. *Neurology, 38,* 1682–1687. http://dx.doi.org/10.1212/WNL.38.11.1682

Diaz, M. T., Rizio, A. A., & Zhuang, J. (2016). The neural language systems that support healthy aging: Integrating function, structure, and behavior. *Language and Linguistics Compass, 10,* 314–334. http://dx.doi.org/10.1111/lnc3.12199

Drumond Marra, H. L., Myczkowski, M. L., Maia Memória, C., Arnaut, D., Leite Ribeiro, P., Sardinha Mansur, C. G., . . . Marcolin, M. A. (2015). Transcranial magnetic stimulation to address mild cognitive impairment in the elderly:

A randomized controlled study. *Behavioural Neurology, 2015*, 287843. Advance online publication. http://dx.doi.org/10.1155/2015/287843

Du, Y., Buchsbaum, B. R., Grady, C. L., & Alain, C. (2016). Increased activity in frontal motor cortex compensates impaired speech perception in older adults. *Nature Communications, 7*, 12241. http://dx.doi.org/10.1038/ncomms12241

Elman, J. A., Oh, H., Madison, C. M., Baker, S. L., Vogel, J. W., Marks, S. M., . . . Jagust, W. J. (2014). Neural compensation in older people with brain amyloid-β deposition. *Nature Neuroscience, 17*, 1316–1318. http://dx.doi.org/10.1038/nn.3806

Festini, S., Zahodne, L. B., & Reuter-Lorenz, P. A. (2018). Theoretical perspectives on age differences in brain activation: HAROLD, PASA, CRUNCH—How do they STAC up? In O. Braddick (Ed.), *Oxford research encyclopedia of psychology*. Oxford, England: Oxford University Press. http://dx.doi.org/10.1093/acrefore/9780190236557.013.400

Fjell, A. M., McEvoy, L., Holland, D., Dale, A. M., & Walhovd, K. B. (2014). What is normal in normal aging? Effects of aging, amyloid and Alzheimer's disease on the cerebral cortex and the hippocampus. *Progress in Neurobiology, 117*, 20–40. http://dx.doi.org/10.1016/j.pneurobio.2014.02.004

Foster, C. M., Kennedy, K. M., & Rodrigue, K. M. (2017). Differential aging trajectories of modulation of activation to cognitive challenge in APOE ε4 groups: Reduced modulation predicts poorer cognitive performance. *Journal of Neuroscience, 37*, 6894–6901.

Franzmeier, N., Duering, M., Weiner, M., Dichgans, M., & Ewers, M. (2017). Left frontal cortex connectivity underlies cognitive reserve in prodromal Alzheimer disease. *Neurology, 88*, 1054–1061. http://dx.doi.org/10.1212/WNL.0000000000003711

Gallen, C. L., Turner, G. R., Adnan, A., & D'Esposito, M. (2016). Reconfiguration of brain network architecture to support executive control in aging. *Neurobiology of Aging, 44*, 42–52. http://dx.doi.org/10.1016/j.neurobiolaging.2016.04.003

Grady, C. L., Haxby, J. V., Horwitz, B., Gillette, J., Salerno, J. A., Gonzalez-Aviles, A., . . . Rapoport, S. I. (1993). Activation of cerebral blood flow during a visuoperceptual task in patients with Alzheimer-type dementia. *Neurobiology of Aging, 14*, 35–44. http://dx.doi.org/10.1016/0197-4580(93)90018-7

Grady, C. L., McIntosh, A. R., Beig, S., Keightley, M. L., Burian, H., & Black, S. E. (2003). Evidence from functional neuroimaging of a compensatory prefrontal network in Alzheimer's disease. *The Journal of Neuroscience, 23*, 986–993. http://dx.doi.org/10.1523/JNEUROSCI.23-03-00986.2003

Gregory, S., Long, J. D., Tabrizi, S. J., & Rees, G. (2017). Measuring compensation in neurodegeneration using MRI. *Current Opinion in Neurology, 30*, 380–387. http://dx.doi.org/10.1097/WCO.0000000000000469.

Grothe, M. J., Heinsen, H., Amaro, E., Jr., Grinberg, L. T., & Teipel, S. J. (2016). Cognitive correlates of basal forebrain atrophy and associated cortical hypometabolism in mild cognitive impairment. *Cerebral Cortex, 26*, 2411–2426. http://dx.doi.org/10.1093/cercor/bhv062

Hartwigsen, G., Saur, D., Price, C. J., Ulmer, S., Baumgaertner, A., & Siebner, H. R. (2013). Perturbation of the left inferior frontal gyrus triggers adaptive plasticity in the right homologous area during speech production. *Proceedings of the National Academy of Sciences of the United States of America, 110,* 16402–16407. http://dx.doi.org/10.1073/pnas.1310190110

Hedden, T., & Gabrieli, J. D. (2004). Insights into the ageing mind: A view from cognitive neuroscience. *Nature Reviews Neuroscience, 5,* 87–96. http://dx.doi.org/10.1038/nrn1323

Hedman, A. M., van Haren, N. E., Schnack, H. G., Kahn, R. S., & Hulshoff Pol, H. E. (2012). Human brain changes across the life span: A review of 56 longitudinal magnetic resonance imaging studies. *Human Brain Mapping, 33,* 1987–2002. http://dx.doi.org/10.1002/hbm.21334

Höller-Wallscheid, M. S., Thier, P., Pomper, J. K., & Lindner, A. (2017). Bilateral recruitment of prefrontal cortex in working memory is associated with task demand but not with age. *Proceedings of the National Academy of Sciences of the United States of America, 114,* E830–E839. http://dx.doi.org/10.1073/pnas.1601983114

Hosseini, S. M. H., Pritchard-Berman, M., Sosa, N., Ceja, A., & Kesler, S. R. (2016). Task-based neurofeedback training: A novel approach toward training executive functions. *NeuroImage, 134,* 153–159. http://dx.doi.org/10.1016/j.neuroimage.2016.03.035

Katzman, R., Terry, R., DeTeresa, R., Brown, T., Davies, P., Fuld, P., . . . Peck, A. (1988). Clinical, pathological, and neurochemical changes in dementia: A subgroup with preserved mental status and numerous neocortical plaques. *Annals of Neurology, 23,* 138–144. http://dx.doi.org/10.1002/ana.410230206

Kennedy, K. M., Rodrigue, K. M., Bischof, G. N., Hebrank, A. C., Reuter-Lorenz, P. A., & Park, D. C. (2015). Age trajectories of functional activation under conditions of low and high processing demands: An adult lifespan fMRI study of the aging brain. *Neuroimage, 104,* 21–34.

Kleerekooper, I., van Rooij, S. J. H., van den Wildenberg, W. P. M., de Leeuw, M., Kahn, R. S., & Vink, M. (2016). The effect of aging on fronto-striatal reactive and proactive inhibitory control. *NeuroImage, 132,* 51–58. http://dx.doi.org/10.1016/j.neuroimage.2016.02.031

Laforce, R., Jr., Tosun, D., Ghosh, P., Lehmann, M., Madison, C. M., Weiner, M. W., . . . Rabinovici, G. D. (2014). Parallel ICA of FDG-PET and PiB-PET in three conditions with underlying Alzheimer's pathology. *NeuroImage. Clinical, 4,* 508–516. http://dx.doi.org/10.1016/j.nicl.2014.03.005

Lenzi, D., Serra, L., Perri, R., Pantano, P., Lenzi, G. L., Paulesu, E., . . . Macaluso, E. (2011). Single domain amnestic MCI: A multiple cognitive domains fMRI investigation. *Neurobiology of Aging, 32,* 1542–1557. http://dx.doi.org/10.1016/j.neurobiolaging.2009.09.006

Li, H. J., Hou, X. H., Liu, H. H., Yue, C. L., Lu, G. M., & Zuo, X. N. (2015). Putting age-related task activation into large-scale brain networks: A meta-analysis of

114 fMRI studies on healthy aging. *Neuroscience and Biobehavioral Reviews, 57,* 156–174. http://dx.doi.org/10.1016/j.neubiorev.2015.08.013

Li, S. C., Lindenberger, U., & Sikström, S. (2001). Aging cognition: From neuromodulation to representation. *Trends in Cognitive Sciences, 5,* 479–486. http://dx.doi.org/10.1016/S1364-6613(00)01769-1

Lin, F., Ren, P., Lo, R. Y., Chapman, B. P., Jacobs, A., Baran, T. M., . . . Foxe, J. J. (2017). Insula and inferior frontal gyrus' activities protect memory performance against Alzheimer's disease pathology in old age. *Journal of Alzheimer's Disease, 55,* 669–678. http://dx.doi.org/10.3233/JAD-160715

Lövdén, M., Bäckman, L., Lindenberger, U., Schaefer, S., & Schmiedek, F. (2010). A theoretical framework for the study of adult cognitive plasticity. *Psychological Bulletin, 136,* 659–676. http://dx.doi.org/10.1037/a0020080

Maillet, D., & Rajah, M. N. (2013). Association between prefrontal activity and volume change in prefrontal and medial temporal lobes in aging and dementia: A review. *Ageing Research Reviews, 12,* 479–489. http://dx.doi.org/10.1016/j.arr.2012.11.001

Mandzia, J. L., McAndrews, M. P., Grady, C. L., Graham, S. J., & Black, S. E. (2009). Neural correlates of incidental memory in mild cognitive impairment: An fMRI study. *Neurobiology of Aging, 30,* 717–730. http://dx.doi.org/10.1016/j.neurobiolaging.2007.08.024

Mason, R. A., Prat, C. S., & Just, M. A. (2014). Neurocognitive brain response to transient impairment of Wernicke's area. *Cerebral Cortex, 24,* 1474–1484. http://dx.doi.org/10.1093/cercor/bhs423

Masten, A. S. (2007). Resilience in developing systems: Progress and promise as the fourth wave rises. *Development and Psychopathology, 19,* 921–930. http://dx.doi.org/10.1017/S0954579407000442

Mattay, V. S., Fera, F., Tessitore, A., Hariri, A. R., Berman, K. F., Das, S., . . . Weinberger, D. R. (2006). Neurophysiological correlates of age-related changes in working memory capacity. *Neuroscience Letters, 392,* 32–37. http://dx.doi.org/10.1016/j.neulet.2005.09.025

McEvoy, L. K., Pellouchoud, E., Smith, M. E., & Gevins, A. (2001). Neurophysiological signals of working memory in normal aging. *Cognitive Brain Research, 11,* 363–376. http://dx.doi.org/10.1016/S0926-6410(01)00009-X

Meinzer, M., Seeds, L., Flaisch, T., Harnish, S., Cohen, M. L., McGregor, K., . . . Crosson, B. (2012). Impact of changed positive and negative task-related brain activity on word-retrieval in aging. *Neurobiology of Aging, 33,* 656–669. http://dx.doi.org/10.1016/j.neurobiolaging.2010.06.020

Meltzer, J. A., Wagage, S., Ryder, J., Solomon, B., & Braun, A. R. (2013). Adaptive significance of right hemisphere activation in aphasic language comprehension. *Neuropsychologia, 51,* 1248–1259. http://dx.doi.org/10.1016/j.neuropsychologia.2013.03.007

Neuropathology Group of the Medical Research Council Cognitive Function and Ageing Study (MRC CFAS). (2001). Pathological correlates of late-onset dementia in a multicentre, community-based population in England and Wales. *The Lancet, 357,* 169–175. http://dx.doi.org/10.1016/S0140-6736(00)03589-3

Nyberg, L., Lövdén, M., Riklund, K., Lindenberger, U., & Bäckman, L. (2012). Memory aging and brain maintenance. *Trends in Cognitive Sciences, 16,* 292–305. http://dx.doi.org/10.1016/j.tics.2012.04.005

Park, D. C., Polk, T. A., Park, R., Minear, M., Savage, A., & Smith, M. R. (2004). Aging reduces neural specialization in ventral visual cortex. *Proceedings of the National Academy of Sciences of the United States of America, 101,* 13091–13095. http://dx.doi.org/10.1073/pnas.0405148101

Perez-Nievas, B. G., Stein, T. D., Tai, H. C., Dols-Icardo, O., Scotton, T. C., Barroeta-Espar, I., . . . Gómez-Isla, T. (2013). Dissecting phenotypic traits linked to human resilience to Alzheimer's pathology. *Brain: A Journal of Neurology, 136,* 2510–2526. http://dx.doi.org/10.1093/brain/awt171

Price, J. L., & Morris, J. C. (1999). Tangles and plaques in nondemented aging and "preclinical" Alzheimer's disease. *Annals of Neurology, 45,* 358–368. http://dx.doi.org/10.1002/1531-8249(199903)45:3<358::AID-ANA12>3.0.CO;2-X

Protzner, A. B., Mandzia, J. L., Black, S. E., & McAndrews, M. P. (2011). Network interactions explain effective encoding in the context of medial temporal damage in MCI. *Human Brain Mapping, 32,* 1277–1289. http://dx.doi.org/10.1002/hbm.21107

Pudas, S., Josefsson, M., Rieckmann, A., & Nyberg, L. (2018). Longitudinal evidence for increased functional response in frontal cortex for older adults with hippocampal atrophy and memory decline. *Cerebral Cortex, 28,* 936–948. http://dx.doi.org/10.1093/cercor/bhw418

Rao, S. M., Bonner-Jackson, A., Nielson, K. A., Seidenberg, M., Smith, J. C., Woodard, J. L., & Durgerian, S. (2015). Genetic risk for Alzheimer's disease alters the five-year trajectory of semantic memory activation in cognitively intact elders. *NeuroImage, 111,* 136–146. http://dx.doi.org/10.1016/j.neuroimage.2015.02.011

Raz, N. (2000). Aging of the brain and its impact on cognitive performance: Integration of structural and functional findings. In F. I. M. Craik & T. A. Salthouse (Eds.), *The handbook of aging and cognition* (2nd ed., pp. 1–90). Mahwah, NJ: Erlbaum.

Raz, N., & Lindenberger, U. (2011). Only time will tell: Cross-sectional studies offer no solution to the age-brain-cognition triangle: Comment on Salthouse (2011). *Psychological Bulletin, 137,* 790–795. http://dx.doi.org/10.1037/a0024503

Reuter-Lorenz, P. A., & Cappell, K. A. (2008). Neurocognitive aging and the compensation hypothesis. *Current Directions in Psychological Science, 17,* 177–182. http://dx.doi.org/10.1111/j.1467-8721.2008.00570.x

Reuter-Lorenz, P. A., & Lustig, C. (2005). Brain aging: Reorganizing discoveries about the aging mind. *Current Opinion in Neurobiology, 15,* 245–251. http://dx.doi.org/10.1016/j.conb.2005.03.016

Reuter-Lorenz, P. A., Marshuetz, C., Jonides, J., Smith, E. E., Hartley, A., & Koeppe, R. (2001). Neurocognitive ageing of storage and executive processes.

European Journal of Cognitive Psychology, 13, 257–278. http://dx.doi.org/10.1080/09541440042000304

Reuter-Lorenz, P. A., & Mikels, J. A. (2006). The aging mind and brain: Implications of enduring plasticity for behavioral and cultural change. In P. B. Baltes, P. A. Reuter-Lorenz, & F. Roesler (Eds.), *Lifespan development and the brain: The perspective of biocultural co-constructivism* (pp. 255–276). Cambridge, England: Cambridge University Press. http://dx.doi.org/10.1017/CBO9780511499722.014

Reuter-Lorenz, P. A., & Park, D. C. (2014). How does it STAC up? Revisiting the scaffolding theory of aging and cognition. *Neuropsychology Reviews, 24*, 355–370. http://dx.doi.org/10.1007/s11065-014-9270-9

Rossi, S., Miniussi, C., Pasqualetti, P., Babiloni, C., Rossini, P. M., & Cappa, S. F. (2004). Age-related functional changes of prefrontal cortex in long-term memory: A repetitive transcranial magnetic stimulation study. *The Journal of Neuroscience, 24*, 7939–7944. http://dx.doi.org/10.1523/JNEUROSCI.0703-04.2004

Sandrini, M., Brambilla, M., Manenti, R., Rosini, S., Cohen, L. G., & Cotelli, M. (2014). Noninvasive stimulation of prefrontal cortex strengthens existing episodic memories and reduces forgetting in the elderly. *Frontiers in Aging Neuroscience, 6*, 289. http://dx.doi.org/10.3389/fnagi.2014.00289

Scarmeas, N., Zarahn, E., Anderson, K. E., Hilton, J., Flynn, J., Van Heertum, R. L., . . . Stern, Y. (2003). Cognitive reserve modulates functional brain responses during memory tasks: A PET study in healthy young and elderly subjects. *NeuroImage, 19*, 1215–1227. http://dx.doi.org/10.1016/S1053-8119(03)00074-0

Scheller, E., Peter, J., Schumacher, L. V., Lahr, J., Mader, I., Kaller, C. P., & Klöppel, S. (2017). APOE moderates compensatory recruitment of neuronal resources during working memory processing in healthy older adults. *Neurobiology of Aging, 56*, 127–137. http://dx.doi.org/10.1016/j.neurobiolaging.2017.04.015

Seidler, R. D., Bernard, J. A., Burutolu, T. B., Fling, B. W., Gordon, M. T., Gwin, J. T., . . . Lipps, D. B. (2010). Motor control and aging: Links to age-related brain structural, functional, and biochemical effects. *Neuroscience and Biobehavioral Reviews, 34*, 721–733. http://dx.doi.org/10.1016/j.neubiorev.2009.10.005

Springer, M. V., McIntosh, A. R., Winocur, G., & Grady, C. L. (2005). The relation between brain activity during memory tasks and years of education in young and older adults. *Neuropsychology, 19*, 181–192. http://dx.doi.org/10.1037/0894-4105.19.2.181

Stern, Y., Moeller, J. R., Anderson, K. E., Luber, B., Zubin, N. R., DiMauro, A. A., . . . Sackeim, H. A. (2000). Different brain networks mediate task performance in normal aging and AD: Defining compensation. *Neurology, 55*, 1291–1297. http://dx.doi.org/10.1212/WNL.55.9.1291

Stoeckel, L. E., Garrison, K. A., Ghosh, S., Wighton, P., Hanlon, C. A., Gilman, J. M., . . . Evins, A. E. (2014). Optimizing real time fMRI neurofeedback for therapeutic discovery and development. *NeuroImage. Clinical, 5*, 245–255. http://dx.doi.org/10.1016/j.nicl.2014.07.002

Sun, F. W., Stepanovic, M. R., Andreano, J., Barrett, L. F., Touroutoglou, A., & Dickerson, B. C. (2016). Youthful brains in older adults: Preserved neuroanatomy in the default mode and salience networks contributes to youthful memory in superaging. *The Journal of Neuroscience, 36,* 9659–9668. http://dx.doi.org/10.1523/JNEUROSCI.1492-16.2016

Teipel, S. J., Meindl, T., Wagner, M., Kohl, T., Bürger, K., Reiser, M. F., . . . Hampel, H. (2009). White matter microstructure in relation to education in aging and Alzheimer's disease. *Journal of Alzheimer's Disease, 17,* 571–583. http://dx.doi.org/10.3233/JAD-2009-1077

Turner, G. R., & Spreng, R. N. (2012). Executive functions and neurocognitive aging: Dissociable patterns of brain activity. *Neurobiology of Aging, 33,* 826.e1–826.e13. http://dx.doi.org/10.1016/j.neurobiolaging.2011.06.005

Tyler, L. K., Shafto, M. A., Randall, B., Wright, P., Marslen-Wilson, W. D., & Stamatakis, E. A. (2010). Preserving syntactic processing across the adult life span: The modulation of the frontotemporal language system in the context of age-related atrophy. *Cerebral Cortex, 20,* 352–364. http://dx.doi.org/10.1093/cercor/bhp105

Vallesi, A., McIntosh, A. R., & Stuss, D. T. (2011). Overrecruitment in the aging brain as a function of task demands: Evidence for a compensatory view. *Journal of Cognitive Neuroscience, 23,* 801–815. http://dx.doi.org/10.1162/jocn.2010.21490

Wierenga, C. E., Benjamin, M., Gopinath, K., Perlstein, W. M., Leonard, C. M., Rothi, L. J., . . . Crosson, B. (2008). Age-related changes in word retrieval: Role of bilateral frontal and subcortical networks. *Neurobiology of Aging, 29,* 436–451. http://dx.doi.org/10.1016/j.neurobiolaging.2006.10.024

Winhuisen, L., Thiel, A., Schumacher, B., Kessler, J., Rudolf, J., Haupt, W. F., & Heiss, W. D. (2005). Role of the contralateral inferior frontal gyrus in recovery of language function in poststroke aphasia: A combined repetitive transcranial magnetic stimulation and positron emission tomography study. *Stroke, 36,* 1759–1763. http://dx.doi.org/10.1161/01.STR.0000174487.81126.ef

8

RISK AND PROTECTIVE FACTORS IN COGNITIVE AGING: ADVANCES IN ASSESSMENT, PREVENTION, AND PROMOTION OF ALTERNATIVE PATHWAYS

ROGER A. DIXON AND MARGIE E. LACHMAN

The chapter presents recent evidence for factors that contribute to aging-related cognitive declines, including both normal and pathological changes. The focus is on nonmodifiable and modifiable risk and protective factors and their independent, multimodal, and interactive effects on trajectories of cognitive change. Findings from long-term longitudinal studies and broad-based epidemiological investigations, as well as short-term experimental and intervention studies, are considered. Moderating factors are reviewed in the context of alternative processes and outcomes, such as cognitive reserve, resilience, and exceptionality. The chapter concludes with a discussion of goals to reduce or delay neurodegenerative risk and associated

Roger Dixon acknowledges support from the National Institutes of Health (National Institute on Aging; R01 AG008235), the Canadian Consortium on Neurodegeneration in Aging (with support from the Canadian Institutes of Health Research), and the Canada Research Chairs program. Margie Lachman acknowledges support from National Institute on Aging grants P30 AG048785, PO1 AG020166, and U19 AG051426. We thank Alec Macdonald for technical contributions to the graphics and Linzy Bohn, Jill Friesen, and Victoria Sorrentino for editorial assistance.

http://dx.doi.org/10.1037/0000143-009
The Aging Brain: Functional Adaptation Across Adulthood, G. R. Samanez-Larkin (Editor)

cognitive declines and ultimately to prevent the onset of cognitive impairment and dementia.

As the world population ages, and the national and global prevalence of Alzheimer's disease (AD) and related dementias (ADRD) increase dramatically, there is growing interest in understanding the processes involved in brain aging and identifying factors that contribute to and protect against cognitive decline and impairment (Alzheimer's Association, 2016; Prince, Comas-Herrera, Knapp, Guerchet, & Karagiannidou, 2016). It was only about a decade ago that a report by the U.S. National Institutes of Health at a State-of-the-Science Conference (Daviglus et al., 2010) summarized their findings in the following way: "Firm conclusions cannot be drawn about the association of any modifiable risk factor with cognitive decline or Alzheimer's disease." In just the past several years, a remarkable amount of progress has been made in identifying the range of risk and protective factors relevant to dementia and selecting the best targets for potential intervention (Barnes & Yaffe, 2011; Livingston et al., 2017; National Academies of Sciences, Engineering, and Medicine, 2017). Given that there are still no effective pharmaceutical interventions for prevention or treatment of AD (Cummings, Morstorf, & Zhong, 2014), there has been a concerted emphasis on identifying and targeting modifiable factors that can be assessed and managed through behavioral and lifestyle changes during the long period of normal or healthy brain aging (Anstey, Eramudugolla, Hosking, Lautenschlager, & Dixon, 2015).

In this chapter, we review the recent evidence on factors that contribute to aging-related cognitive declines, including both normal and pathological changes. The focus is on identifying nonmodifiable (e.g., genotype), modifiable (e.g., lifestyle, exercise), and potentially controllable (e.g., some health conditions) factors and how they may independently or interactively modify trajectories of cognitive change prior to the insidious onset of AD. We present and integrate findings from long-term longitudinal studies and broad-based epidemiological investigations, as well as short-term experimental and intervention studies. Moderating factors (e.g., education, sex and gender) are reviewed in the context of alternative processes and outcomes, such as cognitive resilience and exceptionality. There is a great deal of promise in the recent findings, providing a sense of optimism that we are on the right track towards promotion of healthy brain aging and eventual delay or prevention of cognitive impairment or dementia.

Given the devastating course of ADRD and the projections for large increases in its incidence and the associated health care costs (Hurd, Martorell, Delavande, Mullen, & Langa, 2013; Wimo et al., 2017), there has been an all-out research effort to understand the causes and to develop therapeutics targeting the underlying mechanisms. A recent report by the National Academies of Sciences, Engineering, and Medicine (2017) identified three main areas of promise for prevention of ADRD. Their recommendations were guarded, cautioning there is no clear-cut or conclusive evidence that these interventions can prevent ADRD, yet there are encouraging findings that cognitive training, blood pressure management, and physical activity may slow age-related cognitive decline. Although ADRD has received the bulk of attention and research dollars, there has been some recognition that there are also great costs associated with normal cognitive decline with aging. In 2015, an Institute of Medicine panel embarked on a review to understand normal cognitive aging as distinct from pathological cognitive changes such as those associated with impending ADRD. Their generally accepted premise was that cognitive aging is not a disease, but rather a process that unfolds throughout life and is widely experienced. The group made the following evidence-based recommendations for ways to slow cognitive changes (Institute of Medicine, 2015): Be physically active, reduce and manage cardiovascular disease risk factors, regularly discuss and review health conditions and medications that might influence cognitive health with a health care professional, be socially and intellectually engaged, continually seek opportunities to learn, get adequate sleep, and avoid the risks of cognitive changes due to delirium if hospitalized. Not noted, but of interest in this review, is the complementary premise that understanding pathways to resilience or sustained levels of cognitive change and plasticity in late life can provide new perspectives, targets, and opportunities for promoting healthier cognitive aging. In this chapter, we elaborate on selected recent findings regarding risk and protective factors, consider mitigating and buffering factors for brain aging, and discuss emerging directions of precision assessment and intervention.

RISK AND PROTECTIVE FACTORS

There is growing longitudinal evidence that actual cognitive trajectories associated with normal brain aging (a) vary widely across individuals and domains; (b) include patterns ranging from relatively sustained high levels of performance to steeply accelerating decline; and (c) are influenced by individual differences in biological, health, environmental, and lifestyle factors (Josefsson, de Luna, Pudas, Nilsson, & Nyberg, 2012). Arguably, the rate and extent of individual cognitive decline may not be inevitable or irreversible. In other words, there are things one can do to minimize loss in cognitive functioning and even to reduce the risk of dementia. In general, the results provide substantial evidence for brain and cognitive plasticity with normal aging. We combine the presentation of factors relevant for both dementia and normal cognitive declines, as many of the risk and protective factors are essentially the same. Indeed, given that AD is a neurodegenerative disease with a long preclinical onset period, virtually all known risk factors (e.g., lifestyle, genetic) and biomarkers (e.g., beta-amyloid burden) are actively studied for potential contributions to early detection of elevated AD vulnerability.

Although many studies have identified significant predictors of cognition in middle and later adulthood (Agrigoroaei, Robinson, Hughes, Rickenbach, & Lachman, 2018), the evidence for factors that can delay, reduce, or reverse cognitive decline is still somewhat mixed (Plassman, Williams, Burke, Holsinger, & Benjamin, 2010). For example, in their extensive review of both observational studies and randomized clinical trials, Plassman and colleagues (2010) reported that cognitive training and physical exercise have only limited benefits. They found more consistent evidence for the negative effects of risk factors such as tobacco use and disease. In recent years, this issue has attracted growing attention, with reviewers adding specific risk factors to the list. These include education, cognitive and physical inactivity, social isolation, hypertension, obesity, and environmental toxin exposure (e.g., Barnes & Yaffe, 2011). In addition to systematic reviews regarding single modifiable risk factors, some comprehensive reviews have covered a vast range of risk and protective factors associated with normal cognitive changes, impairment and dementia (Anstey et al., 2015). A 2017 *Lancet* Commissions article reviewed multiple modifiable risk factors and estimated the percentage of risk reduction that would occur if the major ones were eliminated (Livingston et al., 2017). Overall, the authors estimated that approximately 35% of the risk could be attributable to potentially modifiable factors. Figure 8.1 graphically represents their analysis of some of the modifiable risk factors and the fact that they operate in the context of unmodifiable factors. Several risk indexes have been published, some of which are available online (Anstey et al., 2014).

Risk factors and protective factors are often inversely related. For example, physical activity is a protective factor for cognitive functioning. By the same token, sedentary behavior is a risk factor. High social support and integration are beneficial and protective, whereas loneliness and isolation are considered risk factors. Thus, with a prescriptive approach, the focus can be on reducing risk factors or increasing protective factors. In other words, the evidence indicates what to avoid and what to do to promote cognitive health. Risk assessment is an essential tool for promoting healthier brain and cognitive aging, but comprehensive assessment must be linked with strategies for risk management, risk reduction, and protection factor enhancement, strategies that are likely to involve multiple modalities (Anstey et al., 2015).

The modifiability of risk factors for cognitive decline and dementia varies according to onset timing, severity, proximity to brain health, propensity for interactions with other risk and protective factors, and other individualized conditions. However, some risk factors are considered nonmodifiable,

	Nonmodifiable	Modifiable		
		Early Life	**Mid-Life**	**Late Life**
Known	*APOE ε4*	Education	Hearing Loss Hypertension Obesity	Smoking Depression Physical Inactivity Social Isolation Diabetes
Unknown	20 Other GWAS Identified Risk Factors (eg. *TREM2*) **Panel Combinations** Interactions, Intensifications Among Genetic Risk Factors **Potential Protective Factors** *APOE ε2*	**Early Synergies** of Risk-Reducing Lifestyle Factors	**Mid-Life Synergies** of Risk-Reducing Lifestyle Factors	**Late Life Synergies** of Risk-Reducing Lifestyle Factors

Other Potential Modifiable Candidate Risk Factors
Head Injury, Sleep Disorders, Environmental Toxins, Cognitive Activity, Nutrition, Stress

~65%   ~35+%

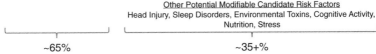

Figure 8.1. Modifiable risk factors for Alzheimer's disease and cognitive impairment, organized by life phase and ordered according to analyses and estimates from a recent review (Livingston et al., 2017, presents full information and further details). GWAS = genome-wide association study. Based on "Dementia Prevention, Intervention, and Care," by G. Livingston, A. Sommerlad, V. Orgeta, S. G. Costafreda, J. Huntley, D. Ames, . . . N. Mukadam, 2017, *The Lancet*, *390*, 2673–2734. Advance online publication. http://dx.doi.org/10.1016/S0140-6736(17)31363-6.

directly linked to brain health, and interactive with other risk factors. Perhaps most prominently are AD genetic risk loci (e.g., apolipoprotein E [*APOE*], and the ε4 allele). In such cases, rather than focusing on direct interventions, it is appropriate to identify ways to moderate the effects, using a person by environment approach. That is, given the vulnerabilities, the focus can be on ways to attenuate the risks or to provide environmental supports to address them. Genetic effects and other nonmodifiable factors will be presented in more detail in the section on modifiers, mechanisms, and alternative pathways.

Some of the most well-known modifiable risk factors for accelerated decline in cognitive, brain, and physical health are smoking, drug use, excessive alcohol use, and obesity. By reducing or eliminating these behaviors and conditions one can expect to improve health, reduce disease such as diabetes and heart disease, and improve cognition, or at least to slow cognitive decline and reduce the likelihood of dementia.

Health

To a large extent, cognitive declines are a manifestation of general poor health (Spiro & Brady, 2011) or multimorbidity (e.g., frailty; Searle & Rockwood, 2015) with much research linking specific health conditions to cognitive performance or change. Those who have diabetes, hypertension, high cholesterol, metabolic syndrome, poor lung function, and other vascular and cardiopulmonary diseases are more likely to show steeper cognitive declines than their healthier counterparts (Livingston et al., 2017). There is also evidence that if treatments for high blood pressure or diabetes and high cholesterol are effective, it can also lead to maintenance of good cognitive functioning. Thus, the longer one can remain in good health, the greater chance for maintaining good cognitive functioning.

Stress and Depression

Stress is a risk factor for poor health and cognition (Lupien, Maheu, Tu, Fiocco, & Schramek, 2007). The mechanisms have been investigated with a focus on the hypothalamic–pituitary–adrenal axis and the brain. Increased stress is associated with the release of cortisol, which has damaging effects on the hippocampus (Lupien, McEwen, Gunnar, & Heim, 2009; Yaffe, Hoang, Byers, Barnes, & Friedl, 2014). Stress is also associated with increased inflammation, which also has known effects on the brain. Higher levels of inflammatory markers such as fibrinogen, C-reactive protein, or interleukin 6 are associated with poorer cognitive performance (Karlamangla et al., 2014). Furthermore, stress is implicated in reduction of telomere (tips of the DNA) length (Epel et al., 2004), which is associated with premature aging. There are many approaches to stress reduction including relaxation training, meditation, and mindfulness, with known cognitive benefits (Grossman, Niemann, Schmidt, & Walach, 2004; Zeidan, Johnson, Diamond, David, & Goolkasian, 2010). Depression, which is often comorbid with stress, has also been associated with increased risk for cognitive decline, and some of the same techniques for reducing stress are effective for treating depression. It is unclear whether depression is a risk factor per se (or an early symptom) of dementia, something that observational research continues to investigate (Dotson, Beydoun, & Zonderman, 2010). There are some promising findings, but the jury is still out on whether these stress-reduction techniques lead to better cognitive functioning or to a reduction in cognitive decline. More work is needed to clarify the mechanisms linking stress and cognitive aging.

Environment

There is growing evidence that air pollution, pesticides, and lead exposure have negative effects on cognition (Anstey et al., 2015; Peters, Peters, Booth, & Mudway, 2015). Weuve and colleagues (2012) found that long-term exposure to particulate air pollution was associated with faster cognitive decline in the Nurses' Health Study. Exposure to toxins in the workplace (Grzywacz, Segel-Karpas, & Lachman, 2016) has been found to have a negative effect on cognitive functioning in middle-aged and older adults. More work is needed to clarify the particular pathways that link environmental pollutants and cognitive decline.

Behavioral and Lifestyle Factors

A number of modifiable behavioral and lifestyle factors show great promise for promoting cognitive health, and may lend themselves to developing effective interventions. Although many of the factors that are good for cognition are widely known, adults do not always behave consistently with the recommendations. For example, a majority of middle-aged and older adults in the United States have poor sleep habits, are overweight or obese, or do not exercise regularly.

Sleep

Many adults have problems with sleep, and this can compromise daily cognitive functioning due to fatigue. There is also evidence for long-term cumulative effects of poor sleep on cognitive functioning, especially memory (Scullin & Bliwise, 2015), and later risk of dementia (Sindi et al., 2018). There has been increased attention to treating sleep disorders and addressing difficulties that increase with age. Pharmacological remedies, both prescription and over the counter, are widely used. Such treatments do not typically solve sleep problems and they may instead contribute to poor cognitive functioning. Thus, cognitive behavioral sleep treatments may be more promising.

Diet

There are many claims about the value of dietary supplements and specific foods (Anstey et al., 2015). For example, vitamin B, antioxidants, and omega-3s are considered helpful for cognitive functioning. Resveratrol and flavonoids, ingredients in red wine and chocolate, have received some attention. Much of this work has been done with nonhuman animals, and the quantities needed to improve functioning in humans are unknown (Kennedy et al., 2010; Macready et al., 2009). Moreover, the large doses of wine and chocolate that would be needed to have significant effects could do more harm than good in terms of brain damage or weight gain. Thus, although these dietary ingredients may be protective, there is also evidence that obesity (body mass index) and large waist circumference are risk factors for cognitive aging and dementia. Diet plans rich in healthy fats, whole grains, legumes, fish, and produce, such as the Mediterranean diet, have also been identified as beneficial for cognitive health (Lourida et al., 2013; Martínez-Lapiscina et al., 2013; Singh et al., 2014; Tangney et al., 2014; Wengreen et al., 2013). This is likely because of their effect on heart health and weight, which in turn have beneficial effects on cognition.

Physical Exercise

There is compelling evidence that an active lifestyle has broad benefits for cognitive, physical, and psychological health (Kohl et al., 2012; Marioni et al., 2015; Powell, Paluch, & Blair, 2011). An active lifestyle can include participation in a wide range of activities—cognitively challenging tasks, social interactions, volunteer or paid work, hobbies, and physical exercise, all of which have some health benefits. Both everyday physical activity (often moderate in extent and degree) and physical exercise (including regimens of aerobic or resistance training) have been linked to numerous health benefits, including improved cardiovascular and respiratory health, enhanced insulin sensitivity, heightened bone and muscle strength, improved positive affect and cognitive function, and increased resistance to Type 2 diabetes, cancers, and depression (e.g., Corder, Ogilvie, & van Sluijs, 2009; Kohl et al., 2012; Powell et al., 2011). Both moderate or everyday physical activity and exercise training have been shown to reduce stress and depression, which affect cognitive functioning. Although the benefits of regular physical exercise are well known, according to a recent report from the U.S. National Center for Health Statistics, only a small percentage of adults engage in regular physical activity (Ashe, Miller, Eng, & Noreau, 2009), and the numbers are lower for middle-aged and older adults (Thorp, Owen, Neuhaus, & Dunstan, 2011). Approximately 20% of adults met the 2008 U.S. Centers for Disease Control and Prevention physical activity guidelines, and in older age groups, the percentage was lower (Clarke, Norris, & Schiller, 2017). Inactivity is a global problem; the World Health Organization (2017) reported that one in four adults were not sufficiently active.

Maintaining physical activity throughout life is an important public health objective (Corder et al., 2009) that is within reach with the right kind of interventions. In fact, physical inactivity has been called a global pandemic and is cited as one of the leading causes of death (Kohl et al., 2012). Physical exercise is perhaps the most well-known protective factor for cognitive aging. This has been substantiated in longitudinal, epidemiological studies as well as in clinical trials (Kramer, Erickson, & Colcombe, 2006). For example, Gow, Pattie, and Deary (2017) found that engagement in leisure physical activities in midlife was positively associated with cognitive ability level (path coefficient = .32), and higher physical activity in later adulthood was associated with less cognitive decline (.27). Moreover, the results of exercise have been found in nonhuman animals as well as humans. More so than other factors, there is promising evidence as to mechanisms linking physical exercise with cognition (Northey, Cherbuin, Pumpa, Smee, & Rattray, 2018). These include increased oxygenation to the brain, brain-derived neurotrophic factor (BDNF; Hillman, Erickson, & Kramer, 2008), and neurovascular integrity (Laitman & John, 2015).

There is limited evidence as to what types or amounts of exercise are needed to produce cognitive benefits, but growing attention to the efficacy of everyday or moderate doses (Thibeau, McFall, Wiebe, Anstey, & Dixon, 2016). Some have suggested that only aerobic activity with cardiovascular benefits is necessary for cognitive benefits (Erickson, Hillman, & Kramer, 2015). In other cases, there is evidence that resistance training has benefits for memory (Neupert, Lachman, & Whitbourne, 2009). In a study by Sofi et al. (2011), subjects who performed at low, moderate, or high levels of physical activity were protected against cognitive impairment to a significant degree. Physical activity has dose–response associations with cognitive function, and even low physical activity frequencies (a few times per month) are positively associated with cognitive function during aging (de Souto Barreto, Delrieu, Andrieu, Vellas, & Rolland, 2016). Low-intensity walking is related to increased hippocampal volume and reduced risk of AD (Varma, Chuang, Harris, Tan, & Carlson, 2015). One type of exercise, tai chi, has been particularly effective, in part because it is a multifaceted regimen that focuses on both body and mind (Wayne et al., 2014). Perhaps the biggest challenge tied to physical exercise is to find ways to motivate adults to engage in it (Sullivan & Lachman, 2017). This is one reason that researchers are also examining everyday, voluntary, and safe forms of physical activity preferred by older adults (Robinson, Bisson, Hughest, Ebert, & Lachman, 2018) that can be integrated into daily routines.

Cognitive Activity

There is evidence that cognitively stimulating activities are associated with better cognitive functioning and less decline (Hertzog, Kramer, Wilson, & Lindenberger, 2008). Some have implemented formal training programs that show effects on the abilities that were trained but little evidence for generalization or transfer across abilities. One exception is the ACTIVE program, which has shown long-term effects of the training over 10 years with an impact on activities of daily living and everyday functioning (Rebok et al., 2014). In other cases, there is a focus on everyday activities (e.g., reading, doing puzzles, using computers) or learning new skills (e.g., quilting, digital photography; Lachman & Agrigoroaei, 2010; Park et al., 2014; Small, Dixon, McArdle, & Grimm, 2012). Regardless of the particular strategy used, what still remains to be determined is how these activities get into the brain to enrich cognitive functioning, and whether they can slow or reverse declines. A plausible alternative explanation is that those who have better cognitive functioning are the ones who are more likely to engage in cognitive activities. Thus, more work is needed to address such directionality issues.

Another approach uses brain-training games that are commercially available. The claims of companies that market these games are often exaggerated and not based on systematic research (Stanford Center on Longevity, 2014). Simon, Yokomizo, and Bottino (2012) concluded that these commercial games have little benefit beyond improvement on the tasks that are specifically practiced. Indeed, the issue of transfer effects (beyond the targeted cognitive process) is a perennial challenge to cognitive intervention studies. Moreover, the evaluations rarely use experimental designs; participants are not blind to conditions and are subject to demand characteristics. One company, Posit Science, incorporated the useful field of view training from the ACTIVE trial into their brain-training program (Ball, Beard, Roenker, Miller, & Griggs, 1988), which has had some promising results, including recent findings tied to reducing the risk of AD (Edwards & Loprinzi, 2017).

Cognitive stimulation in the workplace contributes to good cognitive functioning (Grzywacz et al., 2016). Occupations that involve complex decision-making and greater decision latitude, allowing for control over schedule and priorities, are tied to better cognitive functioning (Andel, Kåreholt, Parker, Thorslund, & Gatz, 2007; Andel, Vigen, Mack, Clark, & Gatz, 2006; Schooler, 1999). More work is needed in this area to tease apart selection effects, as those who have better cognitive functioning are more likely to work in more complex jobs.

Social Activity

Social activity and support have been shown related to cognitive functioning in adulthood and old age (Brown et al., 2016; Foubert-Samier et al., 2014; Fried et al., 2004; Haslam, Cruwys, Milne, Kan, & Haslam, 2016; Seeman et al., 2011). Cognitively stimulating leisure activity was found to be positively related to subsequent cognitive functioning especially among those with lower education (Litwin, Schwartz, & Damri, 2017). Those who have more contact with others as well as have better social support show better cognitive functioning in later life. Moreover, those who experience more strain and conflict in their relationships show worse cognitive functioning

(Liao et al., 2014; Tun, Miller-Martinez, Lachman, & Seeman, 2013). It is emotional not instrumental support that buffers cognitive decline (Ellwardt, Aartsen, Deeg, & Steverink, 2013), yet the mechanisms are still unclear. There is little known as to whether interventions to increase or improve social relationships would have benefits for cognitive aging. Arguably, the apparent benefits of social engagement may operate through (or in conjunction with) the increased cognitive activity (conversation, problem-solving, collaboration) that typically accompanies social interaction.

There is also evidence that the relationship between social contact and memory is moderated by personality (Segel-Karpas & Lachman, 2016). Social contact had more beneficial effects for those high on extraversion than for those who were less extraverted. In contrast, those who were high in neuroticism showed less cognitive benefit from social interaction than those who were less neurotic.

Attitudes and Beliefs

The beliefs one holds about aging make a difference for cognitive performance. Research by Becca Levy and colleagues (Levy, Zonderman, Slade, & Ferrucci, 2012) found that those who hold negative stereotypes about aging in early life are more likely to show declines many years later. There is also evidence that stereotype threat plays a role in cognitive performance (Hess, Auman, Colcombe, & Rahhal, 2003). There is a widespread stereotype that memory declines with age and that older adults have worse memory than younger adults. Under threat conditions—that is, when this stereotype is invoked—older adults perform worse than when they are under nonstereotype conditions (Barber, 2017).

Another important set of beliefs is tied to self-efficacy (Bandura, 1997) and sense of control (Lachman, Neupert, & Agrigoroaei, 2011). Expectancies that one can be successful on a task or that one has the abilities to do well make a difference for outcomes. Those who believe they are in control of outcomes such as cognitive performance show better performance. Moreover, control beliefs are predictive of the course of cognitive change in later life.

Older adults are more likely than younger adults to rate their memory as poor; that is, they have lower memory self-efficacy (Hertzog, Dixon, & Hultsch, 1990) and they are more likely to believe that they do not have control over their memory (Lachman, 2006). Such beliefs are a risk factor for poor memory and for accelerated memory declines (Windsor & Anstey, 2008). Indeed, those with lower control beliefs are less likely to use adaptive strategies for cognitive challenges (Lachman & Andreoletti, 2006). Those who have higher control beliefs improve more on cognitive tests with practice and are less likely to show aging-related declines in cognitive functioning

(Caplan & Schooler, 2003). Most cognitive training studies do not include a focus on expectancies and beliefs. Unfortunately, if beliefs are not directly targeted, they are not likely to change even if performance does improve (Lachman & Leff, 1989; Parisi, Gross, Marsiske, Willis, & Rebok, 2017). Thus, there is a need to directly address beliefs in cognitive interventions to increase the benefits. Addressing the negative stereotypes and low expectancies for cognitive aging can result in increases in persistence and effort in using adaptive strategies in the face of declining abilities.

Subjective age is another construct related to cognitive aging. On average, the older one is, the greater the discrepancy between one's chronological age and how old they feel. Those who feel younger to a greater extent have better health and cognitive performance (Stephan, Caudroit, Jaconelli, & Terracciano, 2014). Moreover, an older subjective age was associated with a higher likelihood of cognitive impairment and dementia, and this association was partially due to physical inactivity and depressive symptoms (Stephan et al., 2017). There is also support for the alternative view that cognitive performance has an impact on subjective age in that if one experiences poor cognitive functioning relative to others one's age, it can lead to an older subjective age (Hughes & Lachman, 2016).

Moderating Variables

Several variables (some qualitative in nature) are thought to play a role in moderating the strength or direction of associations between specific risk factors and cognitive performance or change in aging. Prominent among these moderator variables are education, race, SES, age, sex, and personality. If associations are specific to (for example) males but not females, it implies that sex-specific mechanisms may be operating—and that sex-specific interventions may be required. Failing to investigate such moderators may lead to imprecision in results. In this section we briefly review three such moderators: (a) education, (b) race, and (c) personality. Because of their centrality to brain and cognitive aging, we discuss two other moderators, age and sex, in more detail in a later section.

Education

Educational attainment is strongly related to level of cognitive functioning throughout adulthood. In fact, Langa and colleagues (2017) found that the decreased prevalence of dementia in the United States from 2000 to 2012 was largely attributed to increases in educational attainment. Yet it is not clear whether education is also related to differential changes in cognition. A 12-year longitudinal study showed that higher education was associated with better cognitive performance but not with slowing of decline (Zahodne et al., 2011). Similar results were found in the Midlife in the United

States (MIDUS) study over a 9-year period (Hughes et al., 2018). However, in some cases those with higher education have been found to maintain their functioning longer, and in other cases there are no differences in the onset of cognitive declines as a function of education. Moreover, in some studies, those with higher education have shown delays in declines and steeper slopes of decline than those with less education (Stern, 2012; Zahodne, Sol, & Kraal, 2017). This finding has been linked to the cognitive reserve hypothesis (Stern, 2009), which suggests that those with higher education have more reserve capacity and thus can delay functional declines associated with underlying pathology longer than those with less education. Other aspects of socioeconomic status are also related to cognitive functioning, such as childhood adversity, often operationalized as level of parents' education or degree of financial difficulties in childhood (Richards & Wadsworth, 2004).

Most often education is completed in early adulthood and the focus is on its long-term effects. These effects may be cumulative and indirect in that those with more education are more likely to engage in adaptive and healthy behaviors such as physical exercise, healthy diet, or cognitively stimulating activities. This raises possibilities for interventions that target those who are most vulnerable, i.e., those with lower education levels. In the MIDUS study, Lachman, Agrigoroaei, Murphy, and Tun (2010) found that those with low educational levels who engaged in more frequent cognitively stimulating activities, comparable to those with higher education, had memory performance that was similar to their higher education counterparts. This suggests that there are ways to compensate for lower SES or less education by engaging in lifestyle behaviors that are more consistent with those with more education. Another question of interest is whether obtaining education in middle age or later life would yield similar benefits to those seen with typical education in early adulthood. There is much interest in lifelong learning and adult education and retraining in the workforce. Little is known, however, if the advantages of education obtained later in life will parallel what is found for early life education. To some extent, education is a form of cognitive stimulation and activity. Thus, it is plausible to assume that benefits for cognitive aging will be found no matter when education is obtained.

Race

Although studies show race differences in cognitive performance, these have been largely attributed to differential educational and occupational experiences and differences in environmental exposures (Glymour & Manly, 2008). Moreover, to date there is little evidence for race differences in the trajectories of cognitive aging. Changes in cognition over time seem to follow a similar course for African Americans and Caucasians (Manly, Jacobs,

Touradji, Small, & Stern, 2002), although recent evidence indicates that there may be racial differences in predictors of cognitive impairment (Kaup et al., 2015). African Americans have a higher incidence of AD, but there is little understanding as to why this is the case, although there appear to be potential racial differences in vulnerability to genetic risk factors (Murrell et al., 2006). It is possible that differential health effects (e.g., higher levels of diabetes or heart disease among African Americans) or environmental differences (pollutants, stressors) could help to explain this (Ighodaro et al., 2017). Contextual factors such as segregation, educational resources, and discrimination have been found to contribute to race differences in cognition and cognitive decline (Glymour & Manly, 2008; Zahodne et al., 2017).

Personality

Personality traits have been examined in relation to cognitive aging. There are consistent relationships such that those who have higher neuroticism show lower cognitive functioning, and those who are more conscientious and more open to experience have better cognitive functioning (Graham & Lachman, 2014). The relationships between personality and cognition vary by age, and those who have a more stable personality show better cognitive functioning (Graham & Lachman, 2012). What is still unknown is to what extent personality can serve a protective function. There is some suggestion that those who are higher in neuroticism are more likely to develop AD and those who are more conscientious are less likely to develop AD (Johansson et al., 2014; Terracciano et al., 2014). Personality also is related to resilience in the face of AD pathology. Those with more adaptive personality profiles (i.e., low neuroticism or high conscientiousness) were less likely to show symptoms of AD even with underlying AD neuropathology; and those with high neuroticism or low conscientiousness were less likely to remain asymptomatic. Recent findings suggest that personality change is related to dementia (Terracciano, Stephan, Luchetti, & Sutin, 2018) in that those who have cognitive impairment show less stability of personality traits than those who are of comparable age without evidence of dementia.

INTERACTIONS AMONG RISK AND PROTECTIVE FACTORS: MULTICOMPONENT OBSERVATIONAL AND INTERVENTION APPROACHES

Most research on protective factors for cognitive decline has focused on single factors and their relationship with cognitive health. Another promising approach is to examine multiple factors in concert, as they exist in vivo.

We know that physical activity and social activity are both good for cognitive health, but we know little about how these work together. There is interest in learning more specific information about the recommended dosage and most effective combinations of different protective factors.

Agrigoroaei and Lachman (2011) examined the cumulative contribution of psychosocial and behavioral protective factors (i.e., control beliefs, quality of social support, and physical exercise) to cognitive functioning and decline across 10 years in the MIDUS study. They found that the more protective factors the better the cognitive performance, over and above well-established correlates and risk factors such as functional health, smoking, drug and alcohol use, and engagement in cognitive activities. The particular combination did not matter in that any two of these factors was better than any one factor. Moreover, the episodic memory scores among people with lower education, who engaged in more protective behaviors, were comparable to those of respondents with higher education. Participants with a greater number of protective factors showed lesser decline in reasoning over a 10-year period, especially for those with lower education. These results suggest that educational differences in cognitive performance and change can be attenuated by modifiable psychosocial and behavioral protective factors. Furthermore, this suggests that interventions that are multimodal may be more effective than those that target just one factor.

A 2-year multidomain intervention that included diet, exercise, cognitive training, and vascular risk monitoring with an at-risk group of older adults in Finland found positive results for maintenance of cognitive functioning (the FINGER study; Ngandu et al., 2015). However, some (e.g., Kraft, 2012) have argued that there is not enough evidence to conclude that multimodal interventions are more effective than individual interventions targeting cognitive or physical activity. Much research is examining directly whether combined training (e.g., both physical exercise and cognitive training) is more effective than targeting one component (Livingston et al., 2017). A noteworthy example is the Multidomain Intervention on Cognitive Function in Elderly Adults With Memory Complaints (MAPT) study (Vellas et al., 2014), which examined the contribution of multiple components: omega-3 supplementation alone, multidomain intervention alone (consisting of nutritional counseling, physical exercise, cognitive stimulation), omega-3 plus multidomain intervention, or a placebo on cognitive decline. Like many such studies (Ngandu et al., 2015), the early MAPT results were somewhat mixed (Andrieu et al., 2017). Another example is the INSIGHT Study, a 4-month randomized controlled trial in which healthy adults ages 18–43 were enrolled in one of four conditions: (a) fitness training; (b) fitness training and computer-based cognitive training; (c) fitness, cognitive training, and mindfulness meditation; or (d) active control (Daugherty et al.,

2018). Whereas the combination of fitness and cognitive training produced gains in visuospatial reasoning that were greater than in the active control, this was not the case for other cognitive tasks. The effectiveness of the various combinations of training varied across cognitive outcome measures.

The Experience Corps (Fried et al., 2004, 2013), in which older adults volunteered in Baltimore inner-city schools to tutor elementary school children, found evidence for positive changes in the brain involving increases in hippocampal and cortical volume (Carlson et al., 2015). The positive changes may be attributed to the multimodal nature of the intervention, which included increased physical activity, cognitive stimulation, and social interactions.

A 25% reduction in seven modifiable risk factors including diabetes, hypertension, obesity, depression, physical inactivity, smoking, and education/cognitive inactivity could prevent up to 3 million cases of ADRD worldwide and 492,000 cases in the United States (Yaffe et al., 2014). Given the knowledge we now have regarding modifiable factors that can slow, reduce, or even reverse cognitive declines or reduce the risk of dementia, there is a need to ensure that adults engage in these adaptive behaviors. Thus, there is renewed interest in developing effective behavior change programs to promote a healthy lifestyle that supports good cognitive health. This would involve a focus on behavior changes such as regular exercise, better sleep, improved diet, social interaction, and cognitive stimulation. Interventions can be useful not only for changing behaviors but also for identifying the mechanisms that link cognitive aging with lifestyle factors. Further research is needed to indicate when and how often to intervene. A promising direction for cognitive interventions is to examine whether earlier timing is better and to what extent booster sessions are necessary.

ROLE OF NONMODIFIABLE RISK AND PROTECTIVE FACTORS

Whereas the previous sections reviewed new approaches and recent information on modifiable risk and protective factors, as they influence and differentiate trajectories of normal cognitive aging, in this section, we attend to the main clusters of relatively nonmodifiable risk factors and biomarkers and how they might moderate the influence of other more malleable factors. The effects of nonmodifiable factors can occur in the form of direct associations but also in more complex configurations, such as interactions, panels, risk indexes, and networks. Indeed, they may combine with modifiable factors, even in the direction of cognitive maintenance and positive outcomes. Thus, these nonmodifiable factors serve an important function in identifying risks that may lead to preventive interventions. We provide a brief overview of genetic risk for cognitive decline and dementia, as conveyed by polymorphisms identified in genome-wide association studies (GWAS) for their role in Alzheimer's disease (AD) risk (especially *APOE*) or cognitive aging risk (e.g., *BDNF*). Next, we describe the roles that chronological age and sex can play in moderating observed associations between genetic and other biomarkers, on one hand, and cognitive trajectories and statuses, on the other. Stratification by age or sex can reveal differences in associations and mechanisms, including functions such as magnification of severity and precision of mechanistic pathways. Accordingly, we review new approaches, based on trajectory analyses, to detecting and characterizing subsets of aging adults who have high risk profiles (e.g., for AD) and yet show minimal signs of exacerbated cognitive decline. Furthermore, we review briefly new and objective approaches to identifying subsets of aging adults who demonstrate either superior levels or sustained trajectories of cognitive performance, thus qualifying as "successful" or "exceptional" cognitive agers. For both resilient and exceptional cognitive aging adults, the key effort is in phenotyping them—finding the combinations of protective or risk-reducing factors that promote such healthy brain and cognitive aging. A theme running throughout this section is that of advancing precision assessment and personalized and targeted interventions in the period of brain and cognitive aging before an AD diagnosis.

Genetic Risk

Estimates from prominent behavioral genetic (twin) studies of the heritability of general intelligence (or "g") are typically high, including 60% to 80% for standard intelligence test performance (Harris & Deary, 2011; Kremen, Panizzon, & Cannon, 2016). This suggests that unmodifiable factors (in general) play a substantial role in influencing individual differences in overall cognitive ability in older adults. However, three qualifications relevant to the present review have emerged. The first qualification is that there is indeed considerable room for the influence of other risk factors, some of which may be modifiable, and these may represent aspects of the environment, including risk exposures. The second qualification is that calculations of heritability of cognition are generally less dramatic when the phenotype is not performance level but cognitive change in specific domains (Harris & Deary, 2011; Reynolds & Finkel, 2015; Tucker-Drob, Reynolds, Finkel, & Pedersen, 2014). Trajectories are a crucial target for cognitive aging research. A third qualification is that examination of individual risk genes and their differential associations with specific domains of cognitive level and change may reveal useful information about underlying mechanisms related to subsets (e.g., carriers vs. noncarriers, normal vs. impaired, female vs. male) of aging individuals. Therefore, a key issue for the present review of research on normal cognitive aging is which genotypic influences affect which cognitive functions (and trajectories) in the context of what underlying mechanisms?

Three reasonable points of origin from which to investigate these connections are (a) a small cluster of genotypes that have been extensively explored for their independent associations with cognitive performance and change in nondemented and nonimpaired older adults; (b) *APOE*, the most prominent genetic risk factor for AD; and (c) other AD risk genotypes discovered in GWAS. Note that for (b) and (c), we refer to genetic risk for late-onset or sporadic AD, the most prevalent neurodegenerative disease, and known to be multifactorial in origin. We do not cover the other form of AD, the rare (about 5% of AD cases) early-onset or familial AD (EOAD), for which symptoms typically appear in the 40s and 50s. The incidence of EOAD is determined by inherited mutations in three genes (presenilin 1, presenilin 2, and amyloid precursor protein) controlling corresponding proteins that are associated with beta-amyloid deposition (i.e., plaques) in the brain. In contrast to the genetic determinism of EOAD, the genetic predictors of sporadic AD are probabilistic, likely combining with other risk factors to produce the neurodegeneration typical of transitions from normal to impaired aging and dementia (Fotuhi, Hachinski, & Whitehouse, 2009). The argument for including AD genetic risk factors in studies on nondemented cognitive aging is that the preclinical period of neurodegenerative changes associated with emerging AD can reach back more than a decade before diagnosis. Therefore, AD genetic risk factors may exert their influence on cognitive decline—and especially accelerations in cognitive decline associated with mild cognitive impairment—during a period that appears to be asymptomatic, seemingly normal cognitive aging.

Numerous studies have explored genetic approaches and specific genotypes for their associations with a variety of cognitive phenotypes of normal aging. Several in-depth reviews locate this research direction in its biological, methodological, and theoretical context (e.g., Harris & Deary, 2011; Kremen et al., 2016; Papenberg, Lindenberger, & Bäckman, 2015). An early approach used "candidate genes" to explore associations with cognitive phenotypes potentially linked to underlying mechanistic operations in identified regions of the aging brain. Among the prominently—and most successfully—investigated candidate genes for normal cognitive aging have been *BDNF* and catechol-O-methyl transferase (*COMT*). Because these genes have been linked to functioning within the hippocampus and prefrontal cortex, respectively, they have been investigated with performance on episodic memory and executive function tasks. Although widely investigated in these and other neurocognitive aging contexts, these two candidate genes have produced selectively significant results but inconsistent patterns overall (e.g., Barnett et al., 2008; Mandelman & Grigorenko, 2012). Much more promising has been recent work investigating these two polymorphisms in various combinations (panels, risk scores) or interactions (gene × gene; gene × environment; gene × health) and with specialized outcome measures evaluated longitudinally (e.g., Das et al., 2014; Erickson et al., 2009; Raz, Rodrigue, Kennedy, & Land, 2009; Sapkota, Bäckman, & Dixon, 2017). Notably, this progress fits with the direction of the present review, in which interactions of modifiable and nonmodifiable risk factors are of direct interest.

APOE is the most prominent and commonly studied genetic risk factor for AD. Differentiated by three isoforms, carriers of the ε4 allele (especially homozygotes) are at elevated risk of developing AD, whereas carriers of the ε3 (AD neutral) and ε2 (potentially protective) alleles are at relatively low risk (Liu, Kanekiyo, Xu, & Bu, 2013; Wisdom, Callahan, & Hawkins, 2011). The key question for this review is whether APOE ε4 carriers are also at risk for preclinical impairment and exacerbated but nonimpaired normal cognitive decline. Regarding mild cognitive impairment (MCI), several studies have implicated the predictive role of the ε4 allele (e.g., Brainerd, Reyna, Petersen, Smith, & Taub, 2011; Dixon et al., 2014), with the latter study reporting the intriguing result that COMT contributed complementary prediction patterns to APOE. An early meta-analysis provided an initial assessment of the role that APOE might play in predicting cognitive performance in nondemented older adults (Small, Rosnick, Fratiglioni, & Bäckman, 2004). Since that time, much more research has been reported showing increasingly interpretable patterns of influence, although especially in combinations with other AD genetic risk factors (e.g., Andrews, Das, Anstey, & Easteal, 2017), normal cognitive decline risk genes (Sapkota, Vergote, Westaway, Jhamandas, & Dixon, 2015), as well as with modifiable cognitive aging risk factors (e.g., McFall, Sapkota, McDermott, & Dixon, 2016; McFall et al., 2015; Raz et al., 2009). In an investigation of conversion from MCI to AD, it was the absence of APOE ε4 alleles that best predicted the stability of MCI over a 3-year period (Clem et al., 2017).

In addition to APOE, GWAS have identified 20 genetic loci that are associated with AD (Andrews et al., 2017). Although none of these variants bear the function load of APOE, some may serve purposes useful to the current review. Specifically, these lesser known AD variants may (a) mark coordinated pathophysiological mechanisms of AD, (b) contribute to predictive panels or polygenic risk scores, (c) be applicable in to-be-determined combinations in predicting exacerbated or impaired cognitive decline (or AD progression), or (d) contribute to APOE-based panels that interact with modifiable risk factors in predicting cognitive change (e.g., Carrasquillo et al., 2015; Darst et al., 2017; Sapkota et al., 2017; Zhang & Pierce, 2014). Polygenic risk scores are panels of multiple risk variants with relatively small direct effects on the phenotype of interest, but that may combine to represent coordinated pathways within networks of neurobiological influence. These networks may also include other biomarkers or risk factors (Gaiteri, Mostafavi, Honey, De Jager, & Bennett, 2016), and such networks may vary by age (e.g., magnification among older adults; Papenberg et al., 2015) or sex (differential for females and males; McDermott, McFall, Andrews, Anstey, & Dixon, 2017). Recently, such genetic networks have included sets of risk genes for both normal cognitive aging and AD (Sapkota & Dixon, 2018) in predicting nondemented cognitive trajectories.

In sum, an important point is that in predicting cognitive change, impairment, and dementia, genetic risk interacts with other potentially modifiable risk conferred by a variety of factors of everyday life (activities, exercise, health). Moreover, as we will see in the next subsections, these dynamic associations may also be moderated by age, sex, and even *APOE* ε4 status. Therefore, risk and protective factors may be part of the network of predictors that apply differentially within certain categories of aging demographics.

Age and Sex: Not Just Difference Makers but Tools of Precision Research?

The aptly named *triad* of risk for sporadic AD includes three major elements: (a) chronological age (older is worse), (b) sex (female is worse), and (c) *APOE* (worse for ε4 carriers; Riedel, Thompson, & Brinton, 2016). The simplicity of these three major AD risk factors is remarkable given all the effort expended on discovering hallmarks and biomarkers of AD through invasive or complex procedures such as positron emission tomography scans (for amyloid burden), GWAS (for additional AD-related genotypes), lumbar punctures (for cerebrospinal fluid assays of beta amyloid and phosphorylated tau), brain tissue analyses (for confirmation of AD diagnosis and biomarker analyses), and blood-based biomarker assays (including omics-based unbiased discovery analyses). They are straightforward to measure with accuracy, available as variables in many research studies and data archives, and typically reported at least in background or demographic tables or included as covariates. However, some differences in how these variables are used and interpreted are apparent. We focus on using age and sex advantageously in research on cognitive aging.

Using Age Advantageously

A first question from some observers might be, Why use age at all (or at most as an index)? For other observers, a contrary question might be, What is wrong with using age (e.g., to form groups for comparison)? We will not reprise the decades-long discussions of the status of chronological age in aging research (see Baltes & Willis, 1977; Birren & Cunningham, 1985; Dixon,

2011). Three key points have been enumerated frequently and persuasively: (a) Age may be useful as an index or metric of aging, but it is not a cause or source of theoretical explanations; (b) age is a prominent but not the only way to display time-related trajectories in cognitive aging (e.g., biological age, functional age); and (c) cross-sectional comparisons reveal potentially promising age or group differences in performance and in predictor–performance associations, but their viability as representations of actual change or platforms for testing mechanistic hypotheses cannot be verified and might be considered skeptically under most prevailing assumptions (Baltes, 1968; Baltes, Lindenberger, & Staudinger, 2006; Schaie, 1965, 2012).

Nevertheless, it is true that age per se is the single most predictive biomarker of sporadic AD, and thus it should be useful in some settings and for some purposes. Three such examples of the usefulness of age are relevant in this review. First, a growing number of recently published papers on actual cognitive trajectories (as often displayed in spaghetti plots) reveal the rich variability and differentiation of age changes for many cognitive functions (Dixon et al., 2014; Josefsson et al., 2012). When analyzed appropriately, such trajectories can produce meaningful representations of overall function of cognitive change across a given band of age (Galbraith, Bowden, & Mander, 2017). With (a) relatively large data sets, (b) a broad band of age, (c) well-measured (and even latent) cognitive variables, and (d) application of increasingly available statistical packages for change analyses, these data can highlight the general aging trend but also the vast individual differences in level, slope, and variability of change patterns. Such analyses have the additional advantage of including age directly. Second, contemporary statistical techniques (e.g., parallel process models in latent growth curve analyses) permit the incorporation of theoretically relevant predictor variables in trajectory analyses. These can include nonmodifiable predictors (genotype), modifiable but not changing predictors (baseline education), and modifiable predictors that may change over time (lifestyle or health risk factors; McFall et al., 2016; Sapkota et al., 2017). Moreover, analyses can accommodate single candidate predictors as well as a variety of predictor interactions (e.g., Thibeau, McFall, Camicioli, & Dixon, 2017). Third, given the often-observed heterogeneity of age-related levels of performance (even within older adults) and the intriguing findings of age-related changes in predictor patterns, it is possible to use a reasonable break point of age (in a broad age band sample) to stratify and conduct these analyses separately for two or more age groups. Using similar procedures, researchers have advanced the hypotheses that some biomarkers, including genetic polymorphisms, may have magnified effects for very old, as compared with young-old, adults (Lindenberger et al., 2008; Papenberg et al., 2015).

In sum, age is a major risk factor for AD and cognitive decline but should be used carefully in research. All longitudinal data are, at heart, age-based, but using it as a metric of change, with no assumptions about alleged causal roles, permits analytical and interpretive advantages. As such, age is not just a variable associated with performance differences, but it is also a variable that can provide opportunities for testing mechanistic hypotheses, developing individualized clusters, and leading to precision interventions. This is especially the case given that trajectory groups may demonstrate different patterns of predictions by biomarker and risk or protective factors (McFall et al., 2015; Zahodne et al., 2016). Moreover, the onset and slope of declines vary across persons and cognitive dimensions.

Using Sex and Gender Advantageously

We adopt a standard definition of these two terms but recognize that there are areas of gray (nonbinary, inexact separation, and exceptions) between them. Accordingly, in this discussion *sex* refers to biological and physiological differences in function or mechanisms between males and females, and *gender* refers to differences related to socialization or culture, including associated characteristics, exposures, roles, and identity for women and men. Both sex and gender are of interest in the wider range of brain and cognitive aging, but for present purposes sex and sex-related phenomena are emphasized. Sex differences—and, more importantly, sex-related mechanisms—are of increasing importance in the study of brain and cognitive changes associated with decline, dementia, and mechanisms thereof. The National Institutes of Health has adopted a stringent policy to enhance research on sex as a biological variable. When integrated into research designs, it is possible to examine differences in a variety of areas, including brain and cognitive aging research, as well as research on neurodegenerative diseases (Tierney, Curtis, Chertkow, & Rylett, 2017). One goal is to provide more complete data sets (in terms of sex representation); more generalizable results (to both sexes); and deeper analyses of the biological mechanisms underlying such observations as sex differences in cognitive performance, AD incidence and prevalence, and response to medications (including molecules in AD intervention research). Recently, new and large-scale research programs (e.g., Canadian Consortium on Neurodegeneration in Aging; U.S. National Institute on Aging Research Programs on Alzheimer's Disease and Related Dementias) have emphasized—and in some cases, compelled—the investigation of sex and/or gender differences in basic, clinical, and intervention research.

Thus, the advantageous use of sex and gender in research covered in the present review is predominantly to further investigate sex differences in cognitive performance and change, mechanisms underlying those differences, and how they have differential implications for longer term trajectories and clinical outcomes. For example, among the replicated results pertaining to sex effects in nondemented older adults, cognitive performance is the difference in mean performance levels (Herlitz & Rehnman, 2008; Jack et al., 2015; Weber, Skirbekk, Freund, & Herlitz, 2014). Close inspection usually reveals that these differences are relatively small (in magnitude) and the female–male distributions display considerable overlap. However, they may conceal some important and emerging differences because females may also undergo earlier pathogenic brain changes and steeper declines in performance (Zhao, Mao, Woody, & Brinton, 2016). Moreover, recent research has indicated that female carriers of the *APOE* ε4 risk allele may experience differentially higher risk for AD than do their male counterparts (Altmann, Tian, Henderson, & Greicius, 2014). This and other sex-related neurobiological factors may play a role in the reported greater prevalence of AD for females than males. Moreover, it may indicate the importance of stratifying for sex when AD genetic risk is considered. In sum, an advantageous use of sex as a biological variable includes the possibility of examining many mechanistic analyses separately for males and females. It may also indicate that the importance of including both sexes in AD-related intervention trials should consider the possibility of powering the study so that differential factors and responses can be assessed. We present an example of this in the next subsection.

RISK AND PROTECTIVE FACTORS: ALTERNATIVE PATHWAYS TO COGNITIVE HEALTH

Cognitive Reserve and Resilience to Risk

A pleasantly perplexing issue in the field of brain and cognitive aging is that some older adults seem to retain adaptive, if not relatively high, levels of cognitive performance, despite (a) advancing age, (b) elevated genetic or familial risk for AD, and (c) actual observed AD neuropathology (amyloid deposition). The conceptual framework of reserve has been postulated to account for such intriguing discrepancies in susceptibility to normal or pathological brain changes with aging (Stern, 2002, 2012). Abundantly researched and evaluated, reserve has been differentiated into complementary brain (relatively passive) and cognitive (relatively active) components. The concept of brain reserve reflects the contention that individual differences in neural structure, including ongoing neurodegenerative processes associated with impairment and AD, lead to differences in pathological burden and vulnerability to early or exacerbated cognitive decline. The concept of cognitive reserve refers to a body of epidemiological, neuropsychological, and biomarker evidence that lifelong activities summarized by extent of education, lifestyle engagement, and occupational complexity are associated with sustained cognitive adaptation (Cabeza et al., 2018; Marioni et al., 2012; Stern, 2009, 2012). Reserve has an established position in the lexicon of research and theory in normal cognitive aging, as well as preclinical transitions to AD (Arenaza-Urquijo, Wirth, & Chételat, 2015) and other neurodegenerative diseases (Borroni et al., 2012). Much progress in identifying neuroimaging and lifestyle factors indicative of reserve has been made (e.g., Jones et al., 2011; van Loenhoud et al., 2017). Recent approaches integrate neuroimaging markers with genetic or cognitive markers to capture a flexible and promising model of cognitive reserve (e.g., Ferrari et al., 2013; van Loenhoud et al., 2017).

Although reserve has proven to be a fertile conceptual framework addressed to a salient issue in brain and cognitive aging, as a scientific concept, it is still hypothetical, and its main explanatory devices are only indirectly indicative of its operation. In principle, a full examination of reserve might benefit from (a) direct measures of the dynamics of vulnerability (or risk), (b) the presence of countervailing buffers or protection, and (c) evidence of sustained levels and slopes of cognitive performance beyond that expected for individuals with elevated risk but reduced protection. To be sure, pieces of this dynamic model have been observed. Moreover, that the indirect measures of reserve—for example, higher cumulative levels of life experiences that are cognitive-intensive (education, job complexity)—are associated with cognitive health and dementia delay are suggestive. The process of compensation refers to the recruitment of neural or behavioral resources to address limitations due to cognitive and brain aging especially in high-demand situations (Bäckman & Dixon, 1992; Cabeza et al., 2018; Dixon, Garrett, & Bäckman, 2008). It is likely that the balance between available cognitive reserve and prevailing cognitive deficits (in the context of environmental demands) may determine the extent to which compensatory mechanisms may be recruited and deployed (Dixon & de Frias, 2007; Reuter-Lorenz & Cappell, 2008). The processes per se of reserve and the mechanisms underlying the concept and its effects on cognition may be identifiable and quantifiable. To this extent, specific experiences may be operationally defined, tested experimentally or in interventions, and evaluated for their promise in promoting reserve and healthier brain aging in midlife and beyond.

One corollary concept fulfilling some of these criteria has emerged: the concept of cognitive resilience. A consensus definition refers to actual cognitive maintenance (over time) despite objective evidence for AD risk, such as being a carrier of the ε4 allele of *APOE* (Kaup et al., 2015). It is well known that not all genetic risk carriers convert to clinical diagnosis of AD, and in fact, some of them seem to maintain adaptive, if not high and sustained, levels of performance into late life (Ferrari et al., 2013). If substantial samples of individuals with this combination of characteristics—who are also participants in larger scale longitudinal studies—could be detected and assembled, the process of resilience could be testable. In addition, some studies would likely have variables representing potential risk or protection factors that may be contributing to the emergence of resilience in this subpopulation. A reasonable pool of such potential mechanistic markers of resilience would include both modifiable and nonmodifiable risk and protective factors for cognitive decline and dementia.

Recently, Kaup and colleagues (2015) used longitudinal data from Health ABC Study to examine slope deviations of genetic risk carriers, compared with the remainder of the sample, and classified cognitively resilient individuals as those who were *APOE* ε4 carriers and displayed relatively high cognitive change slopes. Importantly, after classifying a substantial resilient group, the researchers conducted prediction analyses as stratified by race. Different patterns of predictors were observed for White and Black carriers. Using a similar approach and data from the Victoria Longitudinal Study, McDermott and colleagues (2017) focused on episodic memory performance (represented in a latent variable) because memory decline is a cardinal early marker of preclinical AD. The trajectory analyses set the algorithm for comparing both level and slope as determinants of classification for *APOE* ε4 carriers. Their sample lacked racial diversity, but they stratified by sex, reasoning that males and females often perform differently on memory (Herlitz & Rehnman, 2008) and females have higher AD prevalence than males. Their results showed that risk and protective predictors of resilience differed by sex, with more modifiable predictors detected for females. These results were largely replicated for resilience as defined by another AD risk gene, clusterin (*CLU*).

In sum, cognitive reserve and resilience are differentiable conceptually and methodologically but sponsor complementary research goals and activities. Both deserve further attention and perhaps a merging of techniques and issues. Resilience studies feature objective criteria based on dynamic data and sophisticated statistical analyses for classification. Such studies are also amenable to stratification for key group comparisons of predictor patterns. Observing similar phenomena but with different predictors by racial and sex status holds great promise for future mechanistic analyses and precision intervention to promote healthier (resilience) cognitive functioning, even for individuals with substantial and readily measurable AD risk.

Alternative Pathways: A Continuum of Trajectories and Outcomes of Cognitive Aging

How can a continuum of cognitive concepts and phenotypes, including reserve, resilience, normal aging, and exceptional (or "successful") aging, be theoretically differentiated and empirically classified? One way to begin addressing this challenge is presented in the model in Figure 8.2. This figure (based on Dixon, McFall, & McDermott, 2017) shows a flowchart with one common input (normal cognitive aging), two generic mechanisms (AD biomarker risk, brain aging vulnerability risk and protection), and four provisionally distinguishable pathways and clinical outcomes of aging. The model provides a template for discriminating these pathways (Column 2)—theoretically and empirically—as the lead from normal cognitive aging (Column 1) to four alternative trajectory patterns or clinical statuses (Column 3). A brief interpretation of each pathway and outcome is provided in Column 4.

The top pathway (Row 1) is the one that is likely for many middle-aged and aging adults, at least until they accumulate additional risk in advancing age. Low AD genetic risk would be expected, given that the predominant risk gene is *APOE* and its most common genotype is the ε3/ε3 (or nonrisk)

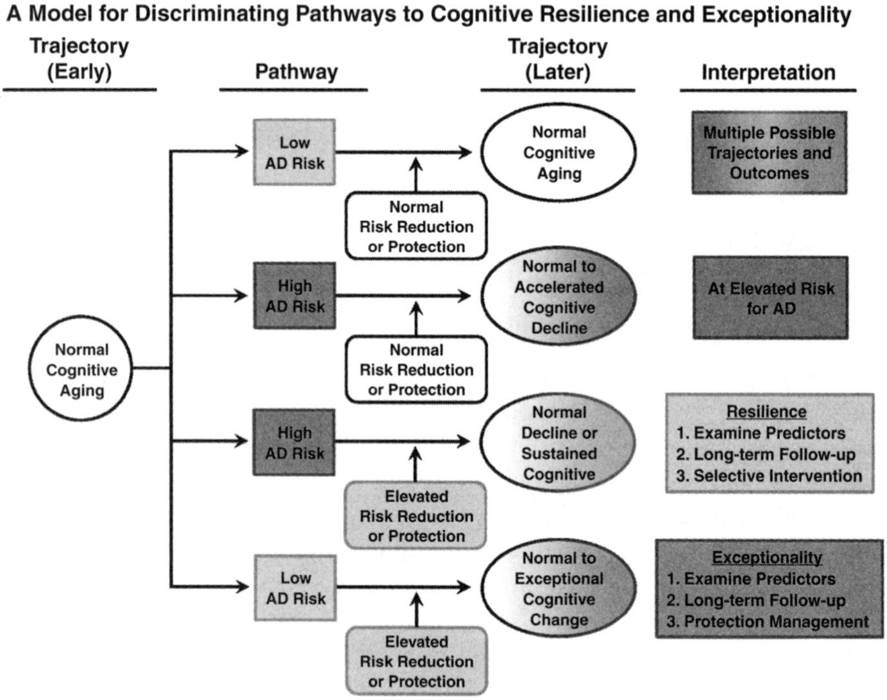

A Model for Discriminating Pathways to Cognitive Resilience and Exceptionality

Figure 8.2. A model for discriminating pathways to (a) normal cognitive aging, (b) impaired or accelerated cognitive decline, (c) resilient cognitive aging, and (d) exceptional cognitive aging. AD = Alzheimer's disease. Adapted from "Discriminating and Predicting Cognitive Exceptionality and Resilience: A Roadmap for Trajectory and Interaction Analyses With Risk and Protection Factors," by R. A. Dixon, G. P. McFall, and K. McDermott, July 2017. Paper presented at Alzheimer's Association International Conference, London, England.

configuration. Nothing conveys immunity to cognitive impairment and dementia, so this group, without further phenotyping, would be expected to follow multiple trajectories leading to multiple potential outcomes. The second row pertains to individuals who have high genetic risk but normal risk reduction from other factors. Initially expected to be in the normal range of cognitive performance (level and slope), these individuals are at elevated risk for early cognitive decline, transition into cognitive impairment, and eventually AD. For these individuals, early detection and implementation of modifiable risk reduction interventions may lead to delayed impairment, if not prevention (Anstey et al., 2014).

The third row pertains to the pathway to resilience, as described earlier. In this pathway, high AD risk is counterbalanced by elevated risk reduction or protective factors with the ensuing range of trajectories encompassing normal to sustained levels and slopes. If resilience is classified, the predictors (reflecting mechanisms) can be identified and targeted in precision interventions. The interventions may be applied to extend the period of resilience, but also potentially to initiate resilience in the previous pathways. Finally, the fourth pathway is one of long-term interest in a variety of fields of aging (Pruchno, 2015). It depicts a potential pathway whereby brain and cognitive exceptionality may be attained and maintained by select individuals. Often referred to as *successful cognitive aging* (Depp & Jeste, 2006) or *superaging* (Rogalski et al., 2013), such an outcome could be promoted by the propitious combination of low AD genetic risk and elevated protective or risk-reducing factors. Again, the research agenda would include determining the phenotype of exceptional brain and cognitive aging and then examining the predictors, both modifiable and nonmodifiable. For those fortunate enough to be following this aging pathway, interventions might still be useful for managing protection, and perhaps sustaining or enhancing it with advancing age. For those following other aging trajectories, it is possible that the modifiable predictors of exceptional brain and cognitive aging could be useful in a risk-reducing capacity in middle to late life.

We emphasize that the model is designed to represent common clusters of pathways and conditions but is broad enough to accommodate many intermediate and changing circumstances. We also note that the outcome trajectories and statuses can be discriminated conceptually and sometimes empirically but that they comprise areas on a continuum of brain and cognitive aging. We note that the model represents the pathways as influenced by genetic and modifiable risk factors, such as those described here, but implies that they may interact to intensify risk or magnify risk reduction. Not specifically included in the model is the fact that some of these mechanisms may vary by important variables of stratification, including sex, race, age, or *APOE* status. To examine these pathways, large-scale and multifaceted longitudinal data are required. To determine underlying mechanisms, experimental work will be useful. To explore interventions for personalized risk reduction or protection enhancement, prevention studies, including multifactorial randomized controlled trials, are the method of choice (e.g., Anstey et al., 2014, 2015; Barnes et al., 2015; Carlson et al., 2015; Ngandu et al., 2015). With these comparative pathways in mind, we turn now to the fourth scenario, that leading to exceptional brain and cognitive aging.

Cognitive Exceptionality: Risk Reduction and Protection Enhancement?

The vast individualized variability of nondemented aging cognitive trajectories is of increasing interest to researchers in both normal aging and AD. For both groups, this diversity of change patterns presents an understudied but promising context for discovery and validation of risk-reducing and protection-enhancing factors in cognitive aging (Depp, Harmell, & Vahia, 2012; Gefen et al., 2014; Yaffe et al., 2009; Zahodne et al., 2016). Traditionally, both cognitive aging and AD researchers have emphasized descriptive and explanatory work on typical and exacerbated decline, impairment, and transitions to AD. A complementary approach focuses on (a) establishing the validity of relatively "healthy," "successful," or "exceptional" phenotypes and (b) exploring their risk predictors to promote healthier brain aging through AD risk management, delay, or even prevention (Anstey, 2014; Barnes & Yaffe, 2011; Daffner, 2010; Dixon, 2010; Pruchno, 2015). Arguably, factors associated with sustained cognitive health may include those that are modifiable through early interventions, operating at a precision or even public health level.

A set of positive concepts of aging—typically known as "successful aging"—have circulated for several decades (Baltes & Baltes, 1990; Pruchno, 2015; Pruchno, Wilson-Genderson, Rose, & Cartwright, 2010; Rowe & Kahn, 1997) and recently benefited from critical reviews (Cosco, Prina, Perales, Stephan, & Brayne, 2014; Depp & Jeste, 2006). New conceptual and empirical applications to cognitive and brain aging have appeared (Depp et al., 2012; Fiocco & Yaffe, 2010) and focused on issues of objective and enriched classification, identification of associated risk and protective factors, and potential application to risk management and prevention. Successful efforts to characterize exceptional brain and cognitive aging have included a variety of methods: single-test averages, multitest distributions, comparisons with younger adults, and, recently, trajectory analyses (Josefsson et al., 2012). Exceptional cognitive performance has been established for multiple domains of cognition, including global cognition (Yaffe et al., 2009), executive function (de Frias & Dixon, 2014; de Frias, Dixon, & Strauss, 2009), and episodic memory (EM; Barral et al., 2013; Dixon & de Frias, 2014; Harrison, Weintraub, Mesulam, & Rogalski, 2012; Josefsson et al., 2012).

Several programs of research have appeared. For example, the North-western SuperAging project defines "SuperAgers" as having EM performance similar to that of adults 20 years their junior. Benefits include maintained performance in other cognitive domains (Gefen et al., 2014) and fewer brain markers of AD pathology (Harrison et al., 2012; Rogalski et al., 2013). Complementary research from the Canadian-based Victoria Longitudinal Study (VLS) identified "cognitively elite" participants from a longitudinal panel as those individuals who scored above the (age × education) mean on a battery of three to five basic cognitive tasks. Whether applied to executive functioning (de Frias & Dixon, 2014; de Frias et al., 2009) or memory (Dixon & de Frias, 2014; Dixon et al., 2012; McFall et al., 2015), objectively classified cognitively exceptional participants performed better on a variety of related tasks. The Swedish Betula Project used longitudinal memory trajectories to separate maintainers (i.e., moderate to high baseline EM score and better-than-average rate of change) from decliners and those with age-typical change (Josefsson et al., 2012). Being a maintainer was predicted by higher education, being female, living with someone, more physical activity, and being a Met carrier of the *COMT* gene. The trajectory approach has recently been applied to classification and determination of modifiable risk factor predictors (McDermott, McFall, Andrews, Anstey, & Dixon, 2017). The latter study stratified by age and found differing predictors for young-old and old-old groups.

In sum, objectively classifying exceptional cognitive aging can be accomplished with several methods. A key goal is to determine clusters of predictors, especially as they discriminate between exceptional groups and normal or declining groups. Such predictors may derive from multiple modalities (brain, genetic, lifestyle) and range in modifiability. Thus far, results indicate that strategies for promoting healthy brain aging may not be just the reverse of strategies for delaying decline or impairment. Precision approaches that target specific modifiable biomarkers may be useful in future intervention strategies to promote or sustain healthy brain and cognitive aging. Moreover, personalized interventions can target specific personal characteristics to maximize the likelihood of effective treatments.

CONCLUSION

As the world population continues to age and the prevalence of AD and related disorders is expected to rise, there is a concerted effort to identify early warning signs of accelerated cognitive decline, transitions to impairment, and impending dementia. There is evidence for wide individual differences in the nature of cognitive aging, and these differences are reflected in variability in onset, level, and slope of trajectories (Dixon et al., 2014). Declines on some cognitive dimensions such as processing speed begin in early midlife for some adults (e.g., Hughes, Agrigoroaei, Jeon, Bruzzese, & Lachman, 2018). As reviewed in this chapter, researchers have identified multiple modalities of both modifiable and nonmodifiable risk factors that hold promise for understanding how, why, and to what extent trajectories of cognitive change are predicted and differentiated with aging. Equally important to detect and catalogue are the risk-reducing or protective factors that predict favorable trajectories and outcomes, such as reserve, resilience, plasticity, and sustained exceptional cognitive performance. In this review, we emphasize the emerging importance of considering multimodal dynamic and network approaches to examining interactions among common risk and protective factors. Such approaches may lead to better precision in both observational and intervention research. Although the ultimate goal is to prevent the onset of cognitive impairment and dementia, a more realistic aim, at least in the short term, may be to reduce or delay neurodegenerative risk and associated cognitive declines.

REFERENCES

Agrigoroaei, S., & Lachman, M. E. (2011). Cognitive functioning in midlife and old age: Combined effects of psychosocial and behavioral factors. *The Journals of Gerontology: Series B. Psychological Sciences and Social Sciences*, 66(Suppl. 1), i130–i140. http://dx.doi.org/10.1093/geronb/gbr017

Agrigoroaei, S., Robinson, S. A., Hughes, M. L., Rickenbach, E. H., & Lachman, M. E. (2018). Cognition at midlife: Antecedents and consequences. In C. D. Ryff & R. F. Krueger (Eds.), *Oxford handbook of integrated health science*. New York, NY: Oxford University Press.

Altmann, A., Tian, L., Henderson, V. W., & Greicius, M. D. (2014). Sex modifies the *APOE*-related risk of developing Alzheimer disease. *Annals of Neurology, 75*, 563–573. http://dx.doi.org/10.1002/ana.24135

Alzheimer's Association. (2016). 2016 Alzheimer's disease facts and figures. *Alzheimer's & Dementia, 12*, 459–509. http://dx.doi.org/10.1016/j.jalz.2016.03.001

Andel, R., Kåreholt, I., Parker, M. G., Thorslund, M., & Gatz, M. (2007). Complexity of primary lifetime occupation and cognition in advanced old age. *Journal of Aging and Health, 19*, 397–415. http://dx.doi.org/10.1177/0898264307300171

Andel, R., Vigen, C., Mack, W. J., Clark, L. J., & Gatz, M. (2006). The effect of education and occupational complexity on rate of cognitive decline in Alzheimer's patients. *Journal of the International Neuropsychological Society, 12*, 147–152. http://dx.doi.org/10.1017/S1355617706060206

Andrews, S. J., Das, D., Anstey, K. J., & Easteal, S. (2017). Late onset Alzheimer's disease risk variants in cognitive decline: The PATH Through Life Study. *Journal of Alzheimer's Disease, 57*, 423–436. http://dx.doi.org/10.3233/JAD-160774

Andrieu, S., Guyonnet, S., Coley, N., Cantet, C., Bonnefoy, M., Bordes, S., . . . Vellas, B. (2017). Effect of long-term omega 3 polyunsaturated fatty acid supplementation with or without multidomain intervention on cognitive function in elderly adults with memory complaints (MAPT): A randomised, placebo-controlled trial. *The Lancet Neurology, 16*, 377–389. http://dx.doi.org/10.1016/S1474-4422(17)30040-6

Anstey, K. J. (2014). Optimizing cognitive development over the life course and preventing cognitive decline: Introducing the Cognitive Health Environment Life Course Model (CHELM). *International Journal of Behavioral Development, 38*, 1–10. http://dx.doi.org/10.1177/0165025413512255

Anstey, K. J., Cherbuin, N., Herath, P. M., Qiu, C., Kuller, L. H., Lopez, O. L., . . . Fratiglioni, L. (2014). A self-report risk index to predict occurrence of dementia in three independent cohorts of older adults: The ANU-ADRI. *PLoS ONE, 9*, e86141. http://dx.doi.org/10.1371/journal.pone.0086141

Anstey, K. J., Eramudugolla, R., Hosking, D. E., Lautenschlager, N. T., & Dixon, R. A. (2015). Bridging the translation gap: From dementia risk assessment to advice on risk reduction. *The Journal of Prevention of Alzheimer's Disease, 2*, 189–198.

Arenaza-Urquijo, E. M., Wirth, M., & Chételat, G. (2015). Cognitive reserve and lifestyle: Moving towards preclinical Alzheimer's disease. *Frontiers in Aging Neuroscience, 7*, 134. http://dx.doi.org/10.3389/fnagi.2015.00134

Ashe, M. C., Miller, W. C., Eng, J. J., & Noreau, L. (2009). Older adults, chronic disease and leisure-time physical activity. *Gerontology, 55*, 64–72. http://dx.doi.org/10.1159/000141518

Bäckman, L., & Dixon, R. A. (1992). Psychological compensation: A theoretical framework. *Psychological Bulletin, 112*, 259–283. http://dx.doi.org/10.1037/0033-2909.112.2.259

Ball, K. K., Beard, B. L., Roenker, D. L., Miller, R. L., & Griggs, D. S. (1988). Age and visual search: Expanding the useful field of view. *Journal of the Optical Society of America: A. Optics and Image Science, 5*, 2210–2219. http://dx.doi.org/10.1364/JOSAA.5.002210

Baltes, P. B. (1968). Longitudinal and cross-sectional sequences in the study of age and generation effects. *Human Development, 11*, 145–171. http://dx.doi.org/10.1159/000270604

Baltes, P. B., & Baltes, M. M. (1990). Psychological perspectives on successful aging: The model of selective optimization with compensation. In P. B. Baltes & M. M. Baltes (Eds.), *Successful aging: Perspectives from the behavioral sciences* (pp. 1–34). New York, NY: Cambridge University Press. http://dx.doi.org/10.1017/CBO9780511665684.003

Baltes, P. B., Lindenberger, U., & Staudinger, U. M. (2006). Life span theory in developmental psychology. In R. M. Lerner & W. Damon (Eds.), *Handbook of child psychology: Theoretical models of human development* (pp. 569–664). Hoboken, NJ: Wiley.

Baltes, P. B., & Willis, S. L. (1977). Toward psychological theories of aging and development. In J. E. Birren & K. W. Schaie (Eds.), *The handbook of the psychology of aging* (pp. 128–154). New York, NY: Van Nostrand-Reinhold.

Bandura, A. (1997). *Self-efficacy: The exercise of control.* New York, NY: Freeman.

Barber, S. J. (2017). An examination of age-based stereotype threat about cognitive decline: Implications for stereotype threat research and theory development. *Perspectives on Psychological Science, 12,* 62–90. http://dx.doi.org/10.1177/1745691616656345

Barnes, D. E., Mehling, W., Wu, E., Beristianos, M., Yaffe, K., Skultety, K., & Chesney, M. A. (2015). Preventing loss of independence through exercise (PLIÉ): A pilot clinical trial in older adults with dementia. *PLoS One, 10*(2), e0113367. http://dx.doi.org/10.1371/journal.pone.0113367

Barnes, D. E., & Yaffe, K. (2011). The projected effect of risk factor reduction on Alzheimer's disease prevalence. *The Lancet Neurology, 10,* 819–828. http://dx.doi.org/10.1016/S1474-4422(11)70072-2

Barnett, J. H., Scoriels, L., & Munafò, M. R. (2008). Meta-analysis of the cognitive effects of the catechol-O-methyltransferase gene Val158/108Met polymorphism. *Biological Psychiatry, 64,* 137–144. http://dx.doi.org/10.1016/j.biopsych.2008.01.005

Barral, S., Cosentino, S., Costa, R., Andersen, S. L., Christensen, K., Eckfeldt, J. H., . . . Mayeux, R. (2013). Exceptional memory performance in the Long Life Family Study. *Neurobiology of Aging, 34,* 2445–2448. http://dx.doi.org/10.1016/j.neurobiolaging.2013.05.002

Birren, J. E., & Cunningham, W. (1985). Research on the psychology of aging: Principles, concepts and theory. In J. E. Birren & K. W. Schaie (Eds.), *Handbook of the psychology of aging* (2nd ed., pp. 3–34). New York, NY: Van Nostrand Reinhold.

Borroni, B., Alberici, A., Cercignani, M., Premi, E., Serra, L., Cerini, C., . . . Bozzali, M. (2012). Granulin mutation drives brain damage and reorganization from preclinical to symptomatic FTLD. *Neurobiology of Aging, 33,* 2506–2520. http://dx.doi.org/10.1016/j.neurobiolaging.2011.10.031

Brainerd, C. J., Reyna, V. F., Petersen, R. C., Smith, G. E., & Taub, E. S. (2011). Is the apolipoprotein e genotype a biomarker for mild cognitive impairment? Findings from a nationally representative study. *Neuropsychology, 25,* 679–689. http://dx.doi.org/10.1037/a0024483

Brown, C. L., Robitaille, A., Zelinski, E. M., Dixon, R. A., Hofer, S. M., & Piccinin, A. M. (2016). Cognitive activity mediates the association between social activity and cognitive performance: A longitudinal study. *Psychology and Aging, 31,* 831–846. http://dx.doi.org/10.1037/pag0000134

Cabeza, R., Albert, M., Belleville, S., Craik, F. I. M., Duarte, A., Grady, C. L., . . . Rajah, M. N. (2018). Maintenance, reserve and compensation: The cognitive neuroscience of healthy ageing [erratum at http://dx.doi.org/10.1038/

s41583-018-0086-0]. *Nature Reviews Neuroscience, 19*, 701–710. http://dx.doi.org/10.1038/s41583-018-0068-2

Caplan, L. J., & Schooler, C. (2003). The roles of fatalism, self-confidence, and intellectual resources in the disablement process in older adults. *Psychology and Aging, 18*, 551–561. http://dx.doi.org/10.1037/0882-7974.18.3.551

Carlson, M. C., Kuo, J. H., Chuang, Y.-F., Varma, V. R., Harris, G., Albert, M. S., . . . Fried, L. P. (2015). Impact of the Baltimore Experience Corps Trial on cortical and hippocampal volumes. *Alzheimer's & Dementia, 11*, 1340–1348. http://dx.doi.org/10.1016/j.jalz.2014.12.005

Carrasquillo, M. M., Crook, J. E., Pedraza, O., Thomas, C. S., Pankratz, V. S., Allen, M., . . . Ertekin-Taner, N. (2015). Late-onset Alzheimer's risk variants in memory decline, incident mild cognitive impairment, and Alzheimer's disease. *Neurobiology of Aging, 36*, 60–67. http://dx.doi.org/10.1016/j.neurobiolaging.2014.07.042

Clarke, T. C., Norris, T., & Schiller, J. S. (2017). *Early release of selected estimates based on data from the 2016 National Health Interview Survey.* Retrieved from https://www.cdc.gov/nchs/data/nhis/earlyrelease/earlyrelease201705.pdf

Clem, M. A., Holliday, R. P., Pandya, S., Hynan, L. S., Lacritz, L. H., & Woon, F. L. (2017). Predictors that a diagnosis of mild cognitive impairment will remain stable 3 years later. *Cognitive and Behavioral Neurology, 30*, 8–15. http://dx.doi.org/10.1097/WNN.0000000000000119

Corder, K., Ogilvie, D., & van Sluijs, E. M. (2009). Invited commentary: Physical activity over the life course—whose behavior changes, when, and why? *American Journal of Epidemiology, 170*, 1078–1081. http://dx.doi.org/10.1093/aje/kwp273

Cosco, T. D., Prina, A. M., Perales, J., Stephan, B. C., & Brayne, C. (2014). Operational definitions of successful aging: A systematic review. *International Psychogeriatrics, 26*, 373–381. http://dx.doi.org/10.1017/S1041610213002287

Cummings, J. L., Morstorf, T., & Zhong, K. (2014). Alzheimer's disease drug-development pipeline: Few candidates, frequent failures. *Alzheimer's Research & Therapy, 6*(4), 37. http://dx.doi.org/10.1186/alzrt269

Daffner, K. R. (2010). Promoting successful cognitive aging: A comprehensive review [erratum at http://dx.doi.org/10.1080/13607863.2016.1231172]. *Journal of Alzheimer's Disease, 19*, 1101–1122. http://dx.doi.org/10.3233/JAD-2010-1306

Darst, B. F., Koscik, R. L., Racine, A. M., Oh, J. M., Krause, R. A., Carlsson, C. M., . . . Engelman, C. D. (2017). Pathway-specific polygenic risk scores as predictors of β-amyloid deposition and cognitive function in a sample at increased risk for Alzheimer's disease. *Journal of Alzheimer's Disease, 55*, 473–484. http://dx.doi.org/10.3233/JAD-160195

Das, D., Tan, X., Bielak, A. A., Cherbuin, N., Easteal, S., & Anstey, K. J. (2014). Cognitive ability, intraindividual variability, and common genetic variants of catechol-O-methyltransferase and brain-derived neurotrophic factor: A longitudinal study in a population-based sample of older adults. *Psychology and Aging, 29*, 393–403. http://dx.doi.org/10.1037/a0035702

Daugherty, A. M., Zwilling, C., Paul, E. J., Sherepa, N., Allen, C., Kramer, A. F., . . . Barbey, A. K. (2018). Multimodal fitness and cognitive training to enhance fluid intelligence. *Intelligence, 66*, 32–43.

Daviglus, M. L., Bell, C. C., Berrettini, W., Bowen, P. E., Connolly, E. S., Jr., Cox, N. J., . . . Trevisan, M. (2010). National Institutes of Health State-of-the-Science Conference statement: Preventing Alzheimer disease and cognitive decline. *Annals of Internal Medicine, 153*, 176–181. http://dx.doi.org/10.7326/0003-4819-153-3-201008030-00260

de Frias, C. M., & Dixon, R. A. (2014). Lifestyle engagement affects cognitive status differences and trajectories on executive functions in older adults. *Archives of Clinical Neuropsychology, 29*, 16–25. http://dx.doi.org/10.1093/arclin/act089

de Frias, C. M., Dixon, R. A., & Strauss, E. (2009). Characterizing executive functioning in older special populations: From cognitively elite to cognitively impaired. *Neuropsychology, 23*, 778–791. http://dx.doi.org/10.1037/a0016743

de Souto Barreto, P., Delrieu, J., Andrieu, S., Vellas, B., & Rolland, Y. (2016). Physical activity and cognitive function in middle-aged and older adults: An analysis of 104,909 people from 20 countries. *Mayo Clinic Proceedings, 91*, 1515–1524. http://dx.doi.org/10.1016/j.mayocp.2016.06.032

Depp, C. A., Harmell, A., & Vahia, I. V. (2012). Successful cognitive aging. *Current Topics in Behavioral Neurosciences, 10*, 35–50. http://dx.doi.org/10.1007/7854_2011_158

Depp, C. A., & Jeste, D. V. (2006). Definitions and predictors of successful aging: A comprehensive review of larger quantitative studies. *The American Journal of Geriatric Psychiatry, 14*, 6–20. http://dx.doi.org/10.1097/01.JGP.0000192501.03069.bc

Dixon, R. A. (2010). An epidemiological approach to cognitive health in aging. In L. Bäckman & L. Nyberg (Eds.), *Memory, aging, and the brain* (pp. 144–166). London, England: Psychology Press.

Dixon, R. A. (2011). Enduring theoretical themes in psychological aging: Derivation, functions, perspectives, and opportunities. In K. W. Schaie & S. L. Willis (Eds.), *Handbook of the psychology of aging* (7th ed., pp. 3–23). San Diego, CA: Academic Press. http://dx.doi.org/10.1016/B978-0-12-380882-0.00001-2

Dixon, R. A., & de Frias, C. M. (2007). Mild memory deficits differentially affect 6-year changes in compensatory strategy use. *Psychology and Aging, 22*, 632–638. http://dx.doi.org/10.1037/0882-7974.22.3.632

Dixon, R. A., & de Frias, C. M. (2014). Cognitively elite, cognitively normal, and cognitively impaired aging: Neurocognitive status and stability moderate memory performance. *Journal of Clinical and Experimental Neuropsychology, 36*, 418–430. http://dx.doi.org/10.1080/13803395.2014.903901

Dixon, R. A., DeCarlo, C. A., MacDonald, S. W. S., Vergote, D., Jhamandas, J., & Westaway, D. (2014). APOE and COMT polymorphisms are complementary biomarkers of status, stability, and transitions in normal aging and early mild cognitive impairment. *Frontiers in Aging Neuroscience, 6,* 236. http://dx.doi.org/10.3389/fnagi.2014.00236

Dixon, R. A., Garrett, D., & Bäckman, L. (2008). Principles of compensation in cognitive neuroscience and neurorehabilitation. In D. T. Stuss, G. Winocur, & I. H. Robertson (Eds.), *Cognitive neurorehabilitation* (2nd ed., pp. 22–38). Cambridge, England: Cambridge University Press. http://dx.doi.org/10.1017/CBO9781316529898.004

Dixon, R. A., McFall, G. P., & McDermott, K. (2017, July). *Discriminating and predicting cognitive exceptionality and resilience: A roadmap for trajectory and interaction analyses with risk and protection factors.* Paper presented at Alzheimer's Association International Conference, London, England.

Dixon, R. A., Small, B. J., MacDonald, S. W. S., & McArdle, J. J. (2012). Yes, memory declines with aging—But when, how, and why? In M. Naveh-Benjamin & N. Ohta (Eds.), *Memory and aging* (pp. 325–347). New York, NY: Psychology Press.

Dotson, V. M., Beydoun, M. A., & Zonderman, A. B. (2010). Recurrent depressive symptoms and the incidence of dementia and mild cognitive impairment. *Neurology, 75*(1), 27–34. http://dx.doi.org/10.1212/WNL.0b013e3181e62124

Edwards, M. K., & Loprinzi, P. D. (2017). The association between sedentary behavior and cognitive function among older adults may be attenuated with adequate physical activity. *Journal of Physical Activity & Health, 14,* 52–58. http://dx.doi.org/10.1123/jpah.2016-0313

Ellwardt, L., Aartsen, M., Deeg, D., & Steverink, N. (2013). Does loneliness mediate the relation between social support and cognitive functioning in later life? *Social Science & Medicine, 98,* 116–124. http://dx.doi.org/10.1016/j.socscimed.2013.09.002

Epel, E. S., Blackburn, E. H., Lin, J., Dhabhar, F. S., Adler, N. E., Morrow, J. D., & Cawthon, R. M. (2004). Accelerated telomere shortening in response to life stress. *Proceedings of the National Academy of Sciences of the United States of America, 101,* 17312–17315. http://dx.doi.org/10.1073/pnas.0407162101

Erickson, K. I., Hillman, C. H., & Kramer, A. F. (2015). Physical activity, brain, and cognition. *Current Opinion in Behavioral Sciences, 4,* 27–32. http://dx.doi.org/10.1016/j.cobeha.2015.01.005

Erickson, K. I., Prakash, R. S., Voss, M. W., Chaddock, L., Hu, L., Morris, K. S., . . . Kramer, A. F. (2009). Aerobic fitness is associated with hippocampal volume in elderly humans. *Hippocampus, 19*(10), 1030–1039. http://dx.doi.org/10.1002/hipo.20547

Ferrari, R., Dawoodi, S., Raju, M., Thumma, A., Hynan, L. S., Maasumi, S. H., . . . Momeni, P. (2013). Androgen receptor gene and sex-specific Alzheimer's disease. *Neurobiology of Aging, 34,* 2077.e19–2077.e20. http://dx.doi.org/10.1016/j.neurobiolaging.2013.02.017

Fiocco, A. J., & Yaffe, K. (2010). Defining successful aging: The importance of including cognitive function over time. *Archives of Neurology, 67,* 876–880. http://dx.doi.org/10.1001/archneurol.2010.130

Fotuhi, M., Hachinski, V., & Whitehouse, P. J. (2009). Changing perspectives regarding late-life dementia. *Nature Reviews. Neurology, 5,* 649–658. http://dx.doi.org/10.1038/nrneurol.2009.175

Foubert-Samier, A., Le Goff, M., Helmer, C., Pérès, K., Orgogozo, J. M., Barberger-Gateau, P., . . . Dartigues, J. F. (2014). Change in leisure and social activities and risk of dementia in elderly cohort. *The Journal of Nutrition, Health & Aging, 18,* 876–882. http://dx.doi.org/10.1007/s12603-014-0475-7

Fried, L. P., Carlson, M. C., Freedman, M., Frick, K. D., Glass, T. A., Hill, J., . . . Zeger, S. (2004). A social model for health promotion for an aging population: Initial evidence on the Experience Corps model. *Journal of Urban Health, 81,* 64–78. http://dx.doi.org/10.1093/jurban/jth094

Fried, L. P., Carlson, M. C., McGill, S., Seeman, T., Xue, Q.-L., Frick, K., . . . Rebok, G. W. (2013). Experience Corps: A dual trial to promote the health of older adults and children's academic success. *Contemporary Clinical Trials, 36,* 1–13. http://dx.doi.org/10.1016/j.cct.2013.05.003

Gaiteri, C., Mostafavi, S., Honey, C. J., De Jager, P. L., & Bennett, D. A. (2016). Genetic variants in Alzheimer disease—molecular and brain network approaches. *Nature Reviews Neurology, 12,* 413–427. http://dx.doi.org/10.1038/nrneurol.2016.84

Galbraith, S., Bowden, J., & Mander, A. (2017). Accelerated longitudinal designs: An overview of modelling, power, costs and handling missing data. *Statistical Methods in Medical Research, 26*(1), 374–398. http://dx.doi.org/10.1177/0962280214547150

Gefen, T., Shaw, E., Whitney, K., Martersteck, A., Stratton, J., Rademaker, A., . . . Rogalski, E. (2014). Longitudinal neuropsychological performance of cognitive superagers. *Journal of the American Geriatrics Society, 62,* 1598–1600.

Glymour, M. M., & Manly, J. J. (2008). Lifecourse social conditions and racial and ethnic patterns of cognitive aging. *Neuropsychology Review, 18,* 223–254. http://dx.doi.org/10.1007/s11065-008-9064-z

Gow, A. J., Pattie, A., & Deary, I. J. (2017). Lifecourse activity participation from early, mid, and later adulthood as determinants of cognitive Aging: The Lothian birth cohort 1921. *The Journals of Gerontology: Series B. Psychological Sciences and Social Sciences, 72,* 25–37. http://dx.doi.org/10.1093/geronb/gbw124

Graham, E. K., & Lachman, M. E. (2012). Personality stability is associated with better cognitive performance in adulthood: Are the stable more able? *The Journals of Gerontology: Series B. Psychological Sciences and Social Sciences, 67,* 545–554. http://dx.doi.org/10.1093/geronb/gbr149

Graham, E. K., & Lachman, M. E. (2014). Personality traits, facets and cognitive performance: Age differences in their relations. *Personality and Individual Differences, 59,* 89–95. http://dx.doi.org/10.1016/j.paid.2013.11.011

Grossman, P., Niemann, L., Schmidt, S., & Walach, H. (2004). Mindfulness-based stress reduction and health benefits. A meta-analysis. *Journal of Psychosomatic Research, 57,* 35–43. http://dx.doi.org/10.1016/S0022-3999(03)00573-7

Grzywacz, J. G., Segel-Karpas, D., & Lachman, M. E. (2016). Workplace exposures and cognitive function during adulthood: Evidence from national survey of midlife development and the O*NET. *Journal of Occupational and Environmental Medicine, 58,* 535–541. http://dx.doi.org/10.1097/JOM.0000000000000727

Harris, S. E., & Deary, I. J. (2011). The genetics of cognitive ability and cognitive ageing in healthy older people. *Trends in Cognitive Sciences, 15,* 388–394. http://dx.doi.org/10.1016/j.tics.2011.07.004

Harrison, T. M., Weintraub, S., Mesulam, M.-M., & Rogalski, E. (2012). Superior memory and higher cortical volumes in unusually successful cognitive aging. *Journal of the International Neuropsychological Society, 18,* 1081–1085. http://dx.doi.org/10.1017/S1355617712000847

Haslam, C., Cruwys, T., Milne, M., Kan, C. H., & Haslam, S. A. (2016). Group ties protect cognitive health by promoting social identification and social support. *Journal of Aging and Health, 28,* 244–266. http://dx.doi.org/10.1177/0898264315589578

Herlitz, A., & Rehnman, J. (2008). Sex differences in episodic memory. *Current Directions in Psychological Science, 17,* 52–56. http://dx.doi.org/10.1111/j.1467-8721.2008.00547.x

Hertzog, C., Dixon, R. A., & Hultsch, D. F. (1990). Metamemory in adulthood: Differentiating knowledge, belief, and behavior. *Advances in Psychology, 71,* 161–212. http://dx.doi.org/10.1016/S0166-4115(08)60158-2

Hertzog, C., Kramer, A. F., Wilson, R. S., & Lindenberger, U. (2008). Enrichment effects on adult cognitive development: Can the functional capacity of older adults be preserved and enhanced? *Psychological Science in the Public Interest, 9,* 1–65. http://dx.doi.org/10.1111/j.1539-6053.2009.01034.x

Hess, T. M., Auman, C., Colcombe, S. J., & Rahhal, T. A. (2003). The impact of stereotype threat on age differences in memory performance. *The Journals of Gerontology: Series B. Psychological Sciences and Social Sciences, 58,* 3–11. http://dx.doi.org/10.1093/geronb/58.1.P3

Hillman, C. H., Erickson, K. I., & Kramer, A. F. (2008). Be smart, exercise your heart: Exercise effects on brain and cognition. *Nature Reviews Neuroscience, 9,* 58–65. http://dx.doi.org/10.1038/nrn2298

Hughes, M. L., Agrigoroaei, S., Jeon, M., Bruzzese, M., & Lachman, M. E. (2018). Change in cognitive performance from midlife into old age: Findings from the Midlife in the United States (MIDUS) Study. *Journal of the International Neuropsychological Society, 24,* 805–820. http://dx.doi.org/10.1017/S1355617718000425

Hughes, M. L., & Lachman, M. E. (2016). Social comparisons of health and cognitive functioning contribute to changes in subjective age. *The Journals of Gerontology: Series B. Psychological Sciences and Social Sciences,* gbw044. Advance online publication. http://dx.doi.org/10.1093/geronb/gbw044

Hurd, M. D., Martorell, P., Delavande, A., Mullen, K. J., & Langa, K. M. (2013). Monetary costs of dementia in the United States. *The New England Journal of Medicine, 368,* 1326–1334. http://dx.doi.org/10.1056/NEJMsa1204629

Ighodaro, E. T., Abner, E. L., Fardo, D. W., Lin, A. L., Katsumata, Y., Schmitt, F. A., . . . Nelson, P. T. (2017). Risk factors and global cognitive status related to brain arteriolosclerosis in elderly individuals. *Journal of Cerebral Blood Flow and Metabolism, 37,* 201–216. http://dx.doi.org/10.1177/0271678X15621574

Institute of Medicine. (2015). *Cognitive aging: Progress in understanding and opportunities for action.* Washington, DC: The National Academies Press.

Jack, C. R., Jr., Wiste, H. J., Weigand, S. D., Knopman, D. S., Vemuri, P., Mielke, M. M., . . . Petersen, R. C. (2015). Age, sex and APOE ε4 effects on memory, brain structure, and β-amyloid across the adult life span. *JAMA Neurology, 72,* 511–519. http://dx.doi.org/10.1001/jamaneurol.2014.4821

Johansson, L., Guo, X., Duberstein, P. R., Hällström, T., Waern, M., Ostling, S., & Skoog, I. (2014). Midlife personality and risk of Alzheimer disease and distress: A 38-year follow-up [erratum at http://dx.doi.org/10.1212/WNL.0000000000001174]. *Neurology, 83,* 1538–1544. Advance online publication. http://dx.doi.org/10.1212/WNL.0000000000000907

Jones, R. N., Manly, J., Glymour, M. M., Rentz, D. M., Jefferson, A. L., & Stern, Y. (2011). Conceptual and measurement challenges in research on cognitive reserve. *Journal of the International Neuropsychological Society, 17,* 593–601. http://dx.doi.org/10.1017/S1355617710001748

Josefsson, M., de Luna, X., Pudas, S., Nilsson, L. G., & Nyberg, L. (2012). Genetic and lifestyle predictors of 15-year longitudinal change in episodic memory. *Journal of the American Geriatrics Society, 60,* 2308–2312. http://dx.doi.org/10.1111/jgs.12000

Karlamangla, A. S., Miller-Martinez, D., Lachman, M. E., Tun, P. A., Koretz, B. K., & Seeman, T. E. (2014). Biological correlates of adult cognition: Midlife in the United States (MIDUS). *Neurobiology of Aging, 35,* 387–394. http://dx.doi.org/10.1016/j.neurobiolaging.2013.07.028

Kaup, A. R., Nettiksimmons, J., Harris, T. B., Sink, K. M., Satterfield, S., Metti, A. L., . . . Yaffe, K. (2015). Cognitive resilience to apolipoprotein E ε4: Contributing factors in Black and White older adults. *JAMA Neurology, 72,* 340–348. http://dx.doi.org/10.1001/jamaneurol.2014.3978

Kennedy, D. O., Wightman, E. L., Reay, J. L., Lietz, G., Okello, E. J., Wilde, A., & Haskell, C. F. (2010). Effects of resveratrol on cerebral blood flow variables and cognitive performance in humans: A double-blind, placebo-controlled, crossover investigation. *The American Journal of Clinical Nutrition, 91,* 1590–1597. http://dx.doi.org/10.3945/ajcn.2009.28641

Kohl, H. W., III, Craig, C. L., Lambert, E. V., Inoue, S., Alkandari, J. R., Leetongin, G., & Kahlmeier, S. (2012). The pandemic of physical inactivity: Global action for public health. *The Lancet, 380,* 294–305. http://dx.doi.org/10.1016/S0140-6736(12)60898-8

Kraft, E. (2012). Cognitive function, physical activity, and aging: Possible biological links and implications for multimodal interventions. *Neuropsychology, Development, and Cognition: Section B. Aging, Neuropsychology and Cognition, 19,* 248–263. http://dx.doi.org/10.1080/13825585.2011.645010

Kramer, A. F., Erickson, K. I., & Colcombe, S. J. (2006). Exercise, cognition, and the aging brain. *Journal of Applied Physiology, 101*, 1237–1242. http://dx.doi.org/10.1152/japplphysiol.00500.2006

Kremen, W. S., Panizzon, M. S., & Cannon, T. D. (2016). Genetics and neuropsychology: A merger whose time has come. *Neuropsychology, 30*, 1–5. http://dx.doi.org/10.1037/neu0000254

Lachman, M. E. (2006). Perceived control over aging-related declines: Adaptive beliefs and behaviors. *Current Directions in Psychological Science, 15*, 282–286. http://dx.doi.org/10.1111/j.1467-8721.2006.00453.x

Lachman, M. E., & Agrigoroaei, S. (2010). Promoting functional health in midlife and old age: Long-term protective effects of control beliefs, social support, and physical exercise. *PLoS ONE, 5*, e13297. http://dx.doi.org/10.1371/journal.pone.0013297

Lachman, M. E., Agrigoroaei, S., Murphy, C., & Tun, P. A. (2010). Frequent cognitive activity compensates for education differences in episodic memory. *The American Journal of Geriatric Psychiatry, 18*, 4–10. http://dx.doi.org/10.1097/JGP.0b013e3181ab8b62

Lachman, M. E., & Andreoletti, C. (2006). Strategy use mediates the relationship between control beliefs and memory performance for middle-aged and older adults. *The Journals of Gerontology: Series B. Psychological Sciences and Social Sciences, 61*, 88–94. http://dx.doi.org/10.1093/geronb/61.2.P88

Lachman, M. E., & Leff, R. (1989). Perceived control and intellectual functioning in the elderly: A 5-year longitudinal study. *Developmental Psychology, 25*, 722–728. http://dx.doi.org/10.1037/0012-1649.25.5.722

Lachman, M. E., Neupert, S. D., & Agrigoroaei, S. (2011). The relevance of control beliefs for health and aging. In K. W. Schaie & S. L. Willis (Eds.), *Handbook of the psychology of aging* (7th ed., pp. 175–190). New York, NY: Elsevier. http://dx.doi.org/10.1016/B978-0-12-380882-0.00011-5

Laitman, B. M., & John, G. R. (2015). Understanding how exercise promotes cognitive integrity in the aging brain. *PLoS Biology, 13*, e1002300. http://dx.doi.org/10.1371/journal.pbio.1002300

Langa, K. M., Larson, E. B., Crimmins, E. M., Faul, J. D., Levine, D. A., Kabeto, M. U., & Weir, D. R. (2017). A comparison of the prevalence of dementia in the United States in 2000 and 2012. *JAMA Internal Medicine, 177*, 51–58. http://dx.doi.org/10.1001/jamainternmed.2016.6807

Levy, B. R., Zonderman, A. B., Slade, M. D., & Ferrucci, L. (2012). Memory shaped by age stereotypes over time. *The Journals of Gerontology: Series B. Psychological Sciences and Social Sciences, 67*, 432–436. http://dx.doi.org/10.1093/geronb/gbr120

Liao, J., Head, J., Kumari, M., Stansfeld, S., Kivimaki, M., Singh-Manoux, A., & Brunner, E. J. (2014). Negative aspects of close relationships as risk factors for cognitive aging. *American Journal of Epidemiology, 180*, 1118–1125. http://dx.doi.org/10.1093/aje/kwu236

Lindenberger, U., Nagel, I. E., Chicherio, C., Li, S.-C., Heekeren, H. R., & Bäckman, L. (2008). Age-related decline in brain resources modulates genetic effects on cognitive functioning. *Frontiers in Neuroscience, 2*, 234–244. http://dx.doi.org/10.3389/neuro.01.039.2008

Litwin, H., Schwartz, E., & Damri, N. (2017). Cognitively stimulating leisure activity and subsequent cognitive function: A SHARE-based analysis. *The Gerontologist, 57*, 940–948.

Liu, C.-C., Kanekiyo, T., Xu, H., & Bu, G. (2013). Apolipoprotein E and Alzheimer disease: Risk, mechanisms and therapy [erratum at http://dx.doi.org/10.1038/nrneurol.2013.32]. *Nature Reviews. Neurology, 9*, 106–118. http://dx.doi.org/10.1038/nrneurol.2012.263

Livingston, G., Sommerlad, A., Orgeta, V., Costafreda, S. G., Huntley, J., Ames, D., . . . Mukadam, N. (2017). Dementia prevention, intervention, and care. *The Lancet, 390*, 2673–2734. Advance online publication. http://dx.doi.org/10.1016/S0140-6736(17)31363-6

Lourida, I., Soni, M., Thompson-Coon, J., Purandare, N., Lang, I. A., Ukoumunne, O. C., & Llewellyn, D. J. (2013). Mediterranean diet, cognitive function, and dementia: A systematic review. *Epidemiology, 24*, 479–489. http://dx.doi.org/10.1097/EDE.0b013e3182944410

Lupien, S. J., Maheu, F., Tu, M., Fiocco, A., & Schramek, T. E. (2007). The effects of stress and stress hormones on human cognition: Implications for the field of brain and cognition. *Brain and Cognition, 65*, 209–237. http://dx.doi.org/10.1016/j.bandc.2007.02.007

Lupien, S. J., McEwen, B. S., Gunnar, M. R., & Heim, C. (2009). Effects of stress throughout the lifespan on the brain, behaviour and cognition. *Nature Reviews Neuroscience, 10*, 434–445. http://dx.doi.org/10.1038/nrn2639

Macready, A. L., Kennedy, O. B., Ellis, J. A., Williams, C. M., Spencer, J. P. E., & Butler, L. T. (2009). Flavonoids and cognitive function: A review of human randomized controlled trial studies and recommendations for future studies. *Genes & Nutrition, 4*, 227–242. http://dx.doi.org/10.1007/s12263-009-0135-4

Mandelman, S. D., & Grigorenko, E. L. (2012). BDNF Val66Met and cognition: All, none, or some? A meta-analysis of the genetic association. *Genes, Brain & Behavior, 11*, 127–136. http://dx.doi.org/10.1111/j.1601-183X.2011.00738.x

Manly, J. J., Jacobs, D. M., Touradji, P., Small, S. A., & Stern, Y. (2002). Reading level attenuates differences in neuropsychological test performance between African American and White elders. *Journal of the International Neuropsychological Society, 8*, 341–348. http://dx.doi.org/10.1017/S1355617702813157

Marioni, R. E., Proust-Lima, C., Amieva, H., Brayne, C., Matthews, F. E., & Dartigues, J. F. (2015). Social activity, cognitive decline and dementia risk: A 20-year prospective cohort study. *BMC Public Health, 15*, 1089. http://dx.doi.org/10.1186/s12889-015-2426-6

Marioni, R. E., Valenzuela, M. J., van den Hout, A., Brayne, C., Matthews, F. E., & the MRC Cognitive Function and Ageing Study. (2012). Active cognitive lifestyle is associated with positive cognitive health transitions and compression of morbidity from age sixty-five. *PLoS One, 7*, e50940. http://dx.doi.org/10.1371/journal.pone.0050940

Martínez-Lapiscina, E. H., Clavero, P., Toledo, E., Estruch, R., Salas-Salvadó, J., San Julián, B., . . . Martinez-Gonzalez, M. Á. (2013). Mediterranean diet improves cognition: The PREDIMED-NAVARRA randomised trial. *Journal of Neurology, Neurosurgery, & Psychiatry, 84*, 1318–1325. http://dx.doi.org/10.1136/jnnp-2012-304792

McDermott, K. L., McFall, G. P., Andrews, S. J., Anstey, K. J., & Dixon, R. A. (2017). Memory resilience to Alzheimer's genetic risk: Sex effects in predictor profiles. *The Journals of Gerontology: Series B. Psychological Sciences and Social Sciences, 72*, 937–946.

McFall, G. P., Sapkota, S., McDermott, K. L., & Dixon, R. A. (2016). Risk-reducing Apolipoprotein E and Clusterin genotypes protect against the consequences of poor vascular health on executive function performance and change in nondemented older adults. *Neurobiology of Aging, 42*, 91–100. http://dx.doi.org/10.1016/j.neurobiolaging.2016.02.032

McFall, G. P., Wiebe, S. A., Vergote, D., Westaway, D., Jhamandas, J., Bäckman, L., & Dixon, R. A. (2015). APOE and pulse pressure interactively influence level and change in the aging of episodic memory: Protective effects among ε2 carriers. *Neuropsychology, 29*, 388–401. http://dx.doi.org/10.1037/neu0000150

Murrell, J. R., Price, B., Lane, K. A., Baiyewu, O., Gureje, O., Ogunniyi, A., . . . Hall, K. S. (2006). Association of apolipoprotein E genotype and Alzheimer disease in African Americans. *Archives of Neurology, 63*, 431–434. http://dx.doi.org/10.1001/archneur.63.3.431

National Academies of Sciences, Engineering, and Medicine. (2017). *Preventing Cognitive Decline and Dementia: A Way Forward.* Washington, DC: The National Academies Press. http://dx.doi.org/10.17226/24782

Neupert, S. D., Lachman, M. E., & Whitbourne, S. B. (2009). Exercise self-efficacy and control beliefs: Effects on exercise behavior after an exercise intervention for older adults. *Journal of Aging and Physical Activity, 17*, 1–16. http://dx.doi.org/10.1123/japa.17.1.1

Ngandu, T., Lehtisalo, J., Solomon, A., Levälahti, E., Ahtiluoto, S., Antikainen, R., . . . Kivipelto, M. (2015). A 2 year multidomain intervention of diet, exercise, cognitive training, and vascular risk monitoring versus control to prevent cognitive decline in at-risk elderly people (FINGER): A randomised controlled trial. *The Lancet, 385*, 2255–2263. http://dx.doi.org/10.1016/S0140-6736(15)60461-5

Northey, J. M., Cherbuin, N., Pumpa, K. L., Smee, D. J., & Rattray, B. (2018). Exercise interventions for cognitive function in adults older than 50: A systematic review with meta-analysis. *British Journal of Sports Medicine, 52*, 154–160.

Papenberg, G., Lindenberger, U., & Bäckman, L. (2015). Aging-related magnification of genetic effects on cognitive and brain integrity. *Trends in Cognitive Sciences, 19*, 506–514. http://dx.doi.org/10.1016/j.tics.2015.06.008

Parisi, J. M., Gross, A. L., Marsiske, M., Willis, S. L., & Rebok, G. W. (2017). Control beliefs and cognition over a 10-year period: Findings from the ACTIVE trial. *Psychology and Aging, 32,* 69–75. http://dx.doi.org/10.1037/pag0000147

Park, D. C., Lodi-Smith, J., Drew, L., Haber, S., Hebrank, A., Bischof, G. N., & Aamodt, W. (2014). The impact of sustained engagement on cognitive function in older adults: The Synapse Project. *Psychological Science, 25,* 103–112. http://dx.doi.org/10.1177/0956797613499592

Peters, R., Peters, J., Booth, A., & Mudway, I. (2015). Is air pollution associated with increased risk of cognitive decline? A systematic review. *Age and Ageing, 44,* 755–760. http://dx.doi.org/10.1093/ageing/afv087

Plassman, B. L., Williams, J. W., Jr., Burke, J. R., Holsinger, T., & Benjamin, S. (2010). Systematic review: Factors associated with risk for and possible prevention of cognitive decline in later life. *Annals of Internal Medicine, 153,* 182–193. http://dx.doi.org/10.7326/0003-4819-153-3-201008030-00258

Powell, K. E., Paluch, A. E., & Blair, S. N. (2011). Physical activity for health: What kind? How much? How intense? On top of what? *Annual Review of Public Health, 32,* 349–365. http://dx.doi.org/10.1146/annurev-publhealth-031210-101151

Prince, M., Comas-Herrera, A., Knapp, M., Guerchet, M., & Karagiannidou, M. (2016). *World Alzheimer's Report 2016: Improving healthcare for people living with dementia: Coverage, quality and costs now and in the future.* London, England: Alzheimer's Disease International.

Pruchno, R. (2015). Successful aging: Contentious past, productive future. *The Gerontologist, 55,* 1–4. http://dx.doi.org/10.1093/geront/gnv002

Pruchno, R. A., Wilson-Genderson, M., Rose, M., & Cartwright, F. (2010). Successful aging: Early influences and contemporary characteristics. *The Gerontologist, 50,* 821–833. http://dx.doi.org/10.1093/geront/gnq041

Raz, N., Rodrigue, K. M., Kennedy, K. M., & Land, S. (2009). Genetic and vascular modifiers of age-sensitive cognitive skills: Effects of COMT, BDNF, APOE, and hypertension. *Neuropsychology, 23,* 105–116. http://dx.doi.org/10.1037/a0013487

Rebok, G. W., Ball, K., Guey, L. T., Jones, R. N., Kim, H. Y., King, J. W., . . . Willis, S. L. (2014). Ten-year effects of the advanced cognitive training for independent and vital elderly cognitive training trial on cognition and everyday functioning in older adults. *Journal of the American Geriatrics Society, 62,* 16–24. http://dx.doi.org/10.1111/jgs.12607

Reuter-Lorenz, P. A., & Cappell, K. A. (2008). Neurocognitive aging and the compensation hypothesis. *Current Directions in Psychological Science, 17,* 177–182. http://dx.doi.org/10.1111/j.1467-8721.2008.00570.x

Reynolds, C. A., & Finkel, D. (2015). A meta-analysis of heritability of cognitive aging: Minding the "missing heritability" gap. *Neuropsychology Review, 25,* 97–112. http://dx.doi.org/10.1007/s11065-015-9280-2

Richards, M., & Wadsworth, M. E. J. (2004). Long term effects of early adversity on cognitive function. *Archives of Disease in Childhood, 89,* 922–927. http://dx.doi.org/10.1136/adc.2003.032490

Riedel, B. C., Thompson, P. M., & Brinton, R. D. (2016). Age, APOE and sex: Triad of risk of Alzheimer's disease. *The Journal of Steroid Biochemistry and Molecular Biology, 160,* 134–147. http://dx.doi.org/10.1016/j.jsbmb.2016.03.012

Robinson, S. A., Bisson, A. N., Hughest, M. L., Ebert, J., & Lachman, M. E. (2018). Time for change: Using implementation intentions to promote physical activity in a randomised pilot trial. *Psychology & Health.* Advance online publication. Retrieved from https://www.ncbi.nlm.nih.gov/pubmed/30596272

Rogalski, E. J., Gefen, T., Shi, J., Samimi, M., Bigio, E., Weintraub, S., . . . Mesulam, M.-M. (2013). Youthful memory capacity in old brains: Anatomic and genetic clues from the Northwestern SuperAging Project. *Journal of Cognitive Neuroscience, 25,* 29–36. http://dx.doi.org/10.1162/jocn_a_00300

Rowe, J. W., & Kahn, R. L. (1997). Successful aging. *The Gerontologist, 37,* 433–440. http://dx.doi.org/10.1093/geront/37.4.433

Sapkota, S., Bäckman, L., & Dixon, R. A. (2017). In non-demented aging, executive function performance and change is predicted by apolipoprotein E, intensified by catechol-O-methyltransferase and brain-derived neurotrophic factor, and moderated by age and lifestyle. *Neurobiology of Aging, 52,* 81–89. http://dx.doi.org/10.1016/j.neurobiolaging.2016.12.022

Sapkota, S., & Dixon, R. A. (2018). A network of genetic effects on non-demented cognitive aging: Alzheimer's genetic risk (CLU + CR1 + PICALM) intensifies cognitive aging genetic risk (COMT + BDNF) selectively for APOE ε4 carriers. *Journal of Alzheimer's Disease, 62,* 887–900. http://dx.doi.org/10.3233/JAD-170909

Sapkota, S., Vergote, D., Westaway, D., Jhamandas, J., & Dixon, R. A. (2015). Synergistic associations of COMT and BDNF with executive function in aging are selective and modified by APOE. *Neurobiology of Aging, 36,* 249–256. http://dx.doi.org/10.1016/j.neurobiolaging.2014.06.020

Schaie, K. W. (1965). A general model for the study of developmental problems. *Psychological Bulletin, 64,* 92–107. http://dx.doi.org/10.1037/h0022371

Schaie, K. W. (2012). *Developmental influences on adult intelligence: The Seattle longitudinal study* (2nd ed.). New York, NY: Oxford University Press. http://dx.doi.org/10.1093/acprof:osobl/9780195386134.001.0001

Schooler, C. (1999). The workplace environment: Measurement, psychological effects, and basic issues. In S. L. Friedman & T. D. Wachs (Eds.), *Measuring environment across the life span: Emerging methods and concepts* (pp. 229–246). Washington, DC: American Psychological Association. http://dx.doi.org/10.1037/10317-008

Scullin, M. K., & Bliwise, D. L. (2015). Sleep, cognition, and normal aging: Integrating a half century of multidisciplinary research. *Perspectives on Psychological Science, 10,* 97–137. http://dx.doi.org/10.1177/1745691614556680

Searle, S. D., & Rockwood, K. (2015). Frailty and the risk of cognitive impairment. *Alzheimer's Research & Therapy, 7*(1), 54. http://dx.doi.org/10.1186/s13195-015-0140-3

Seeman, T. E., Miller-Martinez, D. M., Stein Merkin, S., Lachman, M. E., Tun, P. A., & Karlamangla, A. S. (2011). Histories of social engagement and adult cognition: Midlife in the U.S. study. *The Journals of Gerontology: Series B. Psychological Sciences and Social Sciences*, 66(Suppl. 1), i141–i152. http://dx.doi.org/10.1093/geronb/gbq091

Segel-Karpas, D., & Lachman, M. E. (2016). Social contact and cognitive functioning: The role of personality. *The Journals of Gerontology: Series B. Psychological Sciences and Social Sciences*, gbw079. Advance online publication. http://dx.doi.org/10.1093/geronb/gbw079

Simon, S. S., Yokomizo, J. E., & Bottino, C. M. (2012). Cognitive intervention in amnestic mild cognitive impairment: A systematic review. *Neuroscience and Biobehavioral Reviews*, 36, 1163–1178. http://dx.doi.org/10.1016/j.neubiorev.2012.01.007

Sindi, S., Kåreholt, I., Johansson, L., Skoog, J., Sjöberg, L., Wang, H.-X., . . . Kivipelto, M. (2018). Sleep disturbances and dementia risk: A multicenter study. *Alzheimer's & Dementia*, 14(10), 1235–1242. http://dx.doi.org/10.1016/j.jalz.2018.05.012

Singh, B., Parsaik, A. K., Mielke, M. M., Erwin, P. J., Knopman, D. S., Petersen, R. C., & Roberts, R. O. (2014). Association of mediterranean diet with mild cognitive impairment and Alzheimer's disease: A systematic review and meta-analysis [erratum at http://dx.doi.org/10.17116/jnevro201711741107-111]. *Journal of Alzheimer's Disease*, 39, 271–282. http://dx.doi.org/10.3233/JAD-130830

Small, B. J., Dixon, R. A., McArdle, J. J., & Grimm, K. J. (2012). Do changes in lifestyle engagement moderate cognitive decline in normal aging? Evidence from the Victoria Longitudinal Study. *Neuropsychology*, 26, 144–155. http://dx.doi.org/10.1037/a0026579

Small, B. J., Rosnick, C. B., Fratiglioni, L., & Bäckman, L. (2004). Apolipoprotein E and cognitive performance: A meta-analysis. *Psychology and Aging*, 19, 592–600. http://dx.doi.org/10.1037/0882-7974.19.4.592

Sofi, F., Valecchi, D., Bacci, D., Abbate, R., Gensini, G. F., Casini, A., & Macchi, C. (2011). Physical activity and risk of cognitive decline: A meta-analysis of prospective studies. *Journal of Internal Medicine*, 269, 107–117. http://dx.doi.org/10.1111/j.1365-2796.2010.02281.x

Spiro, A., III, & Brady, C. B. (2011). Integrating health into cognitive aging: Toward a preventive cognitive neuroscience of aging. *The Journals of Gerontology: Series B. Psychological Sciences and Social Sciences*, 66(Suppl. 1), i17–i25. http://dx.doi.org/10.1093/geronb/gbr018

Stanford Center on Longevity. (2014). *A consensus on the brain training industry from the scientific community*. Max Planck Institute for Human Development and Stanford Center on Longevity. Retrieved from http://longevity3.stanford.edu/blog/2014/10/15/the-consensus-on-the-braintraining-industry-from-the-scientific-community/

Stephan, Y., Caudroit, J., Jaconelli, A., & Terracciano, A. (2014). Subjective age and cognitive functioning: A 10-year prospective study. *The American Journal of Geriatric Psychiatry, 22,* 1180–1187. http://dx.doi.org/10.1016/j.jagp.2013.03.007

Stephan, Y., Sutin, A. R., Luchetti, M., & Terracciano, A. (2017). Feeling older and the development of cognitive impairment and dementia. *The Journals of Gerontology: Series B. Psychological Sciences and Social Sciences, 72,* 966–973.

Stern, Y. (2002). What is cognitive reserve? Theory and research application of the reserve concept. *Journal of the International Neuropsychological Society, 8,* 448–460. http://dx.doi.org/10.1017/S1355617702813248

Stern, Y. (2009). Cognitive reserve. *Neuropsychologia, 47,* 2015–2028. http://dx.doi.org/10.1016/j.neuropsychologia.2009.03.004

Stern, Y. (2012). Cognitive reserve in ageing and Alzheimer's disease. *The Lancet Neurology, 11,* 1006–1012. http://dx.doi.org/10.1016/S1474-4422(12)70191-6

Sullivan, A. N., & Lachman, M. E. (2017, January 11). Behavior change with fitness technology in sedentary adults: A review of the evidence for increasing physical activity. *Frontiers in Public Health, 4,* 289. http://dx.doi.org/10.3389/fpubh.2016.00289

Tangney, C. C., Li, H., Wang, Y., Barnes, L., Schneider, J. A., Bennett, D. A., & Morris, M. C. (2014). Relation of DASH- and Mediterranean-like dietary patterns to cognitive decline in older persons. *Neurology, 83,* 1410–1416. http://dx.doi.org/10.1212/WNL.0000000000000884

Terracciano, A., Stephan, Y., Luchetti, M., & Sutin, A. R. (2018). Cognitive impairment, dementia, and personality stability among older adults. *Assessment, 25,* 336–347. http://dx.doi.org/10.1177/1073191117691844

Terracciano, A., Sutin, A. R., An, Y., O'Brien, R. J., Ferrucci, L., Zonderman, A. B., & Resnick, S. M. (2014). Personality and risk of Alzheimer's disease: New data and meta-analysis. *Alzheimer's & Dementia, 10,* 179–186. http://dx.doi.org/10.1016/j.jalz.2013.03.002

Thibeau, S., McFall, G. P., Camicioli, R., & Dixon, R. A. (2017). Alzheimer's disease biomarkers interactively influence physical activity, mobility, and cognition associations in a non-demented aging population. *Journal of Alzheimer's Disease, 60,* 69–86. http://dx.doi.org/10.3233/JAD-170130

Thibeau, S., McFall, G. P., Wiebe, S. A., Anstey, K. J., & Dixon, R. A. (2016). Genetic factors moderate everyday physical activity effects on executive functions in aging: Evidence from the Victoria Longitudinal Study. *Neuropsychology, 30*(1), 6–17. http://dx.doi.org/10.1037/neu0000217

Thorp, A. A., Owen, N., Neuhaus, M., & Dunstan, D. W. (2011). Sedentary behaviors and subsequent health outcomes in adults: A systematic review of longitudinal studies, 1996–2011. *American Journal of Preventive Medicine, 41,* 207–215. http://dx.doi.org/10.1016/j.amepre.2011.05.004

Tierney, M. C., Curtis, A. F., Chertkow, H., & Rylett, R. J. (2017). Integrating sex and gender into neurodegeneration research: A six-component strategy. *Alzheimer's & Dementia, 3,* 660–667. http://dx.doi.org/10.1016/j.trci.2017.10.006

Tucker-Drob, E. M., Reynolds, C. A., Finkel, D., & Pedersen, N. L. (2014). Shared and unique genetic and environmental influences on aging-related changes in multiple cognitive abilities. *Developmental Psychology, 50*, 152–166. http://dx.doi.org/10.1037/a0032468

Tun, P. A., Miller-Martinez, D., Lachman, M. E., & Seeman, T. (2013). Social strain and executive function across the lifespan: The dark (and light) sides of social engagement. *Neuropsychology, Development, and Cognition: Section B. Aging, Neuropsychology and Cognition, 20*, 320–338. http://dx.doi.org/10.1080/13825585.2012.707173

van Loenhoud, A. C., Wink, A. M., Groot, C., Verfaillie, S. C. J., Twisk, J., Barkhof, F., . . . Ossenkoppele, R. (2017). A neuroimaging approach to capture cognitive reserve: Application to Alzheimer's disease. *Human Brain Mapping, 38*, 4703–4715. http://dx.doi.org/10.1002/hbm.23695

Varma, V. R., Chuang, Y. F., Harris, G. C., Tan, E. J., & Carlson, M. C. (2015). Low-intensity daily walking activity is associated with hippocampal volume in older adults. *Hippocampus, 25*, 605–615. http://dx.doi.org/10.1002/hipo.22397

Vellas, B., Carrie, I., Gillette-Guyonnet, S., Touchon, J., Dantoine, T., Dartigues, J. F., . . . Andrieu, S. (2014). MAPT study: A multidomain approach for preventing Alzheimer's disease: Design and baseline data. *The Journal of Prevention of Alzheimer's Disease, 1*, 13–22.

Wayne, P. M., Walsh, J. N., Taylor-Piliae, R. E., Wells, R. E., Papp, K. V., Donovan, N. J., & Yeh, G. Y. (2014). Effect of tai chi on cognitive performance in older adults: Systematic review and meta-analysis. *Journal of the American Geriatrics Society, 62*, 25–39. http://dx.doi.org/10.1111/jgs.12611

Weber, D., Skirbekk, V., Freund, I., & Herlitz, A. (2014). The changing face of cognitive gender differences in Europe. *Proceedings of the National Academy of Sciences of the United States of America, 111*, 11673–11678. http://dx.doi.org/10.1073/pnas.1319538111

Wengreen, H., Munger, R. G., Cutler, A., Quach, A., Bowles, A., Corcoran, C., . . . Welsh-Bohmer, K. A. (2013). Prospective study of Dietary Approaches to Stop Hypertension- and Mediterranean-style dietary patterns and age-related cognitive change: The Cache County study on memory, health, and aging. *The American Journal of Clinical Nutrition, 98*, 1263–1271. http://dx.doi.org/10.3945/ajcn.112.051276

Weuve, J., Puett, R. C., Schwartz, J., Yanosky, J. D., Laden, F., & Grodstein, F. (2012). Exposure to particulate air pollution and cognitive decline in older women. *Archives of Internal Medicine, 172*, 219–227. http://dx.doi.org/10.1001/archinternmed.2011.683

Wimo, A., Guerchet, M., Ali, G.-C., Wu, Y.-T., Prina, A. M., Winblad, B., . . . Prince, M. (2017). The worldwide costs of dementia 2015 and comparisons with 2010. *Alzheimer's & Dementia, 13*(1), 1–7. http://dx.doi.org/10.1016/j.jalz.2016.07.150

Windsor, T. D., & Anstey, K. J. (2008). A longitudinal investigation of perceived control and cognitive performance in young, midlife and older adults. *Neuro-*

psychology, Development, and Cognition: Section B. Aging, Neuropsychology and Cognition, 15, 744–763. http://dx.doi.org/10.1080/13825580802348570

Wisdom, N. M., Callahan, J. L., & Hawkins, K. A. (2011). The effects of apolipoprotein E on non-impaired cognitive functioning: A meta-analysis. Neurobiology of Aging, 32, 63–74. http://dx.doi.org/10.1016/j.neurobiolaging.2009.02.003

World Health Organization. (2017). Fact sheet: Physical activity. Retrieved from http://www.who.int/mediacentre/factsheets/fs385/en/

Yaffe, K., Fiocco, A. J., Lindquist, K., Vittinghoff, E., Simonsick, E. M., Newman, A. B., . . . Harris, T. B. (2009). Predictors of maintaining cognitive function in older adults: The Health ABC study. Neurology, 72, 2029–2035. http://dx.doi.org/10.1212/WNL.0b013e3181a92c36

Yaffe, K., Hoang, T. D., Byers, A. L., Barnes, D. E., & Friedl, K. E. (2014). Lifestyle and health-related risk factors and risk of cognitive aging among older veterans. Alzheimer's & Dementia, 10(Suppl.), S111–S121. http://dx.doi.org/10.1016/j.jalz.2014.04.010

Zahodne, L. B., Glymour, M. M., Sparks, C., Bontempo, D., Dixon, R. A., MacDonald, S. W. S., & Manly, J. J. (2011). Education does not slow cognitive decline with aging: 12-year evidence from the victoria longitudinal study. Journal of the International Neuropsychological Society, 17, 1039–1046. http://dx.doi.org/10.1017/S1355617711001044

Zahodne, L. B., Manly, J. J., Azar, M., Brickman, A. M., & Glymour, M. M. (2016). Racial disparities in cognitive performance across mid and late adulthood: Analyses in two cohort studies. Journal of the American Geriatrics Society, 64, 959–964. http://dx.doi.org/10.1111/jgs.14113

Zahodne, L. B., Sol, K., & Kraal, Z. (2017). Psychosocial pathways to racial/ethnic inequalities in late-life memory trajectories. The Journals of Gerontology: Series B. Psychological Sciences and Social Sciences. Advance online publication. Retrieved from https://www.ncbi.nlm.nih.gov/pubmed/28958051

Zeidan, F., Johnson, S. K., Diamond, B. J., David, Z., & Goolkasian, P. (2010). Mindfulness meditation improves cognition: Evidence of brief mental training. Consciousness and Cognition, 19, 597–605. http://dx.doi.org/10.1016/j.concog.2010.03.014

Zhang, C., & Pierce, B. L. (2014). Genetic susceptibility to accelerated cognitive decline in the US Health and Retirement Study. Neurobiology of Aging, 35, 1512.e11–1512.e18. http://dx.doi.org/10.1016/j.neurobiolaging.2013.12.021

Zhao, L., Mao, Z., Woody, S. K., & Brinton, R. D. (2016). Sex differences in metabolic aging of the brain: Insights into female susceptibility to Alzheimer's disease. Neurobiology of Aging, 42, 69–79. http://dx.doi.org/10.1016/j.neurobiolaging.2016.02.011

INDEX

ABOUT THE EDITOR

Gregory R. Samanez-Larkin, PhD, is an assistant professor in the Department of Psychology and Neuroscience and core faculty member in the Center for Cognitive Neuroscience in the Duke Institute for Brain Sciences at Duke University. He is a founding director of the Scientific Research Network on Decision Neuroscience and Aging and the Summer School in Social Neuroscience and Neuroeconomics. Dr. Samanez-Larkin is on the editorial board of the journal *Psychology and Aging* (APA).

Samanez-Larkin and his lab members (https://www.mcablab.science) conduct research focused on identifying psychological and neurobiological strengths at all stages of adulthood that enhance everyday decision making and improve health and well-being in older age. His laboratory uses a combination of behavioral measures, computational modeling, structural (DTI) and functional (fMRI) brain imaging, and molecular brain imaging (PET) of the dopamine system. He conducted many of the foundational studies on reward processing and decision making in the aging human brain and continues to be a leader in research on decision neuroscience and aging. He has been continuously supported by training and research grants from the National Institute on Aging since 2005.

Dr. Samanez-Larkin teaches undergraduate courses on statistical methods and applications of human brain imaging in everyday life. As a graduate student at Stanford University he received the Albert H.

and Barbara R. Hastorf Prize for Teaching in 2010 and as a junior faculty member at Yale University he received the Poorvu Family Award for Interdisciplinary Teaching in 2015. He was on the Yale College Committee on Teaching and Learning from 2015–2016.

He grew up in Flint, Michigan and was an undergraduate at the University of Michigan–Flint before transferring to the University of Michigan where he received a bachelor's degree in Psychology Honors in 2002. After spending 3 years as a lab manager (and moonlighting as a freelance graphic designer), he completed a PhD in psychology at Stanford University in 2010. He was a post-doctoral fellow at Vanderbilt University and then faculty member at Yale before moving to Duke in 2017. He lives with his spouse, a child clinical psychologist, and three daughters in Durham, North Carolina.